# MAYO CLINIC

## GUIDE TO

# ARTHRITIS

Managing joint pain for an active life

— **LYNNE S. PETERSON, M.D.** —

## MAYO CLINIC

**Medical Editor**
Lynne S. Peterson, M.D.

**Editorial Director**
Paula M. Marlow Limbeck

**Senior Editor**
Karen R. Wallevand

**Managing Editor**
Anna L. Cavallo

**Senior Product Manager**
Daniel J. Harke

**Art Director**
Stewart J. Koski

**Illustration, Photography and Production**
Paul Flessland, Joanna R. King, Michael A. King, Kent McDaniel, Gunnar T. Soroos

**Editorial Research Librarians**
Abbie Y. Brown, Edward (Eddy) S. Morrow Jr., Erika A. Riggin, Katherine (Katie) J. Warner

**Copy Editors**
Miranda M. Attlesey, Alison K. Baker, Nancy J. Jacoby, Julie M. Maas

**Indexer**
Steve Rath

**Contributors**
Andy Abril, M.D.; Brent A. Bauer, M.D.; Joshua S. Bingham, M.D.; Kathryn (Kathy) R. Cieslak, P.T., D.Sc.; Ali A. Duarte Garcia, M.D.; Kostas J. Economopoulos, M.D.; Floranne C. Ernste, M.D.; Alicia M. Hinze, M.D., M.H.S.; Mary L. Jurisson, M.D.; Stephanie N. Kannas, C.H.T., O.T.; Edward R. Laskowski, M.D.; Amir B. Orandi, M.D.; Ashley O. Otto, Pharm.D., R.Ph.; Gregory S. Peterson, M.D.; Christopher D. Sletten, Ph.D., L.P.; Kenneth J. Warrington, M.D.; Katherine A. Zeratsky, RDN, LD

Published by Mayo Clinic Press

© 2020 Mayo Foundation for Medical Education and Research (MFMER)

MAYO, MAYO CLINIC and the Mayo triple-shield logo are marks of Mayo Foundation for Medical Education and Research. All rights reserved. No part of this book may be reproduced, stored in a retrieval system, or transmitted, in any form or by any means, electronic, mechanical, photocopying, recording, or otherwise, without the prior written permission of the publisher.

The information in this book is true and complete to the best of our knowledge. This book is intended only as an informative guide for those wishing to learn more about health issues. It is not intended to replace, countermand or conflict with advice given to you by your own physician. The ultimate decision concerning your care should be made between you and your doctor. Information in this book is offered with no guarantees. The author and publisher disclaim all liability in connection with the use of this book.

From time to time, Mayo Clinic or a Mayo Clinic physician may have a financial interest in an invention, technology, company or product mentioned in Mayo Clinic books. Dr. Kenneth Warrington, a contributing editor of Chapter 5, has received an honorarium and research funding from the manufacturer of the medication tocilizumab, referenced in that chapter.

For bulk sales to employers, member groups and health-related companies, contact Mayo Clinic, 200 First St. SW, Rochester, MN 55905, call 800-430-9699, or send an email to *SpecialSalesMayoBooks@mayo.edu*.

ISBN 978-1-893005-56-3 (hardcover)
ISBN 978-1-893005-55-6 (softcover)

Library of Congress Control Number: 2019957432

Printed in the United States of America

# Contents

III

rheumatica (PMR) · Crystalline arthritis · Septic (infectious) arthritis and infection-related arthritis · Moving forward

Diffuse idiopathic skeletal hyperostosis (DISH) · Herniated disk · Cervical spine disorders · Mechanical low back pain · Scheuermann's (juvenile) kyphosis · Spinal stenosis · Spondylolysis and spondylolisthesis

Juvenile idiopathic arthritis · Other inflammatory joint conditions · Connective tissue diseases · Vasculitis · Orthopedic conditions · Growing pains

What causes pain? · Peripheral pain · Central pain · Fibromyalgia: Example of central pain

Laboratory tests · Procedures · Imaging (radiographic) studies · Specialty evaluations

## Part 2: Treating arthritis

Different treatment strategies · Arthritis medication guide · Pain relievers · Corticosteroids · Conventional disease-modifying antirheumatic drugs (DMARDs) · Biologic DMARDs · Targeted DMARDs

Common types of joint surgery · Choosing the right procedure · Things to know before surgery · New lease on life

Treating acute pain · Professional help for pain

Choosing an integrative therapy · Forms of integrative therapy · Mind-body medicine · Herbs and other dietary supplements · Energy therapies · Hands-on therapies · Alternative medical and healing systems · Evaluating integrative therapies

# From the editor

This book is dedicated to my cousin Susan.

One of the fondest memories from my childhood is of my family's annual trip from Wyoming to Kansas to visit relatives. The best part about these trips was getting to see my cousin Susan. Susan and I formed a close bond at a young age, and whenever our families got together, the two of us were inseparable. When we were about 14 years old, I noticed Susan didn't join the rest of the cousins while we played kick the can. At the time, I just assumed she wasn't fond of the game. But looking back on it now, this is the first memory I have of Susan and her struggles with arthritis.

When Susan was diagnosed, limited treatment options were available for her arthritis. Over the years, I watched as she endured her pain, joint deformities and multiple surgeries with patience and determination. But despite her health struggles, Susan inspires me with her perseverance and dedication to family and her career. Susan served as my inspiration to become a rheumatologist many years ago, and she continues to be one of my role models today.

Fortunately, over the last several decades, significant advances have occurred in the understanding and treatment of arthritis. Doctors now have a host of effective medications, physical therapies, new support systems and more psychological help for people struggling with joint pain. People diagnosed with arthritis today have hope — and a great likelihood — that their disease can be treated and put into remission.

It has been my pleasure to help create the new *Mayo Clinic Guide to Arthritis*, and I'm grateful for the contributions of many colleagues. Mayo Clinic is dedicated to providing the best medical care to everyone, and this is accomplished through an integrated model of clinical practice, education and research. This book will provide you with high-quality, reliable and up-to-date information regarding different types of arthritis, medications used for treatment, surgical options and ways to manage your symptoms to help you lead a more active life.

This book is divided into three sections. Part 1 reviews the different types of arthritis and explores the difference between inflammatory and noninflammatory arthritis. Chapters in Part 1 also discuss common musculoskeletal and spine disorders, childhood arthritis, and pain conditions. In addition, Chapter 9 describes various tests and medical specialists that may be part of the diagnosis and treatment of arthritis.

Part 2 reviews different treatment options. In recent years, many new medications and other treatments have become available for patients with arthritis. Chapters discuss these medications in simple terminology, as well as surgical options, joint injections, pain management and complementary therapies.

Finally, Part 3 is a guide to help people with arthritis live as normally and comfortably as possible through self-care. Chapters in this section focus on being active, eating healthfully, reducing stress, protecting the joints, boosting the immune system and managing the disease in daily life.

Whether arthritis affects you, your family or someone else in your life, this book will leave you with a better understanding of the condition, symptoms and ways to manage life with arthritis. Most importantly, this book aims to provide you and your family with hope. Susan, I am indebted to you and many others like you who demonstrate that, despite the hardships of the disease, arthritis does not have the power to stand in the way of living an exceptional life.

Lynne S. Peterson, M.D.

**Lynne S. Peterson, M.D.,** is a rheumatologist at Mayo Clinic in Rochester, Minnesota, and an assistant professor of medicine at Mayo Clinic College of Medicine and Science. A graduate of Tulane University School of Medicine, she completed a residency in internal medicine and a fellowship in rheumatology at Mayo Clinic School of Graduate Medical Education. Dr. Peterson has presented nationally and internationally on her research, focused on adult rheumatology. She has been recognized with multiple Clinical Researcher of the Year awards from the Rheumatoid Arthritis Investigational Network as well as the organization's Clinical Distinction Award. She is also a two-time Arthritis Walk Medical Honoree, conferred by the Arthritis Foundation.

# Understanding arthritis

# Arthritis – Common and complex

When your joints are working smoothly, it's easy to take them for granted. When they begin to ache, you take notice. If you've ever experienced pain, stiffness, swelling and difficulty moving because of arthritis, you're not alone.

Arthritis is a common condition, affecting about 1 in 5 adults in the United States. More than 54 million Americans, including around 300,000 children, have been diagnosed with some form of the disease. And research suggests that the number of people affected by arthritis may be much higher, if you include those who have symptoms but haven't been officially diagnosed.

Arthritis is one of the leading causes of disability in the United States. The costs for medical care and lost productivity due to arthritis amount to more than $300 billion annually. As the population ages, the number of people with arthritis is expected to increase. By 2040, an estimated 78 million adults age 18 and older will have some form of this disease.

Although people often think of arthritis as one disease, it's not. The term refers to many diseases that can cause joint pain or stiffness, damage to the structure of a joint, or loss of joint function. The word arthritis is a blend of the Greek *arthron* + -itis that literally means "joint inflammation." However, the term is commonly used to refer to any disease of the joints.

Arthritis occurs in more than 100 different forms. Some forms develop gradually due to the natural wear of joints, while others appear suddenly and then disappear, recurring at a later date. Other forms of arthritis are chronic and progressive, getting worse over time. Signs and symptoms can vary a great deal from one person to another, even if both individuals have the same form of the disease.

The most common symptoms of arthritis are pain while using the affected joints and joint stiffness after periods of rest or inactivity. But many arthritic disorders affect more than your joints. They can also affect the muscles, tendons and ligaments surrounding and supporting the joints, as well as your skin and other organs, such as the lungs, heart, bowel, brain, liver and kidneys.

Although there's no cure for arthritis, treatment options are far ahead of what was available just a decade ago, and new research offers hope of even better therapies. Getting the right treatment early on can help prevent joint damage and mobility

## WHAT IS RHEUMATISM?

If your grandparents had achy joints, they might have talked about the "rheumatism" in their bones. Rheumatism is an older term used to describe the pain and stiffness of arthritis. Both words — rheumatism and arthritis — are often used in a general way to describe joint problems.

In fact, arthritis is an umbrella term for more than 100 diseases that cause joint pain, swelling and stiffness. The term rheumatic disease has broader significance for any disease of the bones, muscles and joints.

Rheumatology is the branch of medicine devoted to arthritis and other diseases of the musculoskeletal system, which includes the bones, joints, muscles, tendons, ligaments and other connective tissues that provide a framework and support for your body. Rheumatologists are medical doctors who have specialized training in rheumatology and internal medicine.

In addition to treating arthritis, rheumatologists treat certain illnesses in which your immune system attacks your own body tissues (autoimmune diseases), musculoskeletal disorders including back pain and bursitis, and bone diseases such as osteoporosis.

problems. You can also take steps at home to prevent arthritis or minimize its effects. By actively managing your arthritis, you can enjoy a more active, fulfilling life.

## WHO GETS ARTHRITIS?

Arthritis affects people of all ages — nearly two-thirds of people with arthritis are under age 65, and symptoms often begin after age 40. Nevertheless, the risk of getting arthritis increases as you get older. By conservative estimates, half of all adults age 65 and older have some form of arthritis.

Women are at higher risk than men of getting many forms of arthritis, especially after age 40. Researchers believe that female hormones that are naturally produced in the body may play a role in how — and when — arthritis develops. These hormones may

## ANATOMY OF A JOINT

Joints are points of connection between two or more bones. The joints are designed to hold the bones together and allow your skeleton to move. The parts of a bone within your joints are covered with shock-absorbing cartilage. Cartilage is a tough, smooth, slippery material that prevents bone-against-bone contact, allowing for easy movement with little friction.

Synovial joints, found in the neck, shoulders, elbows, wrists, fingers, hips, knees, ankles and toes, are the most mobile form of a joint. These joints are surrounded by a tough, fibrous capsule that attaches to the bone on each side of the joint. The joint capsule helps stabilize and protect the joint. The capsule is lined with a tissue called the synovium. This thin membrane produces synovial fluid, a clear substance that nourishes the cartilage and "oils" (lubricates) the joint so that it can move smoothly.

Ligaments are tough cords of fibrous tissue that attach bone to bone. They help support the joint and keep it properly aligned. Muscles and tendons also hold the joint together. Tendons — which connect muscle and bone — attach to bone just outside the capsule above or below the joint.

Bursae are small, fluid-filled sacs tucked between muscles, tendons and bone. Synovial membrane lines the inside of each bursa, releasing a lubricating fluid to cushion the joint and reduce friction as tendons and muscles glide over bones.

also affect the severity of arthritis symptoms in women.

The likelihood of having arthritis varies by race and ethnicity. For example, white and black Americans and American Indians are more likely to get arthritis than are Hispanics and Asians.

People who are overweight have a higher risk of developing arthritis, especially in the knees. According to one survey, approximately two-thirds of U.S. adults diagnosed with arthritis are either overweight or obese. Excess weight puts more pressure on the joints. In addition, a past joint injury can also increase the risk of arthritis.

## NORMAL JOINT

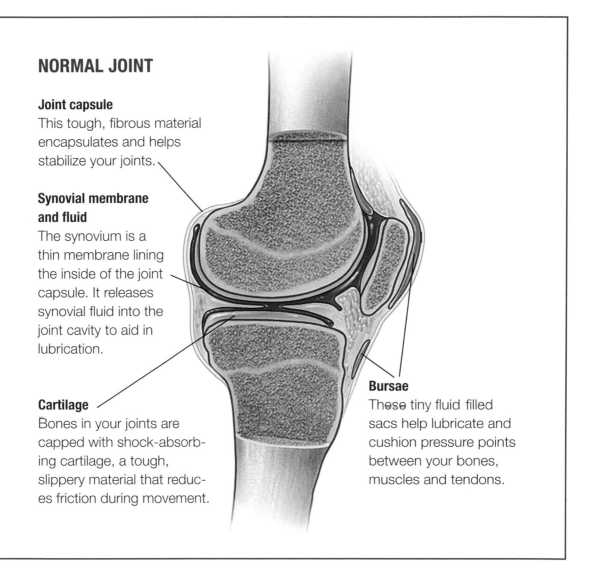

### Joint capsule
This tough, fibrous material encapsulates and helps stabilize your joints.

### Synovial membrane and fluid
The synovium is a thin membrane lining the inside of the joint capsule. It releases synovial fluid into the joint cavity to aid in lubrication.

### Cartilage
Bones in your joints are capped with shock-absorbing cartilage, a tough, slippery material that reduces friction during movement.

### Bursae
These tiny fluid filled sacs help lubricate and cushion pressure points between your bones, muscles and tendons.

## WHAT CAUSES ARTHRITIS?

The pain associated with arthritis is caused by joint damage, but the damage can occur in different ways. Osteoarthritis, the most common form of arthritis, involves a wearing away of the tough, lubricated cartilage that normally cushions the ends of the bones in your joints. Rheumatoid arthritis develops from an uncontrolled response of your immune system, which causes chronic inflammation in the lining of your joints.

Most of the underlying causes of arthritis are unclear, but researchers believe that the condition may result from a complex interplay of multiple factors, including genetics and environment.

While it's true that wear and tear on joints over time can contribute to osteoarthritis, the condition isn't just a normal consequence of aging. Some people never develop it.

There's little doubt that heredity influences whether or not you get arthritis. Scientists have identified specific genes linked to an increased risk of rheumatoid arthritis. Genetic factors that contribute to some cases of osteoarthritis have also been identified. But even people who are genetically predisposed to having arthritis don't necessarily develop it.

Other possible factors that could trigger the onset of arthritis may include infectious agents such as viruses, bacteria, fungi or parasites, toxic materials, or substances in food, water or air. An imbalance of certain hormones or enzymes in the body could possibly play a role as well.

Physical trauma, such as an ankle sprain or knee injury, can set the stage for osteoarthritis and other forms of the disease. Lack of physical activity, excess weight and joint defects such as bowlegs can also lead to arthritis. Stress or other forms of emotional trauma can worsen symptoms.

## TYPES OF ARTHRITIS

While arthritis occurs in many forms, it can generally be divided into two categories: types with inflammatory joint symptoms with joint damage caused by inflammation, or noninflammatory joint symptoms. Dividing arthritis into these two categories is important as the symptoms and treatment options are different.

The vast majority of people who have arthritis have one of two forms — osteoarthritis or rheumatoid arthritis. Osteoarthritis is the most common type of noninflammatory arthritis, and is by far the most common form of arthritis overall (see Chapter 2). Rheumatoid arthritis, the most common inflammatory type, affects fewer people, but its symptoms can be much more debilitating (see Chapter 4).

All forms of arthritis have certain signs and symptoms in common, such as joint pain or tenderness, stiffness, difficulty moving, and joint swelling. However, other musculoskeletal conditions may cause similar joint discomfort. New technology and tests have made it easier to diagnose arthritis. But there still aren't definitive tests that can pinpoint the specific condition.

For these reasons, diagnosing arthritis can sometimes be a challenge. Your doctor will rely on your description of the symptoms and your risk factors, as well as a physical exam and possibly lab tests. Your honest input is key to successfully diagnosing your condition. It may require a series of visits before your doctor can confirm a diagnosis and find a treatment that works best for you. Regardless, the earlier you can start treatment, the better it is for your long-term health.

## HOW ARTHRITIS CHANGES A JOINT

**Normal joint**

Bone

Synovial membrane

Cartilage

**Osteoarthritis**

**Rheumatoid arthritis**

Osteoarthritis, the most common form of arthritis, involves the wearing away of the cartilage that caps the bones in your joints. With rheumatoid arthritis, the synovial membrane that protects and lubricates joints becomes inflamed, causing pain and swelling. Joint erosion may follow.

## CAN ARTHRITIS BE PREVENTED?

Many risk factors for arthritis, such as your heredity, age and sex, aren't under your control. But there are things you can do to help lower your risk of arthritis. Even if you're beginning to experience pain and stiffness, you can influence how the disease affects you.

One of the best ways to prevent pain and joint damage is to see a doctor as soon as you have signs and symptoms such as joint pain, stiffness or swelling. Early diagnosis and proper treatment can limit much of the damage.

To help prevent arthritis or minimize its effects, follow these guidelines:
- Avoid joint injuries. Injuries to joints can lead to arthritis. Make sure to warm up before exercise, and stretch appropriately afterward.
- Treat injuries properly and promptly. This will help the injury heal correctly and limit possible joint damage.
- Stay physically active. Exercise keeps your joints flexible and strong. Aerobic exercise can help you maintain that flexibility. Strength training strengthens the joint muscles.
- Use good body mechanics — in exercise and daily tasks — to avoid joint stress. Use your large joints and largest muscles for tasks such as lifting. Don't lift or move things that are too heavy for you.
- Maintain a healthy weight. Being overweight or obese increases your chance of getting osteoarthritis. If you do have arthritis, the pressure on your joints may make your symptoms a little worse.
- Avoid cigarette smoking. Studies suggest that smoking increases the risk of rheumatoid arthritis and quitting smoking may help prevent it.
- Pay attention to what you eat. Although there's no magic diet that can prevent arthritis, foods containing healthy fats, such as olive oil, certain fish and nuts, may have anti-inflammatory effects. Antioxidants and other compounds in vegetables and fruits also may help fight inflammation. Calcium and vitamin D help keep bones strong, which helps protect against arthritis damage.

## WHEN TO CALL A DOCTOR

Most often, arthritis isn't an emergency. But treatment is usually more effective when symptoms are caught in the early stages of the disease. In addition, some symptoms require immediate attention.

If you experience joint pain and stiffness that disappears within a few days, you probably don't need to call your doctor. But if you experience any of the signs and symptoms listed below, call your doctor:

- You have new pain or persistent symptoms lasting several days or more.
- You have joint pain with a fever, rash, headache or weight loss.
- You have severe or worsening pain in one or more joints.
- You have numbness or pain in your hands or legs or pain that radiates from your neck or lower back.
- You experience joint injury or trauma.

## LIVING IN MOTION

Despite the aches and pains and the joint problems that arthritis causes, most people with arthritis get on with their lives and control their symptoms successfully. The two most common forms of arthritis, osteoarthritis and rheumatoid arthritis, aren't ordinarily life-threatening, and they respond well to medical treatments and self-care.

Start by learning as much as you can about your form of arthritis, your treatment options and, most importantly, the steps you can take to control the condition in partnership with your physician. The following chapters in this book will give you information as well as tools and strategies for living with a chronic disease.

Armed with this information and a positive attitude, you can move forward, adjusting your lifestyle to manage arthritis without compromising your happiness and fulfillment.

# CHAPTER 2

# Osteoarthritis

Osteoarthritis (OA), also called degenerative joint disease or wear-and-tear arthritis, affects more than 30 million adults in the United States. It is the most common form of arthritis.

OA can affect any joint in your body. It most often occurs in the hands, knees, hips and back. Less commonly, it affects the shoulders, elbows, wrists and ankles. It tends to start in only one joint, but it can spread to others.

## UNDERSTANDING THE CONDITION

Osteoarthritis is the primary type of noninflammatory joint disease — meaning it isn't caused by swelling, redness or warmth (inflammation) in the joint. Rather, this condition occurs when the protective cartilage that cushions the ends of bones in your joints deteriorates. With use, the soft, pliable layer of cartilage may start to wear down and its smooth surface becomes rough. At this point many people feel intermittent pain in the joint, especially after strenuous use.

If the cartilage wears away completely, you may be left with bone rubbing on bone, which damages the ends of your bones. This is usually painful.

Your body tries to repair the damage, but lost cartilage typically can't be regenerated. When this protective layer wears away, new bone growth forms spurs (osteophytes) along the sides of existing bones. Prominent lumps can form around the joint as a result. These occur most often with osteoarthritis of the hands and feet. Pain and tenderness over the bony lumps may be most noticeable early in the disease and less noticeable later on.

If cartilage in a joint is severely damaged, the joint lining (synovium), also called the synovial membrane, may become inflamed. A low-grade inflammation (synovitis) can cause episodes of joint swelling.

Many scientists believe cartilage damage may be due to an enzyme imbalance in the cartilage cells or lining of the joint. When balanced, these enzymes allow for the natural breakdown and regeneration of cartilage. But too many enzymes can cause the cartilage to break down faster than it's rebuilt. The exact cause of this enzyme imbalance is unclear.

Early changes to the cartilage and bone don't always result in pain or other symptoms. Many older adults have OA but are unaware of it until their doctors see it on a routine X-ray.

The risk of OA increases with age, with the disease most often developing in people over 40. It's more common in women than men overall, although before the age of 45 it's more prevalent in men. It's relatively rare among younger adults unless they've had a joint injury or they have an underlying secondary cause of OA as discussed on page 22. Those affected often have a family history of the disease.

An active lifestyle may slow the development of osteoarthritis, although almost everyone older than age 65 will experience some joint damage and have mild signs of arthritis that are visible in imaging tests such as X-rays. Still, these mild signs and symptoms may or may not cause pain or affect your activity.

## JOINT CHANGES IN OSTEOARTHRITIS

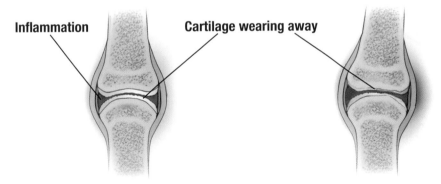

**Inflammation**   **Cartilage wearing away**

A. The first signs of osteoarthritis in a joint are microscopic pits and fissures on the surface of cartilage, which are usually accompanied by mild inflammation.

B. As the cartilage is worn completely through, the contours of the joint are changed and patches of exposed bone appear.

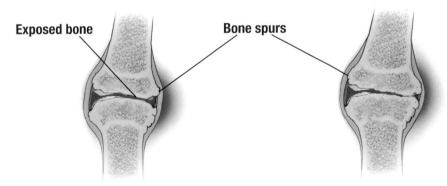

**Exposed bone**   **Bone spurs**

C. The exposed bone thickens and bone spurs (osteophytes) develop. It becomes painful to use the joint.

D. In advanced stages, the space between bones may disappear and ligaments loosen, causing further joint instability. The irregular surface of bones can significantly limit the motion of the joint.

A severe injury to one or more joints at an early age may lead to OA years later. Also, excessively stressful use of joints over many years — such as working at a job that requires repeated knee bending — may cause OA later on. If certain activities are causing joint pain, try to avoid those activities until you've had the joint examined by a doctor.

Being overweight also increases your risk of developing OA, especially in the knees. In one study, women who were heaviest were more than twice as likely to get osteoarthritis and had nearly five times the risk of knee OA. Losing excess weight can help you reduce that risk. (See Chapter 16 for information on weight management.)

## SIGNS AND SYMPTOMS

Osteoarthritis symptoms usually develop slowly and worsen over time. At first, many people notice pain and stiffness when getting out of bed in the morning. This feeling of stiff or creaky joints after a period of inactivity, a phenomenon called "gelling," usually passes within 30 minutes. Others often notice OA pain after strenuous activity. Typically, resting the joint helps relieve the pain.

With osteoarthritis, you may experience:

- Joint pain or tenderness during or after use, or following a period of inactivity
- Joint discomfort before or during a change in the weather
- Joint swelling and stiffness, particularly after use

- Formation of bony lumps on the middle or end finger joints or at the base of the thumb
- Loss of joint flexibility
- Grating sensation in the joint

For example, you may first feel pain and stiffness in the index finger of one hand, but eventually multiple finger joints in both hands may be affected. Your fingers may be stiff and deformed, making it hard to hold a pen or open a jar. Your knees may start to ache after a game of tennis or a jog in the park.

Be aware that the normal wear and tear on your joints doesn't necessarily result in osteoarthritis. OA isn't an inevitable part of aging. But if you develop the condition, the

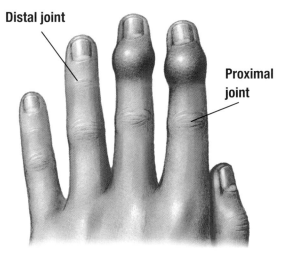

Some people with hand osteoarthritis have bony lumps in the joints near the tips of the fingers (Heberden's nodes). The nodes may be painful at first but are mostly a cosmetic concern once the pain subsides.

symptoms don't go away without treatment. In the early stages, OA pain often fades within a year, but it can return if you overuse an affected joint. Pain tends to increase over the years and, progressively, limits your activity. OA often affects joints on one side of the body at first. Gradually, joints on the opposite side may become involved as well.

Osteoarthritis can affect one joint (localized OA) to many joints (generalized OA). It often affects the hands and the weight-bearing joints of the hips, knees and feet. You may have pain whenever you stand, walk, get up from a chair or climb up stairs. Unless multiple joints are involved, the effects of osteoarthritis are likely to be mild. Keeping active helps prevent problems.

## Hand osteoarthritis

In the hands, osteoarthritis is most common in the joints near the tip and middle of the fingers (distal and proximal joints). The joint at the base of the thumb (carpometacarpal joint) also is often affected. These joints in the hand may be painful or tender and show some redness or swelling, especially in early stages. This discomfort usually lessens over time.

Bone spurs may form in the finger joints with OA. If these growths develop in the joints near your fingertips, they are called Heberden's nodes, while growths in the middle finger joints are known as Bouchard's nodes. This pattern of arthritis (nodal osteoarthritis) tends to run in the family. It often is passed down from the mother or maternal grandmother.

Erosive osteoarthritis, also called inflammatory osteoarthritis, is another type of OA that can affect the hands. It is usually more aggressive than typical hand OA, causing

**Carpometacarpal joint**

This hand of a person with osteoarthrits shows how finger joints have become misaligned and lumpy over time.

more-severe joint damage more quickly. It affects the distal finger joints, like nodal OA, but is often associated with swelling and warmth. Because of this, it can be confused with an underlying inflammatory arthritis such a rheumatoid arthritis. X-rays will show erosions or "bites" out of the bone.

## Knee osteoarthritis

When OA affects the knees, both knees are usually involved, although the condition may be more severe on one side. People who have knee OA often describe a feeling

This X-ray image of knees affected by OA shows the uneven spaces and the points of contact between the thighbone (femur) and shinbone (tibia) on the inside of the joints.

of giving way and may be prone to falls. The knee may be stiff and swollen, and you may feel a grating or catching sensation when you move it. The joint sometimes makes a sound with use.

## Hip osteoarthritis

Pain from hip OA usually occurs deep in the groin area. Pain is worse with activities such as standing from a seated position and starting to walk after being seated for a while. Unlike knee OA, hip OA frequently affects only one hip.

Hip joint damaged by OA

## Big toe osteoarthritis

Osteoarthritis in the foot develops most often where the big toe attaches to the foot. This joint gets less flexible and larger with bony swelling. With this type of OA you may find it uncomfortable to wear shoes, and it may be painful to walk or stand. When this joint bulges out to the side of your foot, it is called a bunion deformity. Usually, both big toes are affected.

## Spine osteoarthritis

Osteoarthritis commonly occurs in the neck or back when the cartilage in your spine wears down. Disks of cartilage normally cushion the bones (vertebrae) of your spine. But they can wear down over time, making spaces between the bones narrower. Bony outgrowths called spurs may form. When bone surfaces rub together, those areas of the vertebrae become inflamed, causing stiffness and pain. Gradually your spine stiffens and loses flexibility. If several disks are involved, you may notice a loss of height. Specific spine conditions are discussed in more detail in Chapter 6.

### Normal spine

### Osteoarthritic spine

This X-ray image of advanced osteoarthritis of the spine shows vertebrae that have become misaligned and unevenly spaced.

Elastic structures called disks cushion the vertebrae in a normal spine, keeping the spine flexible. In OA, disks may narrow and bone spurs can form. Pain and stiffness may occur where bone surfaces rub together, and the spine becomes less flexible.

### Generalized osteoarthritis

When multiple joints are affected with osteoarthritis, it's called generalized osteoarthritis. It's also known as polyarticular arthritis. Usually the distal joints in the hands, the joint at the base of the thumbs, and the big toes, neck, low back, knees and hips are involved. The symptoms usually first appear in one or two joints and gradually appear in others.

### Secondary osteoarthritis

The term secondary osteoarthritis refers to arthritis that develops after a known cause, such as a previous joint injury. Other physical factors that can lead to osteoarthritis include obesity, legs of different lengths, previous joint diseases, surgery or fracture. Certain bone disorders, metabolic conditions and very loose (hypermobile) joints

also can predispose someone to developing OA.

## DIAGNOSIS AND TREATMENT

If you have joint pain and stiffness that may be from osteoarthritis, schedule an appointment with your doctor.

A diagnosis of osteoarthritis is usually based on a careful physical examination and your medical history. Your doctor may ask for details about your symptoms, such as pain, swelling or stiffness. The nature of the joint pain and specific joints that are affected can help your doctor distinguish between different forms of arthritis.

Your doctor may also want to know whether the symptoms started gradually or suddenly, how they've changed over time, and how they're affected by certain types of ac-

## JOINT PAIN: MANY POSSIBILITIES TO CONSIDER

A number of musculoskeletal diseases — disorders affecting the bones, muscles and joints — are associated with arthritis. These might cause joint pain and stiffness or occur alongside arthritis, or they may be a result of arthritis. The pain may stem from problems in the joint itself or from problems in nearby bones, ligaments, tendons, muscles, nerves and other tissues. The symptoms often overlap with arthritis symptoms, which can make diagnosis a challenge. Some of the more common musculoskeletal diseases are discussed in more detail in Chapter 3.

tivity. For example, mild morning stiffness is common in osteoarthritis and usually gets better after a few minutes of activity. In contrast, morning stiffness that lasts for hours is more likely to be a symptom of rheumatoid arthritis or another type of inflammatory disorder.

Your doctor may ask whether you have other symptoms, such as fever, fatigue or skin problems. It's important to alert your doctor to any events or changes that occurred just before your symptoms began and whether you have a family history of arthritis.

During a physical exam, your doctor will check your joints for tenderness, swelling and redness. He or she will look for bony outgrowths (bone spurs) along the sides of existing bones and listen for a crunching or grating sound (crepitation), which indicates that the joint cartilage surface has become rough. Your doctor may also move your

joints through their range of motion to check for pain in certain positions and see if you have limited motion.

Your doctor may recommend an X ray to confirm the diagnosis, rule out other causes of pain and determine the extent of joint damage. Although soft tissue such as bone cartilage doesn't show up on X-ray images, a narrowing of the space between bones can indicate cartilage loss. X-rays may also show bone spurs developing on the affected joint.

Magnetic resonance imaging (MRI) provides detailed images of bone and soft tissue, which can help determine exactly what's causing the pain.

There's no blood test for osteoarthritis, but doctors sometimes request a blood sample to help rule out rheumatoid arthritis and other forms of arthritis.

## QUESTIONS YOUR DOCTOR MAY ASK

To diagnose any form of arthritis, a doctor relies heavily on your description of signs and symptoms and other relevant information. It's a good idea to make a list of your signs and symptoms and when and where they occur. Keeping a pain record or diary for two weeks to share with your doctor can help in making a diagnosis. Keep track of the intensity of your pain, how long it lasts, what it feels like, and whether anything makes it better or worse.

Following are some questions you may be asked about your arthritis signs and symptoms:

- Which joints are painful?
- Do the same joints on both sides of your body hurt at the same time, or is the pain just on one side?
- Has the pain moved from one joint to another?
- Did pain start in just one joint and then progress to include others? How quickly did this happen?
- Did your symptoms start gradually or all at once? Have they gotten worse over time or stayed about the same?
- Do you have stiffness in the morning or after a period of inactivity, such as when watching TV? How long does morning stiffness last?
- What time of day is the pain most severe?
- If you have pain in your hands, which joints hurt the most?
- Have you had times of feeling weak and uncomfortable all over? Have you been unusually tired?
- Does anything make your pain better or worse?
- Does pain or difficulty moving interfere with your work, sleep or daily activities?
- Do you have any other symptoms besides joint problems? Have you had fever, loss of appetite, changes in vision or any other physical changes?
- Does arthritis or rheumatic disease run in your family?
- Before your symptoms first appeared, did you have a viral or bacterial illness, injury, vaccination, or new medication?

Keep in mind that the presence of osteoar-thritis in a joint doesn't in itself indicate a serious problem. Many people have no symptoms or disability from the condition. They may not even realize that they have osteoarthritis and experience little, if any, discomfort.

While there's no known cure for osteoar-thritis, you and your doctor can develop a treatment program that helps you reduce pain, preserve joint movement and main-tain a high quality of life.

Your doctor may recommend an all-around approach that includes medications, physi-cal exercise and splints. In addition, physi-cal therapy and occupational therapy may help you learn how to change certain be-haviors, such as gripping objects, to protect your joints. In some cases, surgery may be necessary. Specific treatments are described more in Part 2: Treating Arthritis. These treatments have long-lasting benefits that can help you control the disease and live an active, independent life.

# Other noninflammatory musculoskeletal disorders

Musculoskeletal disorders are problems with the body's muscles, bones, tendons and ligaments. Osteoarthritis and other forms of arthritis are types of musculoskeletal disorders. But muscle and joint pain can result from many other conditions. This chapter reviews some of the most common causes.

While the conditions discussed here often cause pain and inflammation, they are considered noninflammatory. That's because inflammation is typically the result of these conditions, not the cause.

See your doctor if you have any joint pain. Ignoring the pain — and living with inflammation — may lead to more-serious problems. A doctor's careful diagnosis can help you know how to treat the condition, reduce your pain and prevent joint damage.

## ANKLE SPRAINS

Ankle sprains are a common injury. They're usually due to the ankle joint turning too far in a particular direction, especially inward. The ligaments that hold the ankle bones together stretch or tear, causing pain and swelling. A sprain often makes it difficult to bear weight on the affected ankle because of pain and unsteadiness.

Initial treatment of an ankle sprain involves rest, ice, compression and elevation (R.I.C.E.). Rest the ankle and stay off your feet. You may need crutches to get around and take pressure off the ankle. Ice the ankle every one to two hours, for 15 minutes each time, to help ease pain and inflammation. Wrapping the ankle in an elastic bandage (compression) reduces swelling and gives the joint support. Elevating the foot above the level of your heart also helps keep swelling down. Anti-inflammatory medications may help as well.

Most ankle sprains heal with these conservative therapies. Rarely, surgery is needed to repair a torn ligament. People who have had an ankle sprain are typically at higher risk of future sprains, so it's important to perform ankle strength and stability exercises to help prevent injuries in the future.

## AVASCULAR NECROSIS

Avascular necrosis (AVN) is the death of bone tissue due to a lack of blood supply. It can occur when the blood vessels to a joint are disrupted, for example, from a broken bone or a dislocated joint. AVN can affect any joint, but it's usually most severe when the hip or knee is involved. People who have avascular necrosis of the hip or knee typically develop pain in the joint, especially when walking, and may limp.

Factors that may raise your risk of AVN include alcoholism, steroid use, trauma such as a major bone or joint injury, and smoking. Your risk may also be higher after radiation therapy for cancer.

To diagnose AVN, a doctor will examine the joint and look at imaging tests such as an X-ray or CT scan, which can show changes to the bone. Treatment typically includes bed rest, crutches and anti-inflammatory medications. For advanced AVN, your doctor might recommend surgery.

## BAKER'S CYST (POPLITEAL CYST)

**Baker's cyst**

A Baker's cyst, also called a popliteal cyst, is a fluid-filled sac behind the knee. It usually results from an abnormality or injury in the knee such as arthritis or a cartilage tear. This may cause your knee to produce fluid, which can pool and form a cyst. The cyst can lead to pain or stiffness, or it may not cause any symptoms. You may notice swelling or a bulge at the back of the knee, especially when the leg is straight. The pain and stiffness might feel worse if you stand for a long time. Occasionally, the cyst may tear open, causing the calf to swell and become red. Sometimes a bruise will form in the ankle.

Usually, treating a painful Baker's cyst involves draining (aspirating) the synovial fluid in the knee joint, injecting a steroid into the joint and treating any related arthritis. Rarely, surgery is necessary to remove or repair a cartilage tear that's causing the cyst.

## BUNION

A bunion is a bump that may form along the joint at the base of the big toe. The bump develops when the big toe angles toward the next toe. The joint begins to stick out, which can lead to swelling, redness and soreness. Bunions occur in women more often than in men, and they tend to run in the family. They can be associated with wearing tight shoes, such as dress shoes that crunch the toes. A foot deformity from birth also may lead to a bunion.

Most bunions are treatable without surgery. To treat or prevent bunions, it's important to wear properly fitting shoes that don't constrict the toes. A toe spacer placed between the big toe and the second toe can help reduce a bunion deformity, and medial bunion pads — worn on the outside of the big toe joint — may help lessen the pain and other symptoms. When discomfort isn't getting better with conservative management, surgery may be an option.

Bunion

A similar bump that forms on the outside of the fifth toe is called a bunionette or tailor's bunion. This can lead to a hard corn and, occasionally, painful bursitis. A bunionette is typically caused by tight, poorly fitting shoes. You may need to wear shoes that allow plenty of toe space to decrease pressure on the area and relieve symptoms. As with a bunion, surgery is needed only in rare cases if pain persists.

## BURSITIS

Your body has more than 150 bursae — small, fluid-filled sacs that cushion pressure points between the bones, tendons and muscles near your joints. Overuse of a joint or repeated stress on the joint can lead to painful inflammation of a bursa, called bursitis. Bursitis most often affects your shoulders, elbows and hips. But bursitis can also affect your knee, heel and even the base of your big toe.

If you have bursitis, you may feel an ache or tenderness around a joint. The joint may be stiff and difficult to move, and it may hurt especially when you move the joint or put pressure on it. If the inflamed bursa is near the skin's surface, the area may be red, swollen and warm to the touch.

The most common causes of bursitis are repetitive motions or positions that irritate the bursae around a joint. For example, if you spend a lot of time kneeling, the pressure on the knee could cause inflammation in a bursa at the front of your kneecap. Swinging a golf club or throwing a ball repeatedly can affect a bursa in your elbow or shoulder. Bursitis may also result from joint stress; injury to a joint, tendon or ligament; infection; or gout. Often the cause is unknown. Some forms of arthritis also can lead to bursitis.

Bursitis may be diagnosed from a physical exam if your doctor can identify specific areas of tenderness. To help rule out other possible causes of the discomfort, you may have an imaging test such as an X-ray, MRI or ultrasound. Treatment includes resting the affected area and applying ice and compression to reduce swelling. Bursitis pain usually goes away within about a week of home treatment. Taking anti-inflammatory drugs such as ibuprofen (Advil, Motrin IB, others) or naproxen sodium (Aleve) can help relieve pain and reduce inflammation.

To avoid having bursitis become a chronic problem, it's important to prevent flare-ups. This includes protecting the joint and avoiding repetitive activities and positions that put pressure on the bursa. Specific types of bursitis are discussed below.

## Olecranon bursitis

The bursa that sits at the tip of your elbow is called the olecranon bursa. If it becomes inflamed it can cause swelling, often resembling a golf ball on the elbow. Olecranon bursitis is most commonly caused by trauma or irritation to the elbow — for example, leaning on a table or chair or using an elbow to get out of bed. People with certain jobs,

such as carpet laying, are more prone to developing the condition.

When the cause is repetitive trauma, olecranon bursitis usually comes on slowly and the surrounding tissues are normal. The elbow can still fully extend despite the bursa swelling. A doctor may recommend conservative treatments such as elbow pads to prevent ongoing irritation to the joint. Typically, for swelling caused by trauma, a doctor will try to avoid draining the fluid. This is because there isn't a good blood supply to the bursa to fight an infection, on the chance one would occur.

Inflammatory conditions such as gout, rheumatoid arthritis or infection also can lead to olecranon bursitis. When inflammation is the cause, the elbow becomes swollen, red, warm and very painful. Often, inserting a needle into the bursa to analyze the fluid is necessary to find the cause of the swelling. Sometimes surgery is needed to remove the bursa.

**Olecranon bursitis**

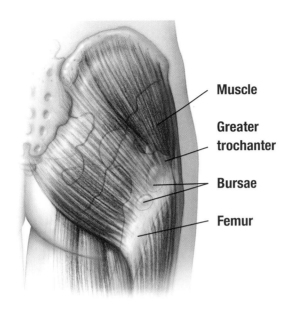

Muscle

Greater
trochanter

Bursae

Femur

## Trochanteric bursitis

Bursitis around the greater trochanter — a portion of the thighbone located just below the hip — is a common cause of hip pain. It may occur from irritation, overuse, early hip arthritis, weak hip muscles or obesity. This type of bursitis usually causes a dull, burning pain. It typically doesn't cause visible swelling or skin redness, because the bursae are located beneath bulky muscles.

Rest and physical therapy are the first therapies for treating bursitis around the hip. If the problem remains painful, steroid injections may help relieve the inflammation.

## DUPUYTREN'S CONTRACTURE

Dupuytren's contracture is a thickening of the tissue in the palm of your hand. Over time, it can pull the fingers into a bent posi-

tion. This condition tends to worsen slowly over years. Initially, the palm of your hand might become thick but not feel painful. In later stages you may develop hard lumps under the skin. Some people have difficulty straightening one or more fingers.

This condition occurs more frequently in men than in women. You may be at higher risk if a family member has the condition, if you have diabetes, or if you use tobacco or alcohol.

There is no treatment to stop Dupuytren's contracture from getting worse, but certain treatments may improve symptoms. Sometimes, a doctor can break up the thick tissue, using either a needle inserted through the skin or a type of enzyme injection. If symptoms are severe, surgery may be needed to break up or remove the tissue.

With mild symptoms, using a cushioned tool handle or padded gloves can reduce pain when gripping or grasping objects.

## MERALGIA PARESTHETICA

A numbness or tingling along the outer thigh may be due to meralgia paresthetica. This condition results when the large nerve in your outer groin (lateral femoral cutaneous nerve) gets pinched, often by a nearby ligament. You might feel tingling in the side of your thigh or burning pain on the surface. However, it doesn't cause any weakness to the muscle.

Meralgia paresthetica often occurs in people who are overweight, have diabetes, are older or are pregnant. Trauma to the area, rapid weight gain and wearing clothing that's tight at the waist also can lead to symptoms.

Most of the time, no specific treatment is needed, but you can learn ways to reduce pressure on the nerve. A doctor may suggest avoiding tight clothing or other measures to help the problem resolve on its own. Occasionally, medications may be used to help reduce persistent symptoms. Surgery is rarely necessary.

Morton's neuroma

## MORTON'S NEUROMA

Morton's neuroma is a thickening of the tissue around one of the nerves that leads to the toes. The condition most frequently develops between the third and fourth toes. It's more common in women and usually occurs in response to irritation, trauma or excessive pressure between the toes.

Symptoms include the feeling of walking on a marble or burning pain in the ball of the foot that may radiate into the toes. Tingling or numbness in the toes also is common. An exam and imaging tests such as an X-ray or ultrasound can confirm the diagnosis.

High-heeled and tight or narrow shoes tend to aggravate Morton's neuroma. You may need to switch to low-heeled or flat shoes with wider toe boxes and use orthotics to relieve pressure on the area. Taking anti-inflammatory medications also can

help. If a neuroma doesn't respond to these types of conservative treatments, a doctor may recommend steroid injections or, eventually, surgery.

## OSGOOD-SCHLATTER DISEASE

Osgood-Schlatter disease causes pain just below the kneecap on the tibia, the large lower leg bone. It usually occurs with swelling or a bump on the front of the knee. Typically, this condition affects children ages 9 to 14. It often occurs in children going through a growth spurt and those who are active in sports that involve running, jumping and fast changes of direction. The repeated stress and activity pulls on the tendon connecting the kneecap and the tibia.

Knee pain from Osgood-Schlatter disease is usually worse with running, jumping or kneeling activities, and it improves with rest. The condition normally goes away after a child's bones stop growing. Icing the area and stretching the quadriceps muscles on the front of the thigh may help the pain. Children with Osgood-Schlatter disease can continue sports and other activities if the pain is manageable.

## OSTEOPOROSIS

Osteoporosis is a bone-weakening disease, caused by the gradual loss of calcium and other minerals from the bones. Over many years, this makes the bones thinner, weaker and more prone to breaking. Unlike osteo-arthritis, which leads to stiffness and pain, osteoporosis causes no symptoms at first. Painful fractures in the spine, hips, wrists or other bones may be the earliest signs of the disease.

Your bones are living tissue that's continuously changing. Over time, old or worn-out bone is broken down and absorbed, and new bone is made to replace it. By the time you reach your mid-30s, more bone tissue is being lost than replaced, so you gradually begin to lose bone strength. Osteoporosis develops if enough bone is lost that portions of your skeleton become porous, brittle and weak. People over age 50 are most likely to develop the disease.

Osteoporosis is common, affecting an estimated 8 million women and 2 million men in the United States. The risk increases with age. Your risk depends in part on your bone mass — how much bone tissue you've developed by the time it peaks during young adulthood. How rapidly you lose it later also affects your risk.

Some risk factors are out of your control. The disease is generally more common among women, people with a parent or sibling with osteoporosis, and men and women who are white or of Asian descent. Those with a small frame also are more likely to get osteoporosis, as they have less bone mass to draw from as they age.

In addition, hormone levels, medications, your diet and other lifestyle choices affect your risk. In women, a sudden drop in estrogen at menopause can speed up bone loss. Lower testosterone levels in older men can do the same. Not getting enough

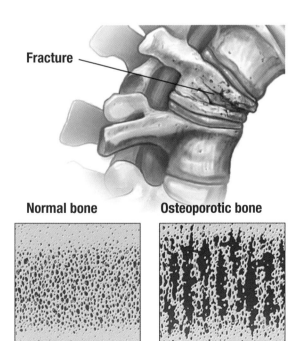

Fracture

Normal bone          Osteoporotic bone

calcium and vitamin D in your diet also can speed up bone loss. Other factors that raise your risk of osteoporosis include an eating disorder such as anorexia, certain diseases, long-term use of some medications, an inactive lifestyle, and use of alcohol and tobacco.

With osteoporosis, bone breaks may happen more easily than expected. In the spine, vertebrae can become compressed and fracture or collapse. You may have back pain, lose height over time and develop a stooped posture. Hip and wrist fractures also are common.

If you have risk factors for osteoporosis, your doctor may recommend diagnostic tests. You'll likely have a bone density scan and a physical exam.

Diagnostic tests are done to:

- Confirm that you have osteoporosis
- Determine the severity of your low bone density
- Establish your baseline values for bone density
- Identify chemical abnormalities that may predispose you to osteoporosis

A bone density test can help your doctor determine if you have osteoporosis and predict your risk of a fracture. Bone density scans are generally simple, fast and painless. They use special X-rays or ultrasound technology to measure how much calcium and other minerals — collectively known as bone mineral content — are packed into your bones. The higher your mineral content, the denser the bone. The denser the

A bone density scan can help identify areas where your bones are growing weaker. The spine, forearm and wrist, fingers, hip, and heel are common areas to have checked.

## WHO SHOULD BE TESTED FOR OSTEOPOROSIS?

Ideally, adults at risk of osteoporosis will have a bone mineral density (BMD) test. Other tools that estimate risk, such as the Fracture Risk Assessment Tool (FRAX), can help determine who should have BMD testing. Early testing gives more time to take steps to prevent bone loss. It's also the first and best step toward receiving a diagnosis and starting treatment. A bone density test is recommended for:

- Women age 65 and older.
- Women over age 50 who are at higher risk of osteoporosis. Risk factors include a family history of fractures, a slender, small frame, lost height, a drop in hormone levels, or being the recipient of a transplant.
- Men who've had an X-ray showing possible low bone density or who've lost height.
- Adults who've had a fragility fracture — when bone becomes so fragile that it breaks much more easily than expected.

- Adults who have a medical condition associated with lower bone mass, such as rheumatoid arthritis, diabetes and hyperparathyroidism.
- Adults who are taking or will soon take a medication associated with lower bone mass, such as corticosteroid drugs and thyroid hormones.
- Anyone being treated for osteoporosis.

Bone density testing is usually not a one-time thing. The frequency of retesting depends on your age and the factors that put you at risk. One to two years is the minimum amount of time for bone affected by osteoporosis to show a noticeable increase or decrease in density. Even if your bone density is normal at the initial test, talk with your doctor about when to repeat the test. Bone density tests over several years can reveal the rate at which you may be losing bone. This rate helps predict your risk of a fracture.

bone, the stronger it is and the less likely it is to break.

Medications such as bisphosphonates are often prescribed to treat osteoporosis. These drugs slow the breakdown of bone. Making healthy lifestyle choices also can help preserve bone strength. To maintain bone density, it's important to eat a diet rich in calcium, avoid smoking and drinking in excess, and stay active, especially with weight-bearing exercise and strength training.

## PATELLOFEMORAL PAIN SYNDROME

Patellofemoral pain syndrome causes pain in the front of the knee, around the kneecap (patella). It's common in runners and others who are active in sports that involve running and jumping. The pain is typically worse with activities that put pressure on the knees, such as squatting, running, going up or down stairs, and sitting for long periods of time. In addition, the knee may make a popping noise while climbing stairs or squatting and standing.

This type of knee pain is more common in women and adolescents or young adults. Experts aren't sure exactly what causes it, but it sometimes occurs when weak or imbalanced muscles around the kneecap don't permit proper movement. It's also associated with overuse of the knee or a previous injury or surgery.

A key part of treatment involves strengthening the core and hip muscles. This helps with proper leg alignment when you're active, permits the kneecap to glide easier and reduces the pressure under the kneecap. Avoiding activities that make the pain worse should also help. Icing the knee, taping around the kneecap, wearing a brace for the kneecap, and using orthotics will usually provide additional relief.

## PLANTAR FASCIITIS

One of the most common causes of heel pain is plantar fasciitis, an inflammation of the connective tissue that runs from the heel to the base of the toes (plantar fascia). This tough layer of fascia supports the arch of the foot. Plantar fasciitis typically causes a sharp pain in the heel when you put weight on it, especially with the first few steps in the morning or after being at rest for a while.

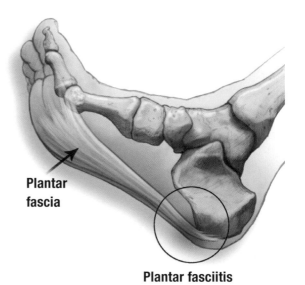

**Plantar fascia**

**Plantar fasciitis**

The pain usually improves as you keep moving.

Plantar fasciitis is often caused by repetitive stress on the connective tissue, which can lead to small tears (microtraumas). The condition is a common injury in runners. Your risk is also higher if you're on your feet for hours at work, if you're overweight or if you don't wear proper foot support.

You can usually manage the pain with rest, acetaminophen (Tylenol, others) and anti-inflammatory medications such as ibuprofen or naproxen sodium, orthotics, heel pads, and physical therapy. Wearing a splint at night also may help. Plantar fasciitis tends to run its course, but it can take months to resolve. If your pain doesn't go away, your doctor may recommend steroid injections or ultrasound-guided procedures to stimulate blood flow or remove damaged tissue.

## SHIN SPLINTS

Shin splints cause pain in the front of the legs along the lower part of the shinbone (tibia). Usually, this pain starts during or after intense exercise such as running or after a rapid increase in activity. The new duration or intensity can overwork the muscles, tendons and bone tissue.

Shin splints typically go away with self-care, including resting, elevating the leg, icing the area and using anti-inflammatory medications. Core and hip strengthening also can help promote proper body me-

chanics during running. However, sometimes shin splints can lead to a stress fracture (see below). You can reduce your chances of getting shin splints by wearing shoes with enough support and increasing your activity gradually.

## STRESS FRACTURE

A stress fracture is a tiny fracture of a bone due to repeated force. These fractures are most common in the weight-bearing foot bones. They tend to occur after a sudden increase in activity — doing too much too soon — and are frequently seen in distance runners, jumping sports or military training.

The pain of a stress fracture develops gradually, becoming more intense with continued activity. At first, rest can relieve the pain. But as the condition worsens, it may be painful even while resting and at night. You may have a specific area of tenderness and swelling, but usually no bruising or discoloration.

To help a stress fracture heal, you'll need to avoid high-impact activities and wear a brace or walking boot or use crutches to decrease stress on the area. With these measures, a stress fracture can generally heal over a period of six to eight weeks.

## TENDINITIS

Tendons are thick, fibrous cords that attach muscles to bones and other structures in the body. Tendinitis is traditionally defined as inflammation of the tendons, though in many cases the degree of inflammation may actually be small. With aging and stressful use, the tendons may become worn, frayed and sometimes torn.

Tendinitis causes pain and tenderness just outside a joint — and over the involved tendon — most often around your shoulders, elbows and knees. Tennis elbow, golfer's elbow, pitcher's shoulder, swimmer's shoulder and jumper's knee are common names for different forms of tendinitis. Pain may also occur in the groin area or above your heel, in the Achilles tendon. Pain is usually worse when you use the muscles attached to the tendon. The location depends on which tendon is affected.

The most common causes of tendinitis are injury and overuse from work or play. Professional athletes and weekend warriors alike may be affected by the condition. It can develop along with rheumatoid arthritis and other inflammatory rheumatic diseases as well. And because of their similar locations in the body, bursitis and tendinitis may occur together. The risk of developing tendinitis increases with age, as your muscles and tendons lose their elasticity. Using proper form and technique while active can help prevent overloading the tendons.

Tendinitis may not require a doctor's care. Treatment usually focuses on resting the tendon, applying ice to reduce swelling, stretching and strengthening the tendon, using proper movement technique, and taking pain relievers as needed. If an elbow or knee is involved, wrapping it with an elastic band may be helpful.

Discomfort from tendinitis may disappear within a few weeks. But if pain interferes with your normal activities or doesn't improve after two weeks, see your doctor. To help rule out other possible problems, you may have an X-ray, MRI or ultrasound.

In older adults and those who continue to use the affected area, tendinitis often heals more slowly and may become chronic. The involved tendon may even tear or rupture.

Several specific tendinitis conditions are discussed below.

## Achilles tendinitis

Achilles tendinitis is an irritation of the Achilles tendon, which connects the calf muscles to the heel bone in the back of the leg. This tendon is used when you walk, run and jump. Achilles tendinitis most often affects people who are physically active, especially in high-impact exercise such as running, but it can occur in anyone.

Your risk of developing this tendinitis is greater if you suddenly increase your exercise or activity, do the same activities over and over, or exercise without warming up the calf muscles. Your risk is also higher if you exercise in shoes that are worn out or not made with the right support. Arthritis or a bone growth on the back of the heel bone can irritate the tendon too.

Typically, Achilles tendinitis causes pain in the back of the leg that gets worse with exercise and better with rest. Occasionally, the tendon becomes swollen and makes noise with motion. Conservative treatment is usually recommended — resting, avoiding painful activities, icing the area, and using an elastic bandage or a heel lift in your shoe for support. Your doctor may also recommend stretches and strengthening exercises. Meanwhile, acetaminophen and anti-inflammatory medications can help relieve symptoms.

Sudden, severe pain in the back of the leg and difficulty putting weight on your foot can be signs of Achilles tendon rupture. With this injury, you may hear a pop or experience a sudden feeling of being kicked in the back of the ankle. A doctor might refer you to an orthopedic surgeon to repair the tear. These tears can also be treated without surgery.

If you've had Achilles tendinitis, it's important to warm up your muscles before exercise to keep it from recurring. You'll want to avoid sudden increases in exercise, easing into a new sport or activity. It also may help to avoid exercising outside in cold weather or on hard surfaces. In addition, keep up strengthening exercises to help the tendons absorb load, and wear supportive shoes.

## De Quervain's tenosynovitis

This form of tendinitis leads to pain in the base of the thumb and wrist, trouble gripping objects and possibly mild wrist swelling. It is caused by irritation of the tendons

**De Quervain's tenosynovitis**

that connect the forearm muscles to the thumb. It also affects the tendons' protective sheaths, a condition called tenosynovitis. De Quervain's tenosynovitis typically is associated with overuse and is more common in manual laborers and during pregnancy.

Treatment includes rest, ice, wearing a splint, and using acetaminophen or anti-inflammatory medications. Sometimes, you may need a steroid injection around the inflamed tendon or surgery for relief. After your symptoms improve, exercises to strengthen the muscles in the wrist, hand and arm will help prevent the condition from coming back.

## Elbow tendinitis

Tendinitis is one of the most common causes of elbow pain. Tennis elbow, one form of

Tennis elbow, a type of tendinitis, causes pain due to tiny tears in a tendon on the outside of the elbow that becomes inflamed.

elbow tendinitis, causes pain on the outside of your elbow as you rotate your forearm or grip an object. The pain of golfer's elbow occurs more on the inside of your elbow, affecting a different tendon. The pain typically spreads into the upper arm or down to the forearm. It can cause forearm weakness and difficulty with activities such as throwing a ball.

Sports other than tennis and golf also can cause these conditions. So can work-related activities that involve heavy use of the wrist and forearm muscles. And as people age, tendons can break down, leading to tendon irritation even with normal use.

Symptoms can often be treated with anti-inflammatory medications. Wearing a forearm brace and icing the area can also help bring relief. Exercises can help to strengthen the muscle and tendon. To avoid another injury, make sure to use proper technique, whether you're swinging a tennis racket or a golf club.

## Rotator cuff tendinitis and subacromial bursitis

Pain in the shoulder may occur when the tendons or bursa of the shoulder joint is irritated. The rotator cuff tendons help hold the arm in place in the shoulder. They may become inflamed with trauma or overuse, such as repeated throwing motion, or as you age.

If a rotator cuff tendon becomes inflamed, it may also irritate the subacromial bursa, which provides a smooth cushion for the tendons to glide along.

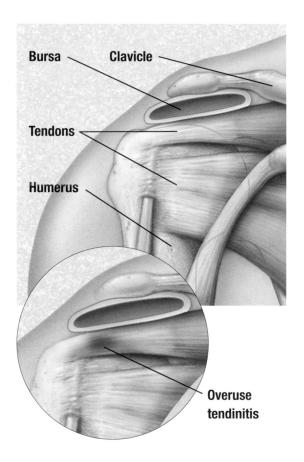

Bursa    Clavicle

Tendons

Humerus

Overuse tendinitis

Rotator cuff tendinitis generally causes shoulder pain that's worse when you move the arm overhead. It may also limit the range of motion of the shoulder. With continued irritation, the tendon may tear.

If your doctor suspects tendinitis without a tear, you may be referred to physical therapy for treatment. Sometimes a steroid injection may be helpful. If the pain persists despite conservative therapy, you may need imaging tests such as an MRI scan to be evaluated for a possible rotator cuff tear.

## TRIGGER FINGER

Trigger finger occurs when a tendon in your hand becomes inflamed or irritated, leading to a finger that's stuck in the bent (flexed) position. The tendon can't glide easily through its inflamed protective sheath, and it becomes "locked" where it connects to the finger in the palm. You may feel a catching or "triggering" upon waking up in the morning. At times you may have to use the other hand to straighten out the finger. Trigger finger occurs most often in the ring finger, thumb and second finger.

Your doctor can diagnose trigger finger by examining your hand. He or she will check for pain, swelling and smooth movement of the tendons as you open and close your hand. To treat the condition, you may try conservative therapies first, including rest, a splint and gentle exercises. Meanwhile, acetaminophen or anti-inflammatory medications can help temporarily relieve pain. If

the triggering continues, a steroid injection may be helpful. In some cases, a needling technique or surgery may be needed to relieve the constriction around the tendon.

Tendon sheath

Tendon

Nodule

# Rheumatoid arthritis

Rheumatoid arthritis (RA) causes painful aching and swelling in your joints and leaves you feeling tired and ill. It's the most common form of inflammatory arthritis — caused by inflammation in the body — and it often occurs at a younger age than osteoarthritis typically does. While its exact cause isn't known, the disease appears to be triggered by an abnormal response from your immune system.

The immune system is your body's primary defense against germs, such as bacteria or viruses, that make you sick. When the immune system identifies a threat, it activates special cells, proteins and chemicals that attempt to seek out and destroy the germs. This battle with foreign invaders often results in inflammation — redness, swelling, warmth and pain at the point of infection.

In rheumatoid arthritis and other forms of inflammatory arthritis, something goes awry with your body's normal immune response. The immune system mistakenly identifies some of your body's own cells as foreign invaders. This triggers an uncontrolled attack on your tissues and organs. Long-term (chronic) inflammation from these misplaced attacks may result in severe damage to parts of your body, including your joints.

Diseases in which the immune system turns against its own body are known as autoimmune disorders. There are more than 80 different autoimmune disorders. Research indicates that some people may be genetically predisposed to develop these diseases. You can find out more about other forms of inflammatory arthritis in Chapter 5.

## UNDERSTANDING THE CONDITION

An estimated 1.5 million Americans have rheumatoid arthritis. The disease is more common among women, affecting two to three times more women than men. It occurs more frequently in older people, often beginning in middle age. But it can also affect children and young adults.

Overall, rheumatoid arthritis occurs in about 0.5% to 1% of people, but it's more common in some geographic regions and ethnic groups than in others.

In rheumatoid arthritis, an immune reaction leads to inflammation, causing the body's joints to swell, ache and throb. Pain, swelling and stiffness can make even simple activities, such as opening a jar or taking a walk, difficult to manage. If the inflammation continues over a long period of time, damage may occur to the joint structure, causing it to become deformed.

The primary target of the immune system is a protective layer lining the joints called the synovial membrane (synovium). White blood cells — whose job it is to attack unwanted invaders — move from the bloodstream into the membrane. The blood cells release potent chemicals that cause the membrane to become inflamed.

As inflammation develops, the body recruits more immune cells to enter the synovial tissues. These cells, along with proteins and other substances they release, cause the normally thin synovium to thicken. As a result, the body's joints become painful, tender and swollen.

If joint inflammation persists, the result is often destruction of cartilage, bone and soft tissues in the joint. Ligaments, muscle and bone also are weakened. This weakening may lead to looseness in the joint and to its eventual destruction. Over time, the involved joints may gradually lose their alignment and shape.

Researchers believe that rheumatoid arthritis begins damaging bones during the first year or two of onset. Because of this, early diagnosis and treatment of the disease are extremely critical.

In contrast to osteoarthritis, which affects primarily bones and cartilage, rheumatoid arthritis can target your whole body. It can affect organs you might not expect to be involved, such as your heart, blood vessels, lungs and eyes. However, the disease most commonly affects your joints.

Rheumatoid arthritis increases your risk of osteoporosis, a bone-thinning disease (see page 37). Taking steroid medications to treat arthritis especially increases the risk.

Some research suggests that people with rheumatoid arthritis also have an increased risk of infections, heart disease and forms of cancer, such as lymphomas. The higher risk of these problems may be due to immune system activity and the effects of inflammation. Medications for rheumatoid arthritis also may play a role.

# JOINT CHANGES IN RHEUMATOID ARTHRITIS

**Synovial membrane**

**Cartilage**

**Bone**

A. In a normal joint, the synovial membrane forms a protective capsule around a joint. Synovial fluid lubricates the joint.

**Pannus formation**

B. Inflammation causes the synovial fluid to thicken, forming a layer called the pannus. The joint becomes swollen and warm.

**Pannus formation**

C. Cells in the pannus release enzymes that destroy cartilage and bone. Space narrows between the bones of the joint as cartilage is eroded.

**Fused joint**

D. Tendons and the joint capsule may become inflamed. The tendons shorten as the joint becomes too painful to move. This results in fusion of the bones of the joint.

# DIFFERENCES BETWEEN OSTEOARTHRITIS AND RHEUMATOID ARTHRITIS

| Osteoarthritis | Rheumatoid arthritis |
|---|---|
| Affects nearly 31 million U.S. adults | Affects 1.5 million U.S. adults |
| Usually begins after age 40 and develops slowly | Usually begins in middle age and may develop suddenly, within weeks or months |
| May occur in a few joints on one or both sides of the body | Usually affects many joints on both sides of the body |
| Typically affects only certain joints, most commonly those of the hips, hands, knees and lower back | Affects many joints, especially small joints of the hands and feet, and the wrists, elbows and shoulders |
| Usually causes minimal warmth and swelling, as well as brief morning stiffness; joints may be hard and bony | Causes warmth, swelling and prolonged morning stiffness, often lasting for hours |
| Can cause Heberden's nodes — bony growths in the end joints of the fingers | Doesn't cause Heberden's nodes |
| Doesn't cause an overall feeling of sickness and fatigue | Often causes an overall feeling of sickness and fatigue and may lead to weight loss |
| Negative blood tests for rheumatoid factor and anti-CCP antibodies; normal sed rate and CRP level | Blood tests often positive for rheumatoid factor and anti-CCP antibodies; sed rate and CRP level sometimes elevated |

## CAUSES

Scientists still don't know exactly what causes an immune system to turn against itself in rheumatoid arthritis. But research has identified several factors that seem to increase the risk or trigger the disease.

Certain genes appear to make you more susceptible to rheumatoid arthritis. How severe your symptoms are also may depend on genetics. This doesn't mean that if you have specific genes you're guaranteed to get rheumatoid arthritis — you're just more likely to do so. People who don't have these genes also can develop RA.

Many researchers suspect that an infection may trigger rheumatoid arthritis, particularly in people whose genes make them more susceptible to the disease. However, many studies have looked for a connection between specific bacteria or viruses and RA. None have been able to prove that an infection contributes to this form of arthritis.

Because women are more likely to get rheumatoid arthritis, researchers believe that reproductive hormones such as estrogen also may play a role. The disease often improves during pregnancy but flares up postpartum. In addition, breast-feeding appears to lower women's risk of RA. However, researchers have a limited understanding of how hormones influence the disease.

Smoking also increases the risk of rheumatoid arthritis, especially if your genes make you more susceptible to the disease. Smoking may also cause more-severe forms of RA. For example, smokers may be more likely to develop nodules or have joint erosion seen on X-rays.

Some studies suggest that gum (periodontal) disease may be another trigger for developing rheumatoid arthritis. As with smoking, a type of gum disease may lead to RA in people who are genetically at higher risk. Researchers are also exploring whether an imbalance of bacteria in the gut microbiome — the organisms that live in your gut — may play a role in triggering this type of arthritis.

Experts believe that rheumatoid arthritis develops when several of these genetic, biological and environmental factors combine. The end result is an autoimmune disease in which your immune system attacks tissue in the joints of your body.

## SIGNS AND SYMPTOMS

Rheumatoid arthritis can affect you in different ways. One common pattern is to have periods when your signs and symptoms are worse, called flares or flare-ups, alternating with periods when you feel better, called remissions.

Some people develop a severe form of the disease that's almost continuously active and lasts for many years. For a few people, the signs and symptoms persist for a certain amount of time — from a few months to a couple of years — and then go away.

The signs and symptoms of rheumatoid arthritis can be more or less severe, and they may be persistent or come and go. Signs and symptoms include:

- Pain in joints, especially the smaller joints of the hands and feet
- Aching or stiffness in joints and muscles, especially in the morning or after periods of rest
- Warmth and swelling in affected joints
- Loss of motion in affected joints
- Weakness in muscles attached to affected joints
- Fatigue, which can be severe during a flare
- Low-grade fever
- General sense of not feeling well

- Weight loss
- Deformity of the joints
- Anxiety or depression

Morning stiffness is common in both osteoarthritis and rheumatoid arthritis. But with osteoarthritis, it usually goes away quickly — within about 30 minutes. In contrast, morning stiffness associated with rheumatoid arthritis generally lasts more than an hour and may even extend for several hours. Stiffness can recur after periods of rest or inactivity.

Rheumatoid arthritis usually causes problems in several joints at the same time. While any joint can be affected, most people

Rheumatoid arthritis often leads to deformity — a change from the usual shape — in the fingers. During flares, your hand may be painful and weak.

experience symptoms of inflammation at first in their wrists, hands and feet. As the disease spreads to other parts of the body, it may also affect the knees, shoulders, elbows, hips, jaw and neck. Usually both sides of the body experience symptoms at the same time, such as the knuckles of both hands.

Rheumatoid arthritis often is more disabling than osteoarthritis. The affected joints are swollen, painful, tender and warm during the initial attack and during the flares that may follow. Swelling or damage to a joint may limit your range of motion in some joints.

Rheumatoid arthritis can affect more than just the joints, too. It may affect all organ systems. This is more common in people who have positive lab tests for rheumatoid arthritis, including rheumatoid factor and CCP antibody tests (see page 57). The disease might involve various organs in the following ways:

**Skin** Small lumps called rheumatoid nodules may form under the skin over bony areas, such as your elbows, hands, knees, toes and the back of your scalp. These nodules are usually painless. They may range in size from smaller than a pea to as large as a walnut.

**Eyes** Many people with RA develop a condition called Sjögren's syndrome, which causes dry eyes and mouth. In addition, some may have inflammation of the eye. An ophthalmologist should evaluate new pain or redness of the eye in people with rheumatoid arthritis.

***Blood vessels*** Very rarely, the disease may result in inflammation of the blood vessels (vasculitis), which can cause red dots to appear on the skin.

***Nerves*** Carpal tunnel syndrome is common in people with active rheumatoid arthritis. This condition causes numbness and tingling in the hand, especially at night. It occurs when inflammation presses on the nerve that runs through the wrist to the fingers. Usually, once the inflammation is controlled, these symptoms improve. However, surgery is sometimes necessary in severe cases.

Long-standing RA may start to affect the bones of the neck (cervical spine). Rarely, joint damage from RA can cause the vertebrae in your neck to shift partly out of place, known as subluxation. This can compress the spinal cord and the nerves connecting into the head and arms. If you need surgery for any reason, your doctor may check X-rays of your cervical spine before the procedure to make sure the vertebrae are not affected. If there is evidence of inflammation, the anesthesiologist also will take special measures so as not to make any nerve damage worse.

***Lungs*** The lining around your lungs may become inflamed and cause pain when you take deep breaths, a condition called pleurisy. In rare cases, scar tissue in the lungs may lead to problems within the lung tissue (interstitial lung disease). Your doctor will refer you to a pulmonologist if these complications develop.

**Heart** In a few people with RA, the lining around the heart (pericardium) may become inflamed. This condition, called pericarditis, typically causes chest pain or shortness of breath.

**Liver** The liver is rarely involved in rheumatoid arthritis. However, many of the medications used to treat RA can affect the liver, so you'll likely have liver function tests done regularly while being treated.

## DIAGNOSIS

It's challenging to diagnose rheumatoid arthritis in its early stages, especially in older people. No single test can confirm the diagnosis, and the signs and symptoms vary from one person to another. Even an experienced rheumatologist may find it hard to tell whether a person has rheumatoid arthritis or another disease that causes similar signs and symptoms.

Doctors use a variety of tools to diagnose rheumatoid arthritis and to rule out other conditions. An important starting point is your medical history, including a description of your signs and symptoms and when and how they began. For example, your doctor may want to know about the morning stiffness you experience and how long it lasts.

A physical exam also can give helpful information. Your doctor will look at your joints, skin, reflexes and muscle strength. He or she will check for typical features of rheumatoid arthritis, such as joint swelling and tenderness, and limited motion of joints or joints out of alignment. The doctor may also test you on certain physical functions to check on factors such as your grip strength and walking time.

## Blood tests

If you have signs and symptoms of rheumatoid arthritis, your doctor will likely order certain lab tests. No test offers proof that you have RA, but several different blood tests can provide useful clues. Along with the physical exam, these tests usually provide enough information for your doctor to make a diagnosis.

**Complete blood count** A complete blood count (CBC) measures different components of your blood to evaluate your overall health and assess a variety of symptoms. For example, a low red blood cell count (anemia) often is associated with rheumatoid arthritis. The white blood cell count is usually normal in people with rheumatoid arthritis.

**Erythrocyte sedimentation rate** Sometimes referred to as the sed rate, this test can reveal inflammation in your body. When a sample of your blood is placed in a tall, thin tube, the test determines the rate at which red blood cells (erythrocytes) fall to the bottom of the tube. Cells that settle quickly may indicate the presence of inflammation, which is typical of active rheumatoid arthritis. In contrast, the sed rate in someone with osteoarthritis tends to be normal.

This test is easy and inexpensive. However, it may be less useful for older people. Everyone's sed rate increases with age, making it harder to determine a "normal" level.

**C-reactive protein** When you have inflammation, your liver quickly manufactures higher amounts of C-reactive protein (CRP), which is released into your blood. A C-reactive protein test measures the level of this protein in your system. In people with rheumatoid arthritis, the CRP level is usually high.

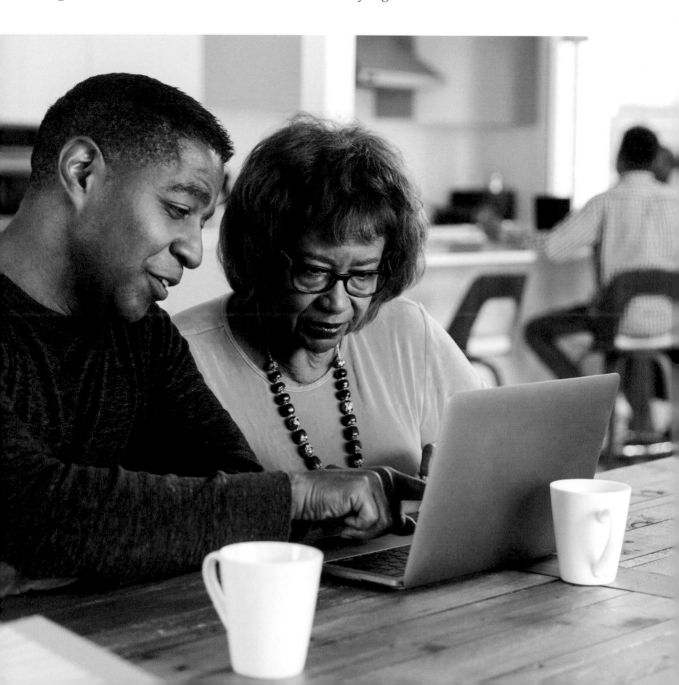

The CRP test is very sensitive, and it generally measures small degrees of inflammation better than the sed rate does. But sometimes, even during a flare-up of rheumatoid arthritis, the CRP level isn't high. Researchers don't know why this is.

The sed rate and CRP tests are often used to help monitor the degree of inflammation at any given point.

***Rheumatoid factor*** This test identifies an antibody in your blood called rheumatoid factor. Antibodies are proteins made by your immune system. They normally attach to foreign substances, such as germs, that enter the body. This allows your body to deactivate and eliminate these foreign substances. But the rheumatoid factor antibody acts abnormally. Instead of targeting an outside agent, it targets your body's own proteins.

Around 80% of people with rheumatoid arthritis develop this abnormal antibody in their bloodstream at some point. But rheumatoid factor doesn't appear to be a cause of arthritis symptoms, and it isn't specific to RA. While the antibody typically isn't found in people with osteoarthritis, it can be present in some people with other inflammatory diseases or infections.

***Anti-cyclic citrullinated peptide (anti-CCP) antibody*** The anti-CCP test identifies anti-citrulline antibodies in your blood. Like rheumatoid factor, these antibodies are proteins made by the immune system in response to a perceived threat from your own body. In this case, the perceived threat is from a protein component called citrulline.

This test can help in diagnosing RA early on, since anti-CCP antibodies are in the blood of half or more of people with early rheumatoid arthritis (having the disease for less than two years). And someone who tests negative for rheumatoid factor may have an elevated anti-CCP test, which is a more sure sign of RA. Eventually, 60% to 70% of people with rheumatoid arthritis will have anti-CCP antibodies.

## Synovial fluid testing

If the cause of the joint swelling isn't clear, your doctor may draw (aspirate) some of the synovial fluid from one of the swollen joints to be analyzed in a lab. In someone with RA, the fluid should have a high white blood cell count — a sign of inflammation. If the result is noninflammatory, the joint swelling may be due to causes such as osteoarthritis or a joint injury. The lab will also look for markers of other conditions, such as gout, pseudogout or infection, to rule out those diseases.

## Imaging tests

In addition to lab tests, your doctor may order X-rays to examine damage to affected joints. X-rays taken from multiple visits over time can show the progression of rheumatoid arthritis. As the disease progresses, many people develop small holes (erosions) near the ends of the bones and a narrowing of the space around the joint from cartilage loss.

It often takes several months of active inflammation before damage appears on an X-ray. So your doctor may not order the test if your symptoms have just developed. Magnetic resonance imaging (MRI) may be more useful in detecting rheumatoid arthritis because it can show early inflammation and cartilage damage that isn't seen on an X-ray. Ultrasound imaging also can help your doctor to see early joint damage and assess the degree of inflammation.

This X-ray image shows two knees affected by rheumatoid arthritis. The cartilage covering the joint surfaces has been eroded, but more severely on one side of each joint.

## TREATMENT

Although there's no cure for rheumatoid arthritis, it's best to start treating the condition as early as possible in its course. The goal is to reduce or stop inflammation during the window of opportunity at the disease's onset before irreparable damage occurs to the joints. To this end, treatment strategies in recent years have shifted to earlier use of powerful prescription medications that can modify the disease rather than simply treat its symptoms. The medications inhibit an overactive immune system, giving you better control of the disease.

Specific drugs used for treatment of rheumatoid arthritis are discussed in more detail in Chapter 10. Medications can be divided into four main categories:

***Nonsteroidal anti-inflammatory drugs (NSAIDs)*** These medications help with day-to-day pain and swelling, and they work quickly. Examples include ibuprofen (Advil, Motrin IB, others) and naproxen sodium (Aleve). However, these do not help to slow or stop RA disease activity.

***Steroids*** Steroids such as prednisone can be very effective in controlling inflammation quickly to treat pain and prevent joint damage, but they have a significant risk of side effects. Often they are used to help control RA symptoms temporarily until slower acting agents, such as DMARDs or biologics, can take effect. Steroids may be taken in pill form or may be given by injections into the joint.

**Disease-modifying antirheumatic drugs (DMARDs)** These medications broadly suppress the immune system to halt the inflammation of RA and stop further progression of the disease. They can take three to six months to kick in, which is why low-dose steroids may be used to control symptoms until these medications have had time to work. In addition, these drugs carry the risk of various side effects, including liver damage and lung infections. Common conventional DMARDs include methotrexate (Trexall, Rasuvo, others), leflunomide (Arava), hydroxychloroquine (Plaquenil) and sulfasalazine (Azulfidine).

**Biologics** In the last few decades, many new options for treating rheumatoid arthritis have become available. Biologics, also known as biologic response modifiers, target specific parts of the immune system that cause inflammation. These medications include tumor necrosis factor inhibitors, such as adalimumab (Humira); interleukin inhibitors, such as tocilizumab (Actemra); the B cell blocker rituximab (Rituxan) and the T cell blocker abatacept (Orencia). Most of these drugs are given by self-injection or infusion through an IV. Your doctor may pair a biologic with a conventional DMARD to be most effective. Because of the way they work, biologics can increase the risk of infections.

Also available are targeted DMARDs, recently developed medications that block specific inflammatory pathways in immune cells. These drugs include Janus kinase (JAK) inhibitors, such as baricitinib (Olumiant) and tofacitinib (Xeljanz).

With the availability of these newer medications, doctors have many more options to aggressively treat rheumatoid arthritis and put it into remission.

In addition to medications, a variety of other treatments may be used, including exercise, physical therapy, joint injections, self-care, and assistive devices and modified behaviors to help protect your joints. In some cases, surgery may be necessary.

With proper treatment, many people with rheumatoid arthritis can avoid the most severe, disabling consequences of the disease.

## A CHRONIC DISEASE

When you're first diagnosed with rheumatoid arthritis, it's impossible to predict how severe your condition may become. It may remain mild, or it may progressively worsen. For most people, the disease is chronic, although its symptoms may be more or less severe at different times. Painful flares may alternate with periods of relative remission.

If the symptoms of rheumatoid arthritis are fairly persistent for four or five years, the condition is more likely to pose long-term issues such as heart disease. Your doctor will likely need to monitor your RA with regular tests and periodic examinations of your joints.

In some people with RA, the symptoms of inflammation, especially joint swelling, may subside after a number of years. However, joint damage from the previous inflammation may remain along with some pain.

According to past research, rheumatoid arthritis may reduce life expectancy by up to 10 years. In most cases this is due to the complications of the disease, such as a weakened immune system or the effects of chronic inflammation. But recent developments in treatment are leading to lower disease activity and long-term well-being in people with RA, so further research is needed.

The prognosis of rheumatoid arthritis has improved significantly, even in the last decade. Doctors can diagnose the disease earlier and begin therapies sooner to more rapidly target inflammation and prevent damage to the joints. Diagnosis and vigorous treatment at the earliest stages of the disease may help you avoid persistent pain and permanent joint damage.

The degree to which rheumatoid arthritis affects your daily life depends in part on how well you cope with the disease. But with continuing advances in treatment and early detection, many people are able to live long, active lives.

# Other inflammatory arthritis

In addition to osteoarthritis and rheumatoid arthritis, more than 100 other forms of arthritis (arthropathies) can affect the joints. Many of these conditions are uncommon. Some forms are mild and resolve quickly with treatment. Others are widespread throughout the body, affecting multiple organs and blood vessels.

The signs and symptoms can vary considerably, even among people with the same type of arthritis. At the same time, the signs and symptoms of different forms often overlap, making it difficult to diagnose a specific condition.

As with rheumatoid arthritis, genetics play a role in other forms of arthritis. Some genes have been identified that are associated with particular types of arthritis. But even if you inherit a tendency to develop arthritis, other factors are involved in triggering the disease.

Many forms of arthritis are inflammatory disorders, such as rheumatoid arthritis, with signs and symptoms caused by inflammation in the body. Some are autoimmune disorders, while others are related to infections or how the body processes food. This chapter will discuss some of the more common inflammatory joint disorders apart from rheumatoid arthritis.

## SPONDYLOARTHRITIS

Spondyloarthritis (spon-duh-loe-ahr-THRI-tis) refers to a group of autoimmune disorders that cause inflammation in the spine, especially in the sacroiliac joints of the pelvis. It may also affect the joints of the arms,

**Front view**

**Back view**

Vertebra

Ilium

Sacroiliac joint

Sacrum

The sacroiliac (SI) joint is the place where two bones — the sacrum and the ilium — come together in your pelvis, forming one SI joint on each side.

legs and toes. Unlike other types of arthritis, it tends to cause pain at the points where tendons and ligaments attach to bones, called entheses.

Diseases in this group include ankylosing spondylitis, reactive arthritis, psoriatic arthritis and arthritis associated with inflammatory bowel disease (enteropathic arthritis). In addition, some people experience common symptoms of spondyloarthritis but don't have all the distinctive symptoms of one of these four conditions. In this case, the disease is classified as undifferentiated spondyloarthritis.

Like other forms of arthritis, spondyloarthritis appears to stem from a combination of genetic and environmental factors. The human leukocyte antigen HLA-B27 is strongly associated with spondyloarthritis, although most people with this gene never develop the disease.

People with spondyloarthritis often have low back pain and stiffness from inflammation that causes pain at night, doesn't improve with rest and does improve with exercise. Often, the back pain starts before age 40 and gradually worsens. The knees or ankles may become inflamed, but any joint can be involved. Swelling of the fingers or toes may cause very mild pain or tenderness. Other signs and symptoms of spondyloarthritis may include eye inflammation with a painful red eye that's light sensitive, a skin rash and bowel inflammation (bloody stools).

Your doctor will base a diagnosis on your symptoms and a physical exam. An X-ray or an MRI scan may help. For example, an X-ray of your pelvis may show changes typical of this condition. If an X-ray appears normal, an MRI may show earlier evidence of the disease. Blood tests can help rule out other forms of arthritis. You may be tested for the HLA-B27 gene. However, having the gene doesn't confirm a diagnosis.

Physical therapy, stretching and range-of-motion exercises can help maintain flexibility in joints and good posture. Several types of medications may be used to control inflammation. These include nonsteroidal anti-inflammatory drugs (NSAIDs), corticosteroids, disease-modifying antirheumatic drugs (DMARDs) and biologic agents, discussed in Chapter 10.

The main types of spondyloarthritis are discussed below.

## Ankylosing spondylitis

Ankylosing spondylitis (ang-kuh-LOE-sing spon-duh-LIE-tis) is a chronic disease that primarily causes inflammation in the sacroiliac joints and vertebrae of your spine. It may also affect areas where tendons and ligaments attach to bones (entheses), the joints of your hips, shoulders, knees and feet, and the joints between your ribs and spine. Your eyes, heart and lungs can be affected as well.

Ankylosing spondylitis is more common in men than in women and typically begins in early adulthood. Many people with this condition carry the HLA-B27 gene. Having this gene doesn't mean you'll get the disease — in fact, HLA-B27 is present in about 6% of the general population in the United States, and most people with the gene never get ankylosing spondylitis. There's often a family history with this condition, and other genes likely play a role.

***Signs and symptoms*** Many people with ankylosing spondylitis have mild forms that involve only the sacroiliac joints. In others, inflammation involves the entire spine or peripheral joints — or both — leading to physical deformities and other complications.

Early signs and symptoms often include pain and stiffness in your lower back and hips, or a dull aching deep in your buttocks. The pain may come and go at first and is often worse in the morning and after periods of inactivity.

Losing flexibility in the lower spine is an early sign of ankylosing spondylitis. Over time, the pain and stiffness may progress up your spine into your ribs and neck.

Ankylosing spondylitis is a chronic condition. As inflammation persists, new bone forms as part of the healing process. The vertebrae may grow or fuse together, forming bony outgrowths and leading to a stiff, inflexible spine. Fusion can also stiffen your rib cage, restricting lung capacity and function.

Many people with ankylosing spondylitis experience eye inflammation (uveitis) and

## ARTHRITIS AND INFLAMMATORY BOWEL DISEASE (ENTEROPATHIC ARTHRITIS)

An estimated 1.4 million Americans have Crohn's disease or ulcerative colitis, two common forms of inflammatory bowel disease (IBD). These diseases cause chronic inflammation of the digestive tract. Along with this inflammation, arthritis also develops in certain joints in as many as 25% of people with IBD. This is known as enteropathic arthritis.

Some researchers believe this form of arthritis may result from an immune response to intestinal bacteria in the inflamed bowel. Because people often experience pain and swelling in multiple joints, especially the knees and ankles, as well as stiffness in the spine, the condition is considered a form of spondyloarthritis.

bowel inflammation. In advanced stages, signs and symptoms may include chronic stooping, fatigue, loss of appetite and weight loss.

***Diagnosis and treatment*** Early diagnosis of ankylosing spondylitis can be difficult if your symptoms are mild, since you may attribute the symptoms to more-common back problems.

If your doctor suspects ankylosing spondylitis, he or she may order X-rays to check for changes in your joints and bones, though the characteristic effects of the disease may not be evident early on. If X-rays don't show changes, your doctor may request an MRI of the sacroiliac joints and lower spine

to get a more detailed look. Blood tests to check for an elevated sedimentation (sed) rate and for the HLA-B27 gene may help confirm the diagnosis.

Many people with ankylosing spondylitis are able to lead normal, active lives. Effective treatment can decrease pain and may help prevent complications and physical deformities. Stretching and breathing exercises, proper posture, and physical therapy are key elements of a treatment program.

Nonsteroidal anti-inflammatory drugs (NSAIDs) can help relieve pain and inflammation from this disease, and medications that block tumor necrosis factor (TNF) are very effective in improving signs and symptoms and quality of life. For more information on medications, see Chapter 10.

## Reactive arthritis

Reactive arthritis is an inflammatory condition that occurs as a reaction to an infection elsewhere in your body. Many different types of infectious organisms can trigger the joint inflammation. This type of arthritis was formerly known as Reiter's syndrome.

What's considered the classic form of reactive arthritis is caused by a bacterial infection in the intestines (GI tract), genitals or urinary (GU) tract. The intestinal form is typically caused by foodborne infections from salmonella, campylobacter, shigella or yersinia. Chlamydia, a sexually transmitted infection, can cause the genital form. Reactive arthritis occurs most often in adults between the ages of 20 and 40. While men and women are equally likely to get it from foodborne bacteria, men are more likely to develop this form of arthritis in response to a sexually transmitted infection.

Having a bacterial infection does not mean you'll get arthritis. Reactive arthritis is thought to occur in people who are genetically predisposed to it — many people with the condition carry the HLA-B27 gene. But again, having this gene doesn't guarantee that you'll get reactive arthritis when you experience an infection.

***Signs and symptoms*** Reactive arthritis typically involves pain and swelling in the knees, ankles, feet and hips. Other joints, such as wrists and fingers, are affected less often. Inflammation of the tendons (tendinitis) or at places where tendons attach to bones (enthesitis) is common. This often results in pain at the heel or back of the ankle (Achilles tendinitis). There may be pain in the lower back and buttocks.

Although joint symptoms are a defining feature of reactive arthritis, the condition can also cause inflammation in your eyes, skin and the tube that carries urine from your bladder (urethra). This can lead to eye conditions, skin rashes, increased frequency of urination and a burning sensation during urination. Signs and symptoms generally start one to four weeks after exposure to a triggering infection. Pain and discomfort may come and go over a period of several weeks or months. In some people, signs and symptoms subside within a few days. Most people recover within a year. Others may redevelop signs and symptoms after their initial condition disappears.

***Diagnosis and treatment*** Reactive arthritis can go undetected for some time because signs and symptoms may be mild. Your doctor might run tests to see if you have any of the infections associated with reactive arthritis. Blood tests, such as the sed rate, rheumatoid factor and antinuclear antibodies tests, can help determine what type of arthritis you have. You may be tested for the HLA-B27 gene.

Treatment may include antibiotics if your doctor suspects a bacterial infection that's ongoing. NSAIDs and corticosteroid medications can help relieve the joint pain and inflammation of reactive arthritis. DMARDs such as sulfasalazine and methotrexate or drugs that inhibit a protein called tumor necrosis factor also may be prescribed. For more information on medications, see Chapter 10.

## Psoriatic arthritis

Approximately 7.5 million Americans have the skin disease psoriasis, causing red patches of scaly skin. Among these, as many as 30% to 40% develop a chronic, inflammatory arthritis known as psoriatic (sor-ee-AT-ick) arthritis. People with psoriatic arthritis have swollen, painful joints, especially in their fingers and toes, usually in addition to the typical red, scaly skin of psoriasis. They may also develop inflammatory eye conditions.

Psoriatic arthritis affects men and women equally. Most people with the condition have psoriasis long before they develop arthritic symptoms, although sometimes joint symptoms can occur first. Psoriasis typically develops in adults in their 20s or 30s, while psoriatic arthritis may show up 20 years later. Children also can get psoriatic arthritis.

Both psoriasis and psoriatic arthritis are autoimmune conditions. Most people with psoriatic arthritis have a close relative with the disease, and researchers have identified certain gene mutations that may be associated with it. Among people with a genetic predisposition for psoriatic arthritis, something in the environment, such as a viral or bacterial infection or physical trauma, may trigger the disease.

***Signs and symptoms*** Psoriasis is a skin condition marked by a buildup of rough, dry, dead cells that form thick scales. These patches (plaques) of thick, red skin often appear on your elbows, knees, scalp or the lower part of your spine. Your fingernails may become pitted and discolored and may separate from the nail beds.

**Psoriasis patches on the elbow and scalp**

Psoriasis most commonly develops on the elbows, knees, trunk and scalp. Dry, red patches of skin are covered with silvery scales. Affected joints may become swollen and stiff.

Arthritic symptoms include pain, redness, swelling and reduced motion in your joints, especially the small joints of your fingers and toes. It's common to have morning stiffness lasting more than 30 minutes. You might also feel stiff following periods of inactivity. Different patterns of psoriatic arthritis cause varying symptoms. The disease might involve joints on one or both sides of your body. Your sacroiliac joints and your spine may be affected, causing inflammatory back pain. Psoriatic arthritis may also cause "sausage-like" swollen fingers or toes.

***Diagnosis and treatment*** To be diagnosed with psoriatic arthritis, you have to have symptoms of both psoriasis and arthritis. Diagnosis can be tricky because in adults, skin problems and joint problems rarely begin at the same time.

Your doctor may order blood tests to check your sed rate and test for rheumatoid factor to rule out rheumatoid arthritis. X-rays may show changes in the joints that develop in psoriatic arthritis but not in other arthritic conditions.

If you have a mild form of the disease, your doctor may recommend NSAIDs. If these medications don't control inflammation, you may be treated with other drugs, such as DMARDs or biologic agents. For more information, see Chapter 10.

Various treatments, including oral medications, ointments and creams, and ultraviolet light or sunlight (phototherapy) are used to treat skin symptoms.

# CONNECTIVE TISSUE DISORDERS

Connective tissue disorders cover a wide range of autoimmune diseases that are often associated with specific autoantibodies. These conditions often affect multiple organs, including joints. Some of the more common connective tissue disorders are discussed below.

## Sjögren's syndrome

Mild decreases in saliva and tear production are normal with aging. If you have Sjögren's (SHOW-grins) syndrome, your saliva glands and tear glands become inflamed and damaged. The result is a dry mouth and a sandy, gritty feeling in your eyes.

Sjögren's syndrome is an autoimmune condition that may occur by itself or along with rheumatoid arthritis, systemic lupus erythematosus, scleroderma or polymyositis.

In Sjögren's syndrome, the immune system attacks the cells of mucous membranes and glands that produce moisture, primarily in your eyes and mouth. The disease may also cause vaginal dryness in women and problems in the muscles, joints, lungs, kidneys and stomach.

Sjögren's syndrome may affect as many as 4 million Americans. The disease is much more likely to occur in women than in men — and usually diagnosed in people older than age 40. Experts don't know exactly

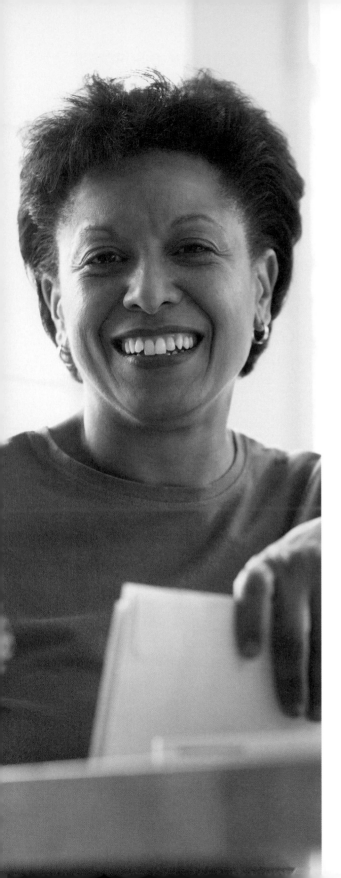

what causes it. They believe that several factors, including genes and environmental triggers, may contribute to the development of Sjögren's syndrome.

***Signs and symptoms*** The classic symptoms are dry mouth and dry eyes. Your eyes may feel as if dirt specks are lodged in them, and you may have difficulty swallowing or chewing. Other signs and symptoms include:

- Dental cavities
- Prolonged fatigue
- Persistent dry cough or hoarseness caused by dry nose, throat and lungs
- Joint pain, swelling and stiffness
- Mucus-like strands in the eyes, especially in the morning
- Enlarged salivary glands behind your jaw and in front of your ears
- Skin rashes, including purple spots
- Shortness of breath
- Change in sense of taste
- Nausea, stomach pain or indigestion
- Vaginal dryness
- Raynaud's phenomenon — numbness, pain or skin color changes brought on by cold or stress (see page 73)

***Diagnosis and treatment*** Your doctor may compile a history of your signs and symptoms and do a physical exam, including an eye exam to measure the dryness of your eyes. You might also have blood tests and a lip biopsy, in which a tissue sample containing small salivary glands is removed for analysis. You may also have an ultrasound or other imaging test of your salivary glands to look for changes associated with the disease.

Most people with Sjögren's syndrome can manage symptoms with a self-care plan that includes using artificial tears, avoiding dry environments, sucking sugarless candy and drinking plenty of fluids.

It's important that your doctor is able to review any medications you take to make sure they aren't contributing to your symptoms. If you have moderate or severe dry eyes, your doctor may recommend prescription eyedrops such as cyclosporine (Restasis) or lifitegrast (Xiidra). Other medications may be prescribed to help increase the production of saliva and tears, including pilocarpine (Salagen) and cevimeline (Evoxac). In addition, your ophthalmologist may recommend sealing the tear ducts with a plug to prevent tear drainage from your eyes.

To relieve arthritis pain and inflammation, your doctor may prescribe NSAIDs or corticosteroids. If those aren't effective, the DMARD medication hydroxychloroquine (Plaquenil) may help treat Sjögren's symptoms systemwide.

## Systemic lupus erythematosus

Systemic lupus erythematosus (er-uh-thee-muh-TOE-sus), often called lupus or SLE, is a chronic inflammatory disease that can affect many parts of your body, including your skin, joints, kidneys, blood cells, heart and lungs. There are several other less common types of lupus, but the term lupus most often refers to SLE.

The most common symptoms include arthritis and skin rashes. Episodes of lupus tend to come and go throughout your life, and they may make you feel tired and achy.

Most people with lupus are women — in fact, the disease affects 7 to 15 times as many adult women as men. It's most commonly diagnosed between the ages of 15 and 45. But it can occur at any age and in either sex. The disease is most common in African American, Hispanic, Asian and Native American women.

*Signs and symptoms* No two cases of lupus are exactly alike. Symptoms may come on suddenly or develop slowly. They may be mild or severe, and there may be times when there are no signs or symptoms.

Fatigue, often severe and prolonged, is the most common symptom of lupus, affecting almost everyone who has the disease. You may feel tired even when no other symptoms are present. Arthritis symptoms, including joint pain, stiffness and swelling, especially in your fingers, hands, wrists and knees, are common and may be the earliest indications of the disease.

Other signs and symptoms include:

- Fever
- Butterfly-shaped rash across the bridge of your nose and cheeks, or rash on your face, neck or arms
- Sensitivity to sunlight, resulting in rashes, fatigue, fever or joint pain
- Raynaud's phenomenon (see page 73)

- Mouth sores (ulcers)
- Chest pain or cough
- Hair loss
- Swollen glands
- Swelling in your legs or around your eyes

***Diagnosis and treatment*** If your doctor suspects lupus based on your symptoms, the diagnosis may be confirmed with blood tests. One test checks for antinuclear antibodies (ANA), which are proteins produced by the immune system and found in the blood of nearly all people with lupus.

A positive ANA result means you have an active immune system — but not necessarily that you have lupus. People with other autoimmune diseases as well as some healthy individuals also may test positive. Your doctor may advise further testing for antibodies that are more specific to lupus to confirm the diagnosis.

In addition to ordering blood tests, your doctor may evaluate how well your kidney, liver, lungs and heart are functioning.

In the past lupus was often considered fatal. However, modern treatments have dramatically improved life expectancy with the disease. Your treatment plan will depend on your symptoms and how severe they are. Most treatments aim to reduce inflammation, control joint pain and fatigue, and avoid complications.

Medications used to control inflammation include NSAIDs, the antimalarial drug hydroxychloroquine (Plaquenil), corticosteroids, immunosuppressants such as mycophenolate (Cellcept) and azathioprine (Imuran), and biologics such as belimumab (Benlysta). See Chapter 10 for more discussion of medications. More-aggressive therapies may be needed for severe symptoms.

## Scleroderma (systemic sclerosis)

Scleroderma (sklair-oh-DUR-muh) means "hard skin." The term refers to a group of rare, progressive disorders that cause hardening and tightening of your skin and connective tissues.

Systemic scleroderma is an autoimmune condition that can affect multiple organs. It occurs when your body produces too much collagen, a fibrous protein that makes up connective tissues, including your skin. Researchers aren't sure what causes this abnormal production of collagen. The disease is more common in women than in men and typically affects middle-aged adults. It usually doesn't run in families.

***Signs and symptoms*** Signs and symptoms of scleroderma vary, depending on which form of the disease you have. Skin abnormalities, such as hardening and thickening, are a common feature.

Often one of the earliest signs of scleroderma is Raynaud's phenomenon, an exaggerated response to cold temperatures or to emotional distress. Small blood vessels in your hands constrict, causing color changes in the skin of the areas affected — typically from a white to blue to red coloration. Some people may develop pitting or sores (ulcers) on the finger tips.

Scleroderma usually causes puffy or tight skin over the fingers. Your skin may lose its elasticity and become shiny as it stretches across underlying bone. In some people, the skin thickens on the hands, arms, chest, face, feet and legs.

The disease can also affect your blood vessels and internal organs such as the heart, lungs and kidneys, as well as the digestive tract. Symptoms may include stiffness or pain in your joints, curling of your fingers, and shortness of breath. You might develop

In Raynaud's phenomenon, blood flow to the fingers is reduced when muscle in the artery walls contracts. Skin coloration typically changes from white to blue to red.

digestive problems such as heartburn or constipation if the esophagus or intestines are affected.

***Diagnosis and treatment*** Typically, your doctor will review your symptoms and medical history and check your skin for thickened and hardened areas. He or she may also look for changes in your joints and tendons.

You may also have blood tests and other imaging or organ-function tests, such as an echocardiogram or a pulmonary function test. These can help determine whether your digestive system, heart or lungs are affected.

There's no cure for scleroderma. However, many treatments can help control symptoms and slow the overproduction of collagen.

For skin changes, anti-itch medications, moisturizers and drugs that suppress the immune system may be used. Raynaud's symptoms may be treated with medications such as calcium channel blockers and phosphodiesterase-5 inhibitors, which help keep blood vessels open. Medications also can treat high blood pressure in the arteries in your lungs (pulmonary arterial hypertension), and some may help prevent scarring of the lung tissue (interstitial lung disease). To control joint pain, stiffness and inflammation, your doctor may prescribe NSAIDs and DMARDs.

Because scleroderma can take a toll on your self-esteem, you may also find it helpful to join a support group or talk with a counselor.

## Polymyositis and dermatomyositis

These two rare conditions are forms of myositis, a disease that causes inflammation within muscle tissues. Myositis is also known as inflammatory myopathy (my-OP-uh-thee).

Polymyositis (pol-e-my-o-SY-tis) can cause inflammation and weakness in your muscles. If muscle inflammation occurs along with a skin rash, the disorder is called dermatomyositis (dur-muh-toe-my-uh-SY-tis).

Adults between the ages of 30 and 60 are most likely to have these disorders. Dermatomyositis can also affect children, usually between the ages of 5 and 15. Both disorders are more common in women than in men.

It's not known what causes either disease, but they're both thought to be autoimmune disorders.

***Signs and symptoms*** Muscle weakness is the most common symptom of both disorders. Usually, the weakness begins gradually and gets worse over several months. It typically affects muscles on both sides of your body, particularly the muscles closest to the trunk, such as those in the hips, thighs, shoulders, upper arms and neck. You may also have pain and swelling in your joints.

Weakness can make it hard to do things such as comb hair, put on clothes, climb stairs, and get in and out of a bed, chair or car. Weakness in the throat muscles can make swallowing difficult. Lung problems also may develop.

Dermatomyositis causes several types of rashes. Violet or dusky red patches of skin may form on the knuckles, elbows, knees, ankles or face, including on the eyelids with swelling. Rashes may also appear on the hips, back, neck and arms.

***Diagnosis and treatment*** Polymyositis and dermatomyositis can be difficult to diagnose. You may have a variety of tests, and your doctor may need to see you several times before pinpointing the diagnosis. A physical exam will be done to check for skin changes and test muscle strength. Blood tests are used to check for elevated levels of certain muscle enzymes, which can indicate muscle damage.

Other tests you may need include electromyography, which measures the electrical activity in your muscles, and magnetic resonance imaging (MRI), which can show areas of muscle inflammation. Your doctor may do a biopsy of muscle tissue to determine the amount and type of damage.

There's no cure for either condition, but treatment can improve muscle strength and function. Treatment usually begins with a high dose of a corticosteroid medication to suppress your immune system. The dosage is gradually lowered as signs and symptoms improve, generally within one to three months.

Your doctor may also recommend a DMARD medication such as azathioprine, methotrexate or mycophenolate mofetil. These can help control the disease and decrease the side ef-

fects of the corticosteroid. If symptoms don't improve, the drug rituximab or an IV of immunoglobulin — a purified blood product containing antibodies — may be effective.

Medications initially used to treat malaria, such as hydroxychloroquine (Plaquenil), can help resolve the skin rash of dermatomyositis if the rash is mild. However, they don't treat muscle inflammation.

Exercise and physical therapy also are helpful. In addition, people with dermatomyositis should protect themselves from sunlight exposure by using sunscreen, wearing a hat and avoiding the sun during the middle of the day.

## VASCULITIS

Vasculitis occurs when there is inflammation of your blood vessels — your veins, arteries and capillaries. There are many types of vasculitis, and most are quite rare. Sometimes vasculitis can cause joint pain. Joint pain is a common symptom of the conditions discussed below.

### Giant cell arteritis (GCA)

If you develop new headaches, your temples are tender or painful, and you're more than 50 years old, you may have giant cell arteritis (ahr-tuh-RYE-tis).

This is an inflammation in the lining of your arteries, the blood vessels that carry blood rich in oxygen from your heart to the rest of your body. Giant cell arteritis may also be associated with symptoms of arthritis — pain and stiffness in your neck, arms or hips.

Giant cell arteritis occurs most often in the arteries of your head and especially in your temples. For this reason, the disorder is also known as temporal arteritis or cranial arteritis. It can also cause inflammation in your neck, upper body and arms, or other parts of the body.

Older adults are at greatest risk of giant cell arteritis. The disease most often occurs in people in their 70s, and it's more common in women than in men. About half of people with giant cell arteritis also have a related inflammatory condition called polymyalgia rheumatica (see page 77).

As with other autoimmune disorders, the inflammation in giant cell arteritis stems from an abnormal immune response. The exact cause isn't known, but researchers believe that both genetic factors and aging play a role. An unknown factor may trigger the onset.

***Signs and symptoms*** Giant cell arteritis frequently causes headache, weight loss, fever and fatigue. Most people with the condition develop a new, severe headache. Other signs and symptoms include:

- Double vision or sudden, painless loss of vision in one or both eyes that can be permanent.
- Tender, thickened artery in the temple.
- Scalp tenderness.
- Jaw pain when chewing (claudication).
- Throat or tongue pain.
- Pain and stiffness in shoulders, neck, arms or hips (symptoms of polymyalgia rheumatica). Pain is usually worse in the morning and improves with activity.

If giant cell arteritis is left untreated, it can lead to permanent blindness, a stroke or an aneurysm because of arteries that are narrowed or blocked from inflammation.

***Diagnosis and treatment*** To diagnose GCA, your doctor may start with your medical history and do an exam. He or she may also order blood tests, including tests for sed rate and C-reactive protein. These levels are usually high in people with GCA. If your doctor suspects that arteries in your chest, arms and neck are affected, you might have an imaging test. Advanced imaging tests such as color Doppler ultrasound or posi-

Giant cell arteritis often involves the arteries of the scalp and head, especially those over the temple.

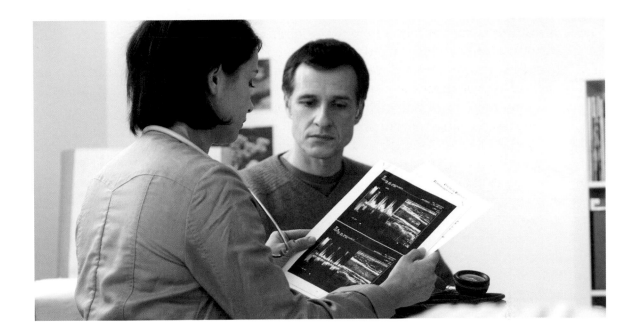

tron emission tomography (PET) can produce detailed images of your larger blood vessels and show areas of inflammation.

To confirm the diagnosis, a small tissue sample (biopsy) may be taken of a temple artery. If you have giant cell arteritis, the sample usually shows signs of inflammation and abnormally large cells (giant cells), which give the disease its name.

Treatment of GCA consists of high doses of a corticosteroid drug. Because GCA can cause vision loss, immediate treatment is needed. Your doctor may start medication even before a biopsy confirms the diagnosis. The biologic medication tocilizumab (Actemra) also has been shown to be effective in treating GCA. This reduces the risk of a disease flare and may allow you to take lower doses of steroids. Once your inflam-

mation is under control, your doctor will gradually reduce the steroid dosage to the lowest dose needed to keep inflammation down.

People who take steroids long term should be counseled on protecting their bones, as steroids can make bones brittle, leading to osteoporosis. Talk with your doctor about calcium, vitamin D and weight-bearing exercise. Occasionally, your doctor might prescribe other medications for osteoporosis or to reduce the risk of complications from swollen blood vessels.

## POLYMYALGIA RHEUMATICA (PMR)

Polymyalgia rheumatica (pol-e-my-AL-juh rue-MAT-ih-kuh) is an inflammatory disorder that occurs in people over the age of 50.

The name of this condition comes from the Greek words that mean "pain in many muscles." It causes widespread muscle aches and joint stiffness, especially in your neck, shoulders, thighs and hips. You might have inflammation in other areas of your body as well.

Just what triggers PMR isn't known, but aging and genetic and environmental factors probably play a role. PMR affects older adults almost exclusively — the age at onset is most often in your 70s. Women are more likely than men to develop PMR, and people of northern European and Scandinavian descent are at higher risk.

**Signs and symptoms** PMR typically causes pain and stiffness in the muscles of your shoulders, neck, upper arms, lower back, thighs and hips. Stiffness is usually worse in the morning or after sitting or lying down for long periods. A slight fever, fatigue and unexplained weight loss also may occur.

Symptoms may come on abruptly or gradually. In some people, pain may appear almost overnight. Other people might develop a gradual worsening of aches, stiffness and fatigue over weeks or longer.

About 10% to 15% of people with PMR may also have giant cell arteritis (see page 75) either before or after having PMR. The two disorders can also occur at the same time.

**Diagnosis and treatment** If your symptoms suggest that you may have polymyalgia rheumatica, your doctor might order blood tests. The sed rate and C-reactive protein levels are usually elevated in people with PMR, while rheumatoid factor usually isn't present.

Aspirin and NSAIDs such as ibuprofen can help treat mild symptoms. However, the usual treatment is a low, daily dose of a corticosteroid drug, which generally provides immediate and complete relief from symptoms. Even without treatment, PMR usually goes away after a year or two.

## CRYSTALLINE ARTHRITIS

Some forms of arthritis are related to how the body breaks down (metabolizes) food. When certain substances build up in the body after food is metabolized, they can form crystals that lead to inflammation of the joints. The two most common crystal diseases that cause joint problems are discussed in the following sections.

### Gout

Gout is a painful form of arthritis that's been recognized since ancient times. It causes sudden, severe attacks of pain, tenderness, redness, warmth and swelling in some joints. It usually affects one joint at a time — typically the large joint of the big toe. But it can also occur in your feet, ankles, knees, hands and wrists. Fortunately, gout is treatable, and there are ways to reduce the risk that it will recur.

Gout occurs when you have an excessive amount of uric acid in your system. Tiny crystals form in the joints, commonly in your feet, and can cause intense pain, inflammation and redness.

The prevalence of gout has been increasing over the last few decades, now affecting more than 8 million people in the United States. Although men are generally more likely than women to get gout, women become more susceptible to it after going through menopause.

Gout is caused by an excessive level of uric acid in your bloodstream. Normally, uric acid — a waste product — dissolves in blood and is filtered through the kidneys. From there, it enters into your urine and is excreted from your body. But sometimes your body produces too much uric acid, or, more commonly, your kidneys don't filter it adequately. When uric acid builds up in your blood, it can form microscopic urate crystals in a joint or surrounding tissue. The crystals are sharp and needle-like. This sets off an intense inflammatory reaction.

***Signs and symptoms*** Gout attacks usually happen suddenly, often at night. You may go to bed feeling fine, but then wake up in the middle of the night feeling like your big toe is on fire, with severe pain and swelling. The affected joint may be red or purple, hot, and extremely tender. The pain typically lasts five to 10 days, then disappears completely. You may have a period with no symptoms at all, followed by a painful episode. An episode of gout can be triggered by drinking too much alcohol, eating too much of certain kinds of foods, surgery, severe illness or joint injury.

If gout isn't treated, it may lead to persistent swelling, stiffness, pain, and damage in one or more joints after a number of years. The uric acid crystals may build up into large deposits called tophi (TOE-fie), which look like lumps beneath the skin around the joints. A high level of uric acid in the blood can also contribute to many conditions including kidney disease, obesity, diabetes, high blood pressure (hypertension), cardiovascular disease and kidney stones.

***Diagnosis and treatment*** Gout is diagnosed by identifying uric acid crystals in a sample of fluid taken (aspirated) from an inflamed joint. Different treatments can be used during the acute swelling, including medications such as NSAIDs, colchicine and prednisone, and steroid injections into the involved joint.

Once an acute attack is under control, your doctor may prescribe a drug to reduce the risk of future episodes. Preventive medicines include allopurinol (Zyloprim), febuxostat (Uloric) and probenecid. They help keep the level of uric acid within a normal range. The goal level of uric acid in the blood is <6.0 milligrams per deciliter (mg/dL). If your gout cannot be controlled or if the uric acid level does not normalize with these medications, pegloticase (Krystexxa) may be recommended. You may also need to watch your diet by avoiding too much protein from animal sources, limiting alcohol and drinking plenty of water.

## Pseudogout

A second type of crystal also can cause joint problems. Pseudogout (SOO-doe-gout), also known as acute calcium pyrophosphate crystal arthritis, occurs when crystals of calcium pyrophosphate dihydrate (CPPD) build up in the lining of a joint (synovium), setting off an episode of pain and swelling.

Although the symptoms are similar to those of gout, pseudogout typically affects one

## PSEUDOGOUT AND GOUT: WHAT'S THE DIFFERENCE?

| Disease | Cause | Signs and symptoms | Who does it affect? | Treatment |
|---|---|---|---|---|
| Pseudogout | Deposits of calcium pyrophosphate dihydrate crystals in joints | Pain and swelling, usually in large joints such as the knee | Typically older adults | NSAIDs, steroids, colchicine |
| Gout | Deposits of uric acid crystals in joints | Pain and swelling, usually in the big toe | Typically older men | NSAIDs, steroids, colchicine, allopurinol, febuxostat, probenecid, pegloticase |

joint such as your knee, wrist or ankle, whereas gout most often affects the big toe.

Pseudogout occurs most often in adults in their 60s or older. The disease can occur with no obvious cause or during recovery from acute illness or surgery. Genetic factors may play a role. Joint injury, osteoarthritis, hyperparathyroidism, low magnesium levels or excess storage of iron also can contribute.

***Signs and symptoms*** Attacks of pseudogout can occur abruptly, causing severe pain, swelling and warmth in the affected joint.

***Diagnosis and treatment*** Like gout, pseudogout can be diagnosed by examining a sample of fluid from an affected joint to see whether CPPD crystals are present. An X-ray can reveal evidence of joint damage, along with crystal deposits in the joint cartilage, known as chondrocalcinosis.

NSAIDs (ibuprofen, naproxen, indomethacin) can reduce pain and inflammation but will not rid your joint of the CPPD crystals. When large joints are involved, such as the knee, aspirating the joint fluid and injecting the joint with corticosteroid may help relieve pain and pressure. To prevent further attacks, low doses of colchicine or NSAIDs may help.

## SEPTIC (INFECTIOUS) ARTHRITIS AND INFECTION-RELATED ARTHRITIS

As discussed earlier in this chapter, inflammation in your joints can develop in response to a bacterial infection elsewhere in your body (reactive arthritis). Other types of infections can trigger arthritis symptoms too. Sometimes an infection gets into the joint itself, leading to pain, swelling and warmth of one or multiple joints. This is known as infectious arthritis or septic arthritis.

Most often septic arthritis is caused by bacteria, but it can also be due to viruses or fungal infections. Usually the infection travels through the bloodstream into the involved joint. In some cases, a deep wound may allow an infection into the joint. If the infection isn't treated, the joint can become damaged.

Septic arthritis often causes sudden symptoms in the affected joint, including pain, stiffness, swelling, warmth and fevers. The knee, wrist, ankle and hip are most often involved. If a septic joint is suspected, your doctor will use a needle and syringe to draw (aspirate) fluid from the joint. The sample is then sent to the lab to check for infection. If you have a fever, a blood test may be done to see if the infection is in the blood.

Several types of infections that can cause arthritis symptoms are discussed below.

### Bacterial infections

Infectious arthritis can occur if a bacterial infection in your blood vessels spreads through the blood to a joint. It can also develop if a wound or other injury allows bacteria into the joint through the skin.

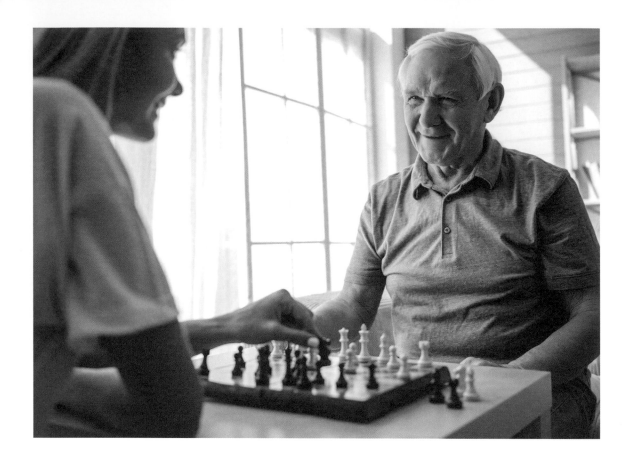

Staph bacteria is the most common type to cause septic arthritis. If not treated promptly, septic arthritis due to this bacteria can destroy a joint. Another type of septic arthritis, a gonococcal joint infection, is caused by the sexually transmitted bacteria that causes gonorrhea. People with this type of infection tend to have painful inflammation in the wrists, fingers, ankles and toes. Often, they have a fever and feel unwell. They may also have a skin rash.

Your risk for septic arthritis is higher if you take medications that suppress the immune system, such as chemotherapy, steroids or

drugs for rheumatoid arthritis. Having an artificial heart valve or joint replacement also raises your risk of developing a joint infection. Only about 0.5% to 1% of people with a replaced joint develop an infection. Unfortunately, artificial joint infections are hard to treat. A structure called a biofilm develops within the joint, which can act as a kind of shield to the bacteria. This makes it difficult for the bacteria to be found and destroyed by the immune system or by medications.

To treat bacterial septic arthritis, antibiotics are typically given through a vein in your arm. Later, you may be able to switch to antibiotic pills. Sometimes, the joint needs to be drained to remove the infected fluid. A severe infection may need surgery to clean out the joint.

## Viral infections

Many viruses may cause joint pain or inflammation. Typically, viruses affect the same joints on both sides of the body. The pain begins suddenly and is often accompanied by a rash and fever. Some viruses can be diagnosed through lab tests.

Common viruses that can cause joint pain include:

**Parvovirus** This virus causes a "slapped cheek" appearance in children (Fifth's disease). In adults, it causes pain in multiple joints that may be confused with rheumatoid arthritis.

**Hepatitis B and hepatitis C** These viruses are transmitted through blood from one infected individual to another.

**Human Immunodeficiency Virus (HIV)** This sexually transmitted infection usually causes flu-like illness within a month or two after the virus enters the body. Symptoms including joint pain may last for a few weeks.

**Epstein-Barr virus** This virus, also known as mononucleosis, causes prolonged fatigue and achiness in young people.

**Mumps** This virus causes swelling of the cheeks and achy joints.

**Chikungunya** This virus causes a high fever, rash, headaches, joint pain and severe pain with walking.

Viral arthritis usually resolves on its own within six to eight weeks. Treatment generally involves pain medications to relieve symptoms. For a few viruses, such as hepatitis C, an antiviral treatment can help to clear the virus from your body.

## Lyme disease

Lyme disease is caused by a type of bacteria that lives in the digestive tract of deer ticks. If you're bitten by a tick that stays attached for 36 hours or more, the bacteria can transfer into your skin.

One of the hallmarks of Lyme disease is a reddish oval- or disk-shaped rash (erythema migrans). This is followed by flu-like symptoms, a fever, chills, sore throat and fatigue.

Without treatment, the bacteria may spread to the joints and other parts of the body. Weeks later, you may develop stiffness, sharp pain and swelling in your joints. The pain may affect one joint for a few days and then go away and reappear in another joint. Or, even if bacteria don't enter the joints, Lyme disease may cause an inflammatory response in your body that leads to joint inflammation.

Your doctor can diagnose Lyme disease with a physical exam and blood and synovial fluid tests. Treatment with antibiotics should start as early as possible. Left untreated, Lyme disease can lead to chronic joint inflammation (Lyme arthritis), particularly in your knee. Other organs, such as your heart or brain, may be affected as well.

## Rheumatic fever

Rheumatic fever is an inflammatory disease that can affect the heart, joints, skin or brain. It can develop if strep throat or scarlet fever isn't properly treated. Strep throat and scarlet fever are both caused by an infection with streptococcus bacteria. While the infection itself doesn't enter the joints, the immune system's reaction in rheumatic fever causes inflammation that can lead to joint pain. Symptoms can occur several weeks after the initial infection.

Anyone can get rheumatic fever, although it primarily affects children between ages 5 and 15. The disease is rare in developed countries, including the United States. But it remains common in many developing countries.

Sometimes rheumatic fever causes heart valve damage and heart failure. This is known as rheumatic heart disease, and it may not be discovered until years later. Treatments can reduce tissue damage and lessen symptoms.

**Signs and symptoms** If rheumatic fever develops after a strep infection, the signs and symptoms usually begin two to four weeks after infection. Signs and symptoms vary and can change during the course of the disease. They may include:

- Fever
- Joint pain and tenderness, most often in the knees, elbows, wrists and ankles
- Red, hot or swollen joints
- Chest pain and feeling short of breath
- A new heart murmur
- Fatigue
- Uncontrollable, jerky movements of your limbs and face or more subtle movement difficulties, such as problems with hand-writing
- Areas of pink rash with clear centers
- Pea-sized lumps under your skin, usually over bony areas

Rheumatic fever usually affects several joints in quick succession, each for a short time. Pain may seem to move from one joint to another.

**Diagnosis and treatment** Diagnosis typically includes a physical exam, listening for abnormal heart rhythms, simple movement tests and blood samples to test for evidence of recent strep infection. Your doctor may also order other blood tests, as well as an electrocardiogram (ECG) of the heart, which checks for abnormal heartbeats.

Penicillin or another antibiotic is typically prescribed to kill the strep bacteria. To control a fever, joint pain and inflammation, your doctor may also prescribe aspirin, an NSAID or a steroid medication. Anticonvulsant medications can help control jerky movements.

## MOVING FORWARD

Even though these inflammatory disorders are chronic diseases, you may be able to avoid their most severe consequences and maintain an active, productive life. Both professional care and self-care are essential elements.

Many people find that they can reduce the impact of these diseases by following a carefully planned, individualized treatment program outlined by their doctor and other health care professionals. Diet, exercise, and knowing when to stop and rest are all important parts of this approach to successfully managing inflammatory joint pain.

# Chapter 6

# Back pain and spine disorders

Most people experience back pain at some point in their lives. Often, this pain lasts just a few days to a few weeks. Pain in the lower part of the back (lumbar region) is the most common, because this area bears the most body weight and stress.

Back pain can have many causes, from poor posture to cancer. The most common cause is an injury to a muscle or ligament (strain), usually the result of putting too much force on your back or overusing the back muscles in repetitive tasks. An injured muscle may "knot up" into a spasm.

Other causes of back pain include osteoarthritis, a ruptured (herniated) disk, spinal stenosis and ankylosing spondylitis.

Most back pain disappears with self-care, although it may take a few weeks. Pain and soreness usually start to improve within the first 72 hours after they begin. If they don't, see your doctor. It's also a good idea to see your doctor for back pain if you are over age 50, if you have a history of back pain or cancer, or if you notice any red flag symptoms listed on page 90.

Your doctor will examine your back and look at how you sit, stand, walk and lift your legs. Diagnostic tests such as blood or fluid tests generally aren't needed to confirm the cause of back pain.

If your doctor suspects a tumor, fracture, infection or other serious problem, he or she may order imaging tests. An X-ray, magnetic resonance imaging scan (MRI), computerized tomography (CT) scan or bone scan can help identify the cause of pain. Another type of test called electromyography (EMG)

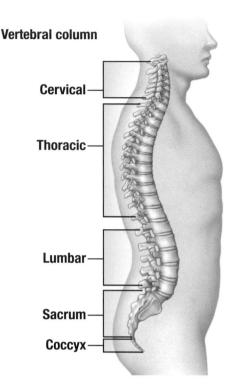

**Vertebral column**

Cervical

Thoracic

Lumbar

Sacrum

Coccyx

can help detect the source of numbness or tingling, often related to underlying nerve disorders.

Many back problems respond well to home treatments such as taking anti-inflammatory medication (ibuprofen or naproxen). Applying ice, heat or gentle massage also can help. Studies show that most cases of back pain improve in a matter of weeks, regardless of the type of treatment you use. If your back pain hasn't resolved within four weeks, your doctor may suggest muscle relaxants, electrical stimulation or physical therapy.

Although back pain is more common as you get older, it's not an inevitable part of aging. You can reduce your risk of developing painful back problems by doing exercises that strengthen the muscles that support your back and practicing good posture and work habits that protect your back. Staying active in general can help to maintain your back strength and function.

## DIFFUSE IDIOPATHIC SKELETAL HYPEROSTOSIS (DISH)

Diffuse idiopathic skeletal hyperostosis (hi-pur-ahs-TOE-sis), or DISH, is a hardening of ligaments and tendons where they attach to bone. The tissue forms bony growths (spurs) at these points, usually around the spine. Bone spurs may also form in the shoulders, elbows, hands, hips, knees, ankles or heels.

DISH often goes undiagnosed until it causes pain or other problems. It's more common in males and people over 50, and it has been associated with obesity and diabetes mellitis. Your risk may also be higher if you've taken retinoid medications such as isotretinoin, used to treat acne and other skin conditions.

### Signs and symptoms

Most people have no symptoms. DISH may be found when having X-rays or other image tests for another condition. When symptoms do occur, they tend to include stiffness and pain, most often in the upper back. Pain can develop when bone spurs begin pressing on the body parts around them. If DISH develops in your neck, you might have difficulty swallowing or a hoarse voice.

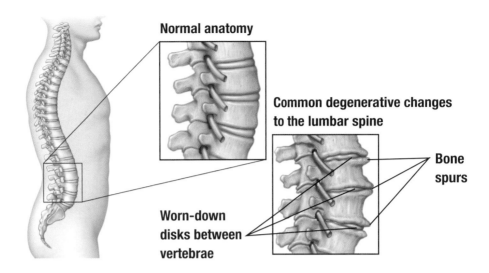

**Normal anatomy**

**Common degenerative changes to the lumbar spine**

**Bone spurs**

**Worn-down disks between vertebrae**

## Diagnosis and treatment

Your doctor can diagnose DISH based on X-rays or other imaging tests of the spine. He or she may begin with a physical exam, pressing lightly on your spine and joints to feel for abnormalities and check your range of motion.

There is no cure for DISH, but you can take steps to reduce pain and stiffness. Treatments may include physical therapy, heat, pain medications and steroid shots. If you have bone spurs on your heels, shoe inserts may help. Staying as active as possible also helps reduce stiffness and keeps your muscles strong.

## HERNIATED DISK

Between the bones of the spine (vertebrae) are disks that act like cushions, with a tough outer covering and a jellylike center. Some-times a tear can develop in the outer covering, allowing the jelly material inside to push out. This is called a herniated disk and is usually the result of age-related wear and tear. It's also sometimes called a slipped disk, or a ruptured disk.

## Signs and symptoms

Herniated disks cause symptoms when the jellylike material pushes out and presses on nearby nerves. The most common symptoms are pain, numbness and tingling that spread down one arm or leg, depending on which disk is affected in the spine. You may also have muscle weakness. However, sometimes a herniated disk doesn't cause any symptoms.

In rare cases, a herniated disk can cause serious complications. Seek emergency care if you have back pain and have a fever, have trouble going to the bathroom or controlling

## RED FLAGS: SIGNS AND SYMPTOMS YOU DON'T WANT TO IGNORE

Most of the time, back pain is an annoying problem that improves over time. But in some cases back pain may be a symptom of a serious problem that needs medical treatment. Get care immediately if you have any of the following:

- Fever with new back pain
- New bowel or bladder problems with back pain
- Pain from a fall or blow to your back

You should also contact your doctor if your pain:

- Is constant or intense, especially at night
- Spreads down one or both legs
- Occurs with weakness, numbness or tingling in one or both legs
- Includes abdominal pain or throbbing
- Is back pain with unexplained weight loss

**Normal anatomy**     **Herniated disk**

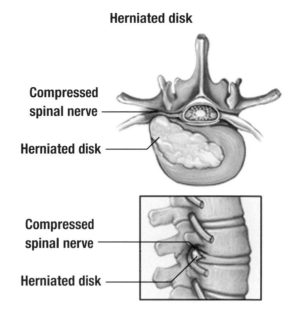

Compressed spinal nerve

Herniated disk

Compressed spinal nerve

Herniated disk

your bowel or bladder, or can't flex your foot (foot drop).

## Diagnosis and treatment

Usually, you doctor can diagnose a herniated disk based on your medical history and a physical exam. He or she will check for tenderness and may also check your reflexes, muscle strength and ability to feel light touches.

Symptoms usually improve on their own within four to six weeks. Meanwhile, conservative treatments such as pain medication, exercise and avoiding painful movements may help. If the symptoms don't improve, imaging tests such as an MRI or CT may be needed to help identify the problem.

Treatment for a herniated disk can include pain medications, muscle relaxants, injections, physical therapy, spinal traction, acupuncture and massage. A small number of people may need surgery to get relief.

Staying as active as possible is an important part of treatment, even if you have some pain or discomfort. Although bed rest was once the recommended treatment, researchers now know that long periods of rest can actually make spine pain worse.

## CERVICAL SPINE DISORDERS

The bones (vertebrae) of the neck make up the upper portion of the spine, called the cervical spine. As in the back, the vertebrae are stacked one on top of another, with disks between them that function as cushions. Ligaments cover the bones and the disks, helping to stabilize and protect the spine. The spinal cord runs down through the vertebrae and connects to other nerves. Muscles surrounding the spine are responsible for holding the head upright.

Neck pain can result from problems with any of these parts, including muscle or ligament irritation, arthritis, or a pinched nerve. Many people — up to half or more of all adults — experience neck pain at some point. Regardless of the cause, most people recover with conservative therapy.

It's often difficult to know for sure what exactly is causing neck pain. Your symptoms and the degree of pain may not correlate with the severity of the problem. In other words, you may have strong pain from a small change in the spine, or you may feel only mild symptoms from a significant problem.

Many of the causes of neck pain, such as changes to the vertebrae, cannot be repaired or undone. So it's important to work on factors you can control. Your posture, muscle strength, sleep habits, proper teeth alignment and the amount of tension in your head can all help relieve neck pain or contribute to it.

Some of the more common causes of neck pain include the following:

***Cervical strain*** An injury to the neck muscles can cause muscle spasms and pain.

**Normal cervical spine anatomy**

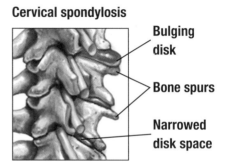

**Cervical spondylosis**

Bulging disk

Bone spurs

Narrowed disk space

***Cervical spondylosis*** This condition involves age-related wear and tear of the bones and disks in the neck (cervical spine).

***Cervical discogenic pain*** A problem with the disks between the vertebrae, such as irritation or degeneration of the disks, is one of the most common causes of neck pain. The pain is worse when the neck is held in one position for long periods of time (for example, while driving).

***Cervical facet joint syndrome*** This type of arthritis affects the facet joints, located on both sides of the vertebrae. You use these joints when moving your neck and head.

**Whiplash injury** This condition is usually caused by the trauma of an abrupt forward or backward movement of the neck, such as from a car accident.

**Cervical myofascial pain** Tight areas of neck muscle may feel tender and painful.

**DISH** See page 88.

**Cervical spondylotic myelopathy** This pinching of the spinal cord in the neck is due to changes from degenerative arthritis, and it keeps the spinal cord from functioning properly. This condition may cause weakness, difficulty walking, inability to empty or control bowel or bladder, and sexual dysfunction.

**Cervical radiculopathy** A nerve root in the neck may become irritated or pinched where it leads out from the spinal cord. When this occurs, it can cause pain or tingling in the shoulder and arm.

## Diagnosis and treatment

Your doctor will examine your neck by moving your head to the left and right, forward and backward, and side to side. Imaging tests also may be needed to confirm a diagnosis, depending on your symptoms.

Most of the time, the pain resolves with conservative treatment such as taking acetaminophen (Tylenol, others) or anti-inflammatory medications. Sometimes your doctor might prescribe a muscle relaxant or antidepressant, which can help treat pain.

Self-care treatments such as ice and heat may also help reduce pain. Massage can help relieve muscle spasms, and stretching exercises may help stretch and strengthen the muscles. Because emotional stress can increase neck tension, reducing stress may help prevent neck pain. In addition, good neck posture can lessen tension across the muscles. Sleeping with a small pillow under the nape of your neck keeps your neck in a neutral position. When carrying heavy items, carrying them close to your body rather than with outstretched arms lowers the risk of straining the neck or back.

Other treatments may include acupuncture, a neck brace, steroid injections, electrical stimulation and a method of learning to regulate your response to pain called biofeedback. Chiropractic therapy, physical therapy, and assisted stretching and lengthening of the neck (cervical traction) are sometimes helpful as well. Surgery isn't usually needed. However, if a nerve is being pinched by a herniated disk and doesn't respond to conservative therapy, surgery may be an option.

## MECHANICAL LOW BACK PAIN

Almost everyone will have back pain at some point in life. In most cases, the back pain isn't serious, and it usually resolves on its own. However, if you have any red flag

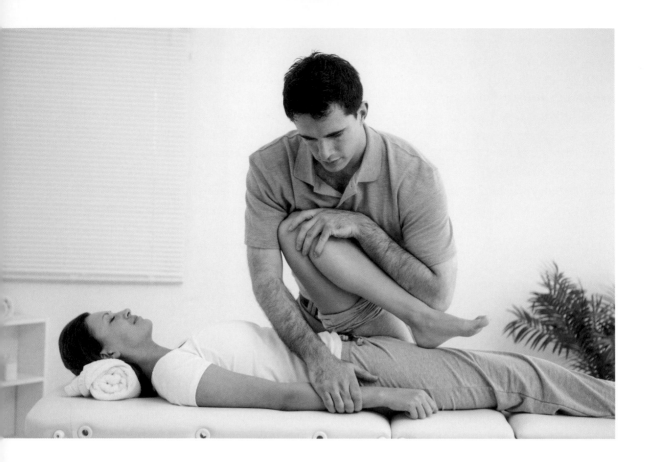

symptoms (see page 90) with persistent pain, see your doctor.

Your low back, like your neck, is made up of vertebrae, shock-absorbing disks, the spinal cord and other nerves, and muscles, tendons and ligaments. One or more of these tissues may become painful when irritated. For example, this can occur with bulging or torn disks, a vertebra out of place, narrowing in the spinal canal, or other changes.

Pain from these issues is called mechanical — due to pain sensors within the mechanical working parts of the spine. Often, it's difficult to determine the specific location and cause of the irritation and pain. Back pain also might be due to arthritis of the spine joints, or rarely, a tumor or infection.

## Diagnosis and treatment

A physical exam may be all your doctor needs to make a diagnosis. Imaging tests usually aren't necessary unless your back pain isn't improving after four to six weeks.

Staying active, even through mild pain, is a key part of treatment. Sometimes treatment will also involve pain medications, physical therapy, low back (lumbar) spine traction, acupuncture, massage, measures to reduce stress or steroid injections.

Low back pain can be a recurring problem, so it's important to stay active and learn exercises that help strengthen and stretch your back. When lifting objects, lift from your legs instead of with your back. And avoid sitting or standing in the same position for too long. Following these tips can help protect you from future injuries.

## SCHEUERMANN'S KYPHOSIS

A humped back (kyphosis) can result from different changes in the spine. Scheuermann's kyphosis, also known as juvenile kyphosis, occurs when the bones of the spine (vertebrae) develop a wedged shape, causing the spine to curve forward. It occurs in some children during a growth spurt, when the growth plates in the spine haven't yet hardened into solid bone. The curve tends to form in the upper or mid back and may sometimes be mistaken for poor posture. However, this curve doesn't disappear when you stand up straight or lie flat on your back.

Evidence shows that genetics can predispose someone to Scheuermann's kyphosis. But other factors likely also affect the bone growth.

### Signs and symptoms

Along with a humped back, this condition often causes back pain around the time of puberty. The pain is typically worse after activities and improves with rest. Later in adolescence, as bone growth slows down, the pain usually improves.

### Diagnosis and treatment

Scheuermann's kyphosis is diagnosed with X-rays. Your doctor will look for at least three vertebrae in a row with a wedge shape to confirm the diagnosis.

Conservative treatment is usually recommended. This may include exercises to stretch and strengthen the muscles around the spine, managing the pain, and avoiding activities that make the pain worse. In rare cases of a significant curve, you may need to wear a back brace or have surgery to correct the spinal curve.

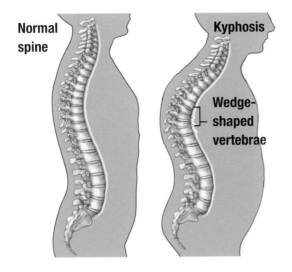

Normal spine

Kyphosis

Wedge-shaped vertebrae

## SPINAL STENOSIS

Spinal stenosis (stuh-NO-sis) is a narrowing of one or more areas in your spine. The narrowing puts pressure on the spinal cord and roots of the spinal nerves.

The spinal cord is a bundle of nerves and nerve cells that extends the full length of your spine. The cord is housed in a canal within the vertebrae. Smaller nerves branch off from the spinal cord, forming an intricate communication network between your brain and the rest of your body.

Spinal stenosis doesn't always cause problems. But when the narrowed spinal canal puts pressure on the spinal cord, it can result in a wide range of symptoms. It may cause pain, cramping, or numbness in your legs, back, neck, shoulders or arms. Inflammation also can contribute to your symptoms.

Spinal stenosis typically affects adults over age 50. Most often, the spinal narrowing results from osteoarthritis. But an injury, cancer or another disease can also lead to it.

As the disks between vertebrae age and bone spurs or other changes of arthritis form, the spaces between the bones may decrease or disappear. These changes can cause vertebrae and soft tissue to push inward into the spinal canal.

### Signs and symptoms

Symptoms of spinal stenosis vary, depending on where in the spine the narrowing

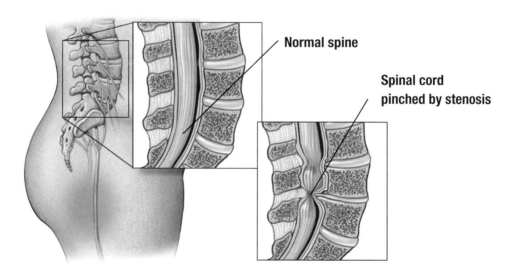

**Normal spine**

**Spinal cord pinched by stenosis**

Spinal stenosis may result when the spinal canal becomes narrowed by osteoarthritis or other changes. It usually affects the neck or low back. If the spinal cord or nerve roots in the low back are pinched, stenosis may cause pain, numbness and tingling in your hips, buttocks and legs.

occurs and which nerves are affected. If the narrowed area does cause symptoms, they often start gradually and get worse over time. They may include:

- Pain that runs down the back of your leg
- Numbness, tingling, cramping or weakness in your hand, arm, foot or leg
- Loss of balance
- Bowel and bladder control problems

The pain of spinal stenosis usually improves if you lean forward, crouch or sit down. You'll likely notice pain more when you walk downhill. This is different from leg pain that occurs as a result of poor circulation, which is usually worse when you walk uphill and improves when you stop walking.

## Diagnosis and treatment

Spinal stenosis can be difficult to diagnose because leg pain is often the main symptom. In addition to a physical exam, you'll also likely undergo imaging tests, such as a spinal X-ray, MRI or CT.

Many people with spinal stenosis find effective relief with pain relievers, rest, physical therapy, exercise and other conservative treatments.

If you have severe pain that interferes with your ability to walk or do other activities, weakness that's getting worse in your legs, or reduced control of your bladder or bowel, your doctor may recommend surgery to relieve the pressure and maintain the strength and integrity of your spine.

# SPONDYLOLYSIS AND SPONDYLOLISTHESIS

Spondylolysis (spahn-duh-LOL-ih-sis) is a crack or separation in the thin section of bone that connects the back and front parts of a vertebra. It affects about 7% of people, most often during adolescence. It's more likely to occur with overuse activities or an injury (trauma). It's more commonly seen in sports that put a lot of stress on the low back, especially by bending backward, during growth spurts in young athletes. For example, dancers, gymnasts, figure skaters, wrestlers, divers and football linebackers are particularly at risk. However, the condition can affect anyone.

Spondylolysis can occur on one or both sides of the vertebra, and in one or more bones. When fractures occur in both sides of a vertebra, the bone may slip forward out of alignment. Spondylolisthesis (spon-duh-loe-lis-THEE-sis) occurs when there is "slippage" (listhesis) of one vertebra on another. This can put pressure on the nerves and lead to more-severe symptoms.

## Signs and symptoms

Children who develop spondylolysis early in life usually have no symptoms. The condition is found when X-rays or other images of the spine are taken for other reasons. In adolescent athletes, symptoms often develop gradually. The most common symptom is low back pain during activities, particularly when bending backward.

A CT scan (left) shows an extreme case of spondylolisthesis in the low back. The L5 vertebra, the lowest bone in the lumbar spine, is almost completely off the S1 vertebra below it. An X-ray (right) shows the corrected spine, with rods and screws in place, after surgery to fuse the L5 with the bones above and below it. In most people with spondylolisthesis, the slippage is less severe and surgery isn't needed.

Children with spondylolisthesis develop pain that spreads across the low back and into the buttocks or the back of the legs. A slipped vertebra can lead to numbness, tingling and weakness if it presses on nerve roots. Athletes may experience sharp pain with back extension during activities — for example, kicking a soccer ball or striking a volleyball.

## Diagnosis and treatment

Spondylolysis is diagnosed with a physical exam and X-rays or other imaging tests. In people with no symptoms, a fracture may be found when imaging tests are done for another reason.

There is limited evidence regarding the best treatment options for these conditions. In addition, treatment varies depending on symptoms and whether the bone has slipped out of alignment. For most adolescents with a fracture or a bone that has slipped only partially, several months of rest from activity may be the most effective way to allow symptoms to improve. Back braces have been used in the past but usually aren't needed for healing.

If someone has a severely slipped vertebra or doesn't respond to nonsurgical therapies, surgery may be needed to fuse the bones of the spine in the correct position.

# Childhood arthritis

Nearly 300,000 children in the United States have some form of juvenile arthritis. As in adults, arthritis in children can take many different forms, with various causes, symptoms and risks. One major difference of juvenile arthritis is that many children can achieve symptom-free periods (remission) that may last months or years at a time, even while off treatments.

Joint pain in children may be caused by inflammation within the joint or other conditions related to the bones and muscles. Some conditions are associated with changes to the bones and joints that occur as children grow. These may even resolve on their own with time.

Whatever the cause, most joint pain in children can be improved with the right diagnosis and modern treatments.

## JUVENILE IDIOPATHIC ARTHRITIS

Juvenile idiopathic arthritis (JIA) is a chronic autoimmune disease that causes joint inflammation in children and youth age 16 and younger. The word *idiopathic* means the cause is unknown — and the exact cause of JIA is unclear. But, like adult rheumatoid arthritis, juvenile idiopathic arthritis seems to involve both genetic and environmental factors.

There are several distinct subtypes of JIA, based on features of the disease. The following sections give information on each type.

### Oligoarticular JIA (pauciarticular JIA)

This is the most common form of JIA, affecting four or fewer joints — typically the larger joints, such as the knees and ankles. Often only one knee is affected, which can make diagnosis challenging, as there are usually no other symptoms. Girls are more likely to have this form of JIA than are boys.

Oligoarticular JIA most commonly occurs in very young children, often before the age of 4. The disease may subside over time. But the longer the disease remains active, the more likely a child is to develop an extended disease that involves multiple joints and lasts into adulthood.

## Polyarticular JIA

*Poly* means many, and this form of arthritis affects five or more joints — typically small joints, such as those in the hands and feet. It often affects the same joint on both sides of the body, such as both wrists. Polyarticular JIA can begin at any age and affects girls more often than boys.

This subtype of JIA resembles adult rheumatoid arthritis more than do other forms of JIA. Certain test results, including a positive rheumatoid factor (RF) or a positive cyclic citrullinated peptide (CCP) antibody count, can help diagnose polyarticular JIA. However, it is the least common subtype and can be the most difficult to treat.

## Enthesitis-related arthritis (ERA)

This subtype of JIA is closely related to adult forms of spondyloarthritis. The main symptom is inflammation that occurs at the sites (entheses) where tendons or ligaments attach to bones near a joint. This inflammation is called enthesitis. It is usually accompanied by arthritis, often involving the ankles, feet, spine and pelvis.

Children with ERA can have back pain and stiffness around their sacroiliac joints, where the spine connects to the pelvis. An MRI may be needed to check for inflammation of the sacroiliac joints. If children have arthritis mainly in these joints, they may be diagnosed with juvenile ankylosing spondylitis. This is often considered a type of ERA with features similar to those of ankylosing spondylitis in adults.

ERA usually occurs in children over age 6 and is more common in boys than in girls. In addition, about 60% of children with ERA have a gene called human leukocyte antigen B27 (HLA-B27). But having this gene doesn't mean you have or will get the disease. About 6% of the general U.S. population has the gene.

## Psoriatic arthritis

Psoriatic arthritis can affect children as well as adults and is more common in girls than in boys. It causes a rash (psoriasis) involving red, scaly and flaky skin and pitted nails, along with pain and swelling of one or multiple joints. Fingers or toes may become swollen, known as "sausage digits." Older children and teens with psoriatic arthritis may have back or hip pain. Rarely, this condition can cause inflammation of the eye (uveitis).

Psoriasis and psoriatic arthritis are strongly linked to family history. Because of this, a child with JIA may be diagnosed with psoriatic arthritis if he or she has a family member with psoriasis. The child doesn't need to have a personal history of psoriasis.

## Systemic JIA

Systemic JIA (formerly called Still's disease) is a unique and rare form of JIA. The disease begins with a recurring high fever that typically appears in the afternoon and evening and is gone in the morning. For a diagnosis, the fever must occur at least three days in a row and intermittently for at least two weeks. A flat, pink rash also may come and go.

The arthritis in systemic JIA usually affects mulitple joints. It may appear along with the initial fevers or rash, or it may not show up until months after the onset of fevers.

True to its name, systemic JIA can affect many areas of the body, not just the joints. It is the only form of JIA that affects internal organs. Children with this condition may develop an enlarged liver and spleen as well as swollen lymph nodes.

## Signs and symptoms

Signs and symptoms of JIA vary from one child to another. They can fluctuate from day to day and even throughout the same day. They may include:

- **Joint swelling with stiffness and achy pain** Children may not complain of joint pain or swelling. Rather, you may notice them limping, being less active than usual, or being reluctant to use an arm or a leg. You may notice difficulty in the way your child crawls, walks, jumps, colors, ties shoes, eats, or holds a cup or spoon. Discomfort may be more pronounced in the morning or after a nap and then improve with some activity.

- **Bone and joint changes** If arthritis in children is severe or goes untreated for a long period of time, a joint may lose its range of motion. This typically improves once the inflammation is treated but may need physical therapy. Joint inflammation in children can also cause growth changes, leading to uneven leg or arm lengths.

- **Eye inflammation** Eye inflammation (uveitis) occurs with several subtypes of JIA, most commonly with oligoarticular JIA. The inflammation often doesn't cause any signs or symptoms. But when it does, it may cause eye pain, redness and increased pain when looking at light. Routine eye examinations are recommended because eye inflammation can be difficult to detect, and it may lead to decreased vision.

- **Rash** Certain forms of JIA can include skin changes. A constant, scaly red rash could be psoriasis, related to psoriatic arthritis. But a faint pink rash that comes and goes (with a fever) could be a sign of systemic JIA.

- **Fever** A recurring high fever is a characteristic sign of systemic JIA. A fever may also occur in other autoimmune diseases that can cause arthritis, including lupus, dermatomyositis, vasculitis and inflammatory bowel disease.

Like other forms of arthritis, JIA includes times when symptoms are present (flares) and times of remission.

## Diagnosis and treatment

The diagnosis of JIA is based on a medical history and physical examination. Blood tests can help rule out other causes of symptoms, pinpoint the type of arthritis and clarify a diagnosis. These tests may include:

- **Complete blood count (CBC)** This important test can suggest an infection, cancer, or certain autoimmune diseases if white blood cell levels are highly elevated or decreased. If the test shows significant anemia, this could suggest inflammatory bowel disease or celiac disease as a cause of arthritis.

- **Erythrocyte sedimentation (sed) rate and C-reactive protein (CRP)** As with adult rheumatoid arthritis, an elevated sed rate or CRP can indicate the presence of inflammation. These tests may be used to determine how severe the inflammation is and to rule out other conditions. In children, these lab tests are not always abnormal, even with active arthritis.

- **Antinuclear antibodies (ANA)** These are proteins produced by the immune system among people with certain autoimmune diseases, including arthritis. Antinuclear antibodies are present in about 40% of children with JIA. This test does not diagnose JIA or show if arthritis or JIA is likely to develop later. However, children with diagnosed JIA who have a positive ANA test are at increased risk for uveitis.

- **Other antibody tests** Rheumatoid factor (RF) and CCP antibody tests are positive in some children with polyarticular JIA, but only in a minority. Abnormal testing isn't required for a diagnosis of JIA.

In addition to lab tests, X-rays may be taken to rule out conditions such as fractures, tumors, infections and birth defects. X-rays may also be used after diagnosis to monitor bone development and possible joint damage. Additional blood tests may be done to look for infections and other conditions associated with bone and joint pain.

The doctor may also remove some fluid from your child's swollen joint to test for an infection that could cause arthritis. Removing fluid may also help relieve pain and improve joint mobility.

Treatment for JIA depends on the type of arthritis your child has and on his or her symptoms. For all children, treatment aims to control the arthritis with the goal of remission — when no arthritis is detectable. With or without remission, the focus is on maintaining a normal level of physical and social activity. Doctors may prescribe a combination of strategies that help relieve pain and swelling, maintain joint movement and strength, and prevent complications. The treatment program may include medications, procedures, exercise, eye care, dental care and good nutrition.

In addition to relieving pain and swelling, medications for JIA can slow the progress of the disease and help with normal bone growth. Initial treatment often includes nonsteroidal anti-inflammatory drugs (NSAIDs), such as ibuprofen or naproxen. Joint injections with corticosteroids also may be used to control inflammation at a specific joint.

Disease-modifying antirheumatic drugs (DMARDs) and biologics are frequently prescribed when the risk of joint damage or disease progression is higher, as in children with polyarticular and systemic JIA. Because these medications suppress the immune system, it's important to talk through the risks and benefits with your child's doctor.

Parents can help children with JIA by encouraging physical activity, normal routines and positive outlooks. Family members should also be prepared to help children cope with the emotional aspects of having a chronic disease.

## OTHER INFLAMMATORY JOINT CONDITIONS

Some types of inflammatory childhood arthritis cause symptoms similar to those of JIA but don't fit under the same umbrella. These diseases may be associated with other chronic conditions, or they may develop as a temporary overactive immune response.

## Enteropathic arthritis

Arthritis that's associated with inflammatory bowel disease (IBD) is called enteropathic arthritis. Children and teens who have IBD, an autoimmune disease, experience inflammation of the intestines and colon. Crohn's disease and ulcerative colitis are the two most common types of IBD.

About 10% to 20% of people with IBD develop enteropathic arthritis. The large joints are most commonly affected, but the pelvis and sacroiliac joints also can be involved. It's not unusual for a child with IBD to develop arthritis first with intestinal symptoms occurring later. Thus, if a child has joint pain and swelling as well as diarrhea, bloody stools, fevers, weight loss or belly cramps, IBD may be the cause. Treating the underlying bowel inflammation often improves the joint symptoms.

## Reactive arthritis

This type of arthritis is not a chronic auto-immune disease. Rather, it usually occurs after an infection of the gut or urinary tract. Inflammation that's part of the immune response can set off a reaction in the joints, causing redness, swelling and stiffness. However, the infection itself is not in the joints, and it can occur even after the initial symptoms of infection are gone.

Reactive arthritis causes pain and swelling of one or just a few joints. The knees and ankles are most commonly affected. This condition can also cause inflammation of the outer layer of the eye (conjunctivitis). It can affect the skin in various ways, but this occurs less often than in adults. Children may have pain with urination if the urinary tract becomes inflamed (urethritis).

Reactive arthritis is often a self-limited condition, meaning it goes away on its own after running its course. Usually NSAIDs are the only treatment needed to control the pain and swelling. The original infection may need to be treated if it hasn't resolved. However, antibiotics usually aren't helpful in improving joint symptoms if there's no lingering active infection.

## Transient synovitis

Transient synovitis is a specific type of reactive arthritis that's isolated to the hip. It occurs most often in children between the ages of 3 and 8 and is more than twice as likely in boys than in girls. Transient synovitis causes relatively sudden pain and a limited range of motion in the hip. Usually only one hip is involved, and a child may limp or refuse to bear weight on the affected side. The cause of the disease isn't clear. But since it typically occurs in close proximity to a mild infection, it's considered a type of abnormal immune response.

When this condition is suspected, imaging tests such as an ultrasound often show extra fluid in the hip joint. Most children with transient synovitis don't seem ill and don't have a fever. NSAIDs are used to reduce inflammation and relieve hip pain. Symptoms resolve within a few days to a few weeks, and most children return to normal activities.

Your doctor may want to rule out an active bacterial hip infection as the cause of pain, especially if the child looks ill, has a fever or has abnormal lab tests. This may be done by drawing (aspirating) fluid from the hip joint.

## CONNECTIVE TISSUE DISEASES

In rheumatology, connective tissue diseases are a group of autoimmune illnesses that tend to affect certain internal organs. They are seen as distinct from other autoimmune illnesses that primarily cause inflammation in the joints, spine and ligaments. The following connective tissue diseases may be a source of joint pain in children.

### Juvenile dermatomyositis

An autoimmune response in the body can cause inflammation of the muscles. This is called inflammatory myopathy, and it typically leads to muscle weakness. When it affects children, it's usually caused by dermatomyositis, which occurs with characteristic skin rashes. When children have muscle weakness, you may notice them having difficulty getting up off the floor, getting into and out of a vehicle, or climbing stairs. Activities such as washing their

hair or feeding themselves also may become difficult. In more severe cases, dermatomyositis can affect the child's voice and ability to swallow or breathe comfortably.

There are several classic skin signs of dermatomyositis in children. These include raised red spots over the knuckles, elbows or knees (Gottron's papules); redness over the chest (shawl sign); redness around the base of the fingernails; and a bluish purple discoloration around the eyes (heliotrope). The rashes are typically worse after sun exposure.

Blood tests can help diagnose dermatomyositis by showing evidence of inflammation and elevated levels of muscle enzymes. Sometimes a doctor may order a nerve test called electromyography (EMG), or a small sample of the muscle (biopsy) may be taken for testing to confirm the diagnosis. An MRI may be a less invasive way to check for muscle inflammation. There's no cure for this disease, but DMARDs and biologics can control symptoms in the muscles and skin. Some children may experience prolonged remission even without therapy.

### Systemic lupus erythematosus

Systemic lupus erythematosus, or lupus, is a systemic autoimmune disease. It can occur at any age, but in children it's most likely to occur after puberty and is more common in girls than boys. Lupus can cause many signs and symptoms in children. A rash, sores in the mouth, hair loss, skin sensitivity in the sun, and color changes in the hands and feet are common. Lupus can also affect internal organs and cause arthritis.

Diagnosis and treatment of lupus are similar for both children and adults, involving different tests and medications based on symptoms. See page 71 for more information on lupus.

## VASCULITIS

Vasculitis is inflammation of the blood vessels from autoimmune activity. It can cause blood vessels to become weak, narrowed, blocked, enlarged or scarred. A damaged blood vessel may not function normally, affecting blood flow to the tissues. This can lead to joint problems and other symptoms.

Several forms of vasculitis occur in children, and all may lead to arthritis. The two most common conditions are discussed below.

### Henoch-Schönlein purpura (HSP)

This type of vasculitis primarily affects children. It causes inflammation and bleeding in the small blood vessels in the skin, joints, intestines and kidneys. This leads to abdominal and joint pain and a rash of purplish

**Childhood arthritis    109**

marks. If the kidney is affected, urine may appear bloody or darkly colored, like tea or coffee. Most commonly, the large joints may develop arthritis and can be quite swollen.

A diagnosis of Henoch-Schönlein purpura (HEN-awk SHURN-line PUR-pu-ruh), or HSP, is based on the symptoms and exam. The doctor will do blood and urine tests and may also do imaging tests. Occasionally, a skin or kidney biopsy is done to rule out other possibilities.

The disease frequently goes away on its own within several weeks. Resting, drinking enough water, eating a healthy diet and controlling blood pressure may help symptoms improve.

## Kawasaki disease (KD)

This vasculitis occurs almost universally in children and is most common in young children between the ages of 1 and 3. It can affect all sizes of blood vessels, but most notably it can cause inflammation of the arteries in the heart. These arteries supply blood to the heart muscle.

Features of Kawasaki disease include a high fever that lasts more than five days; redness and pain of the eyes (conjunctivitis); red, dry lips and a swollen tongue; swollen lymph nodes in the neck; and red palms and soles. Up to 1 in 4 children with the disease also complains of joint pain, although this usually won't lead to joint damage. Peeling skin is another sign of the disease as it advances.

The most concerning symptoms occur when the heart vessels are involved. One of the first signs may be an increased heart rate. The disease can also cause bulges in the artery walls (aneurysms), raising the risk of a heart attack or internal bleeding.

A doctor can diagnose KD based on the symptoms and by ruling out other diseases with similar symptoms. He or she will likely order an ultrasound imaging test of the heart (echocardiogram) to determine if the heart vessels are inflamed. Once a diagnosis of KD is made, the doctor will start the child on intravenous immune globulin (IVIg), a potent anti-inflammatory treatment. This significantly reduces the risk of an aneurysm. Steroids are usually avoided, as they may worsen bulging arteries.

## ORTHOPEDIC CONDITIONS

Often, when children have joint pain, it's not from autoimmune causes. Rather, it's due to abnormalities of the bones or joints as their skeletons are growing and changing. These conditions may cause discomfort, a limp or limited range of motion. Some of the common orthopedic causes of joint pain in children are discussed below.

### Congenital hip dysplasia

Hip dysplasia is the medical term for a hip socket that doesn't fully cover the ball portion of the upper thighbone. Most children with this condition are born with it. As the hip joint develops, the socket part of the joint doesn't form normally and the hip joint is too loose. The ball of the hip can then slip out of the joint easily.

In younger infants, hip dysplasia doesn't usually cause any symptoms since the joints are not weight bearing. It may be found on routine examination. Signs and symptoms may occur as children start to walk. They may have pain, or they may limp or walk in an uneven manner. Milder cases may not cause symptoms until the teenage years.

When this condition is suspected, an X-ray may be taken to look directly at the hip joint. Treatment depends on the child's age. Loose hips are expected in babies less than 2 weeks old. But if the looseness continues, the baby may need to wear a soft brace to hold the hip joint in place so that the bones can grow normally. The brace is usually worn for two to three months. For babies older than 6 months, surgery may be necessary to correct the hip joint position, followed by a cast for three to four months. If the hip joint isn't positioned correctly, pain or damage in the joint may develop as children get older.

### Legg-Calvé-Perthes disease

Legg-Calvé-Perthes (LEG-kahl-VAY-PER-tuz) disease occurs when the blood supply to the ball part (femoral head) of the hip joint is temporarily interrupted and the bone begins to deteriorate. This condition usually affects children between 3 and 12 years of age and is more common in boys. As the bone weakens, it breaks apart and can lose its round shape. The bone eventually heals itself, but if it has changed shape, it can cause pain and stiffness. Children may start having hip pain or a limp that can begin either suddenly or slowly.

The loss of blood supply to the hip joint, called avascular necrosis, is sometimes due to an underlying medical condition such as obesity, infection or steroid use. There may be a family history. But many times, the underlying cause isn't clear.

Early in the disease, X-rays of the hip may appear normal. Other imaging studies such as a bone scan or MRI may help identify changes in the bone.

Treatment involves keeping the ball in the joint socket so that it can heal in its round shape. This may require activity restrictions or crutches for younger children or a cast or surgery in older children. The long-term outcome depends on the damage to the joint as well as the child's age. Children less than 6 to 8 years of age have a better prognosis.

## Osgood-Schlatter disease

Osgood-Schlatter disease causes pain on the front of the knee, in the area just below the kneecap (tibial tuberosity). It usually affects children ages 9 to 14, often after a growth spurt. It's also seen in children who are involved in activities with a lot of running or jumping. Pain may occur in one or both knees. It usually gets worse over time and

can be severe. The pain is typically worse with running, kneeling, jumping, climbing stairs and walking up hills, while it improves with rest.

The condition can usually be diagnosed during a physical exam. Ice or over-the-counter medications such as ibuprofen (Advil, Motrin) or acetaminophen (Tylenol, others) may help ease the pain. A physical therapist can recommend stretches and strengthening exercises for the leg muscles to help with pain, too. Most children can continue their normal activities, including sports, as long as the pain is not severe and improves with rest. Occasionally, a knee-pad or brace may be needed to cushion the front of the knee.

Symptoms tend to resolve on their own as the child's growth slows, which may take six to 18 months. Knee problems from this disease don't usually continue into adulthood.

## Slipped capital femoral epiphysis (SCFE)

Slipped capital femoral epiphysis (SCFE) is the most common hip disorder in adolescence. It usually occurs in children 12 to 13 years of age who are overweight. Most children with SCFE will complain of groin pain, but sometimes it causes knee or thigh pain.

This condition limits the range of motion of the hip. It's caused by changes in the head of the femur — the ball-shaped top of the thighbone — which sits in the hip socket. Normally the femoral head sits atop a growth plate that connects it to the rest of the bone. In SCFE, it slips out of position on the growth plate, like ice cream slipping off a cone. This causes pain in the hip joint and a limp. SCFE may occur after minor trauma.

If your doctor suspects SCFE, X-rays usually can confirm the diagnosis. Most children with SCFE will need surgery to stabilize the slipping bone.

## GROWING PAINS

Growing pains often occur in children, usually between ages 3 and 12. They are the most common cause of intermittent joint pain in children. The pain is most often felt deep in the legs, in the muscles and joints on both sides of the body. Typically, a child will wake up at night or during naps with pain but won't have any symptoms of other musculoskeletal conditions. The pain usually occurs at least once a month for three months or more. It may be worse after days when the child is more active.

The cause of growing pains isn't clear. Possible factors include bone density, overuse of the muscles and emotional disturbances. Often, there is a family history of similar pains.

Your doctor can diagnose growing pains with a physical exam and by ruling out other causes. With growing pains, the physical exam and any lab tests and X-rays taken will be normal. Sometimes, the diagnosis can be made based on the history of symptoms, as growing pains characteristically cause pain late in the day or during sleep.

Massage, heat or over-the-counter pain medications can help relieve the pain. If symptoms keep recurring, stretching or in some cases physical therapy may help. Growing pains usually resolve within a year or two. Meanwhile, children should be encouraged to continue normal activities.

# Different causes of pain: Peripheral and central pain

Pain is a common experience. If you have arthritis, you already likely know how debilitating pain can be. But other conditions list pain as a leading symptom, too.

Pain is a significant cause of disability and a major contributor to health care costs. Long-term (chronic) pain affects up to 2 out of every 5 Americans, while short-term (acute) pain affects millions more. Acute pain is the most common reason people seek medical care — ankle sprains are a good example. Chronic pain, on the other hand, is seen as a health condition in itself.

Because pain is a major problem in the United States and worldwide, research, education and support are dedicated to understanding it and finding the best ways to treat it. In recent years, for example, experts have learned much more about fibromyalgia and other conditions that are like arthritis in that they involve pain, but have a different cause. This new understanding, in turn, has changed the way some types of pain are managed.

This chapter offers insight into what's known today about pain, both in arthritis and in other conditions.

## WHAT CAUSES PAIN?

Pain can have many different causes. It can be short term (acute) or last longer than three months (chronic). Everyone has acute pain from time to time, whether it's from a broken bone, a cut or scrape, or surgery. In time, acute pain goes away. But chronic pain doesn't go away, and many things can cause it.

Chronic pain is broken down into one of two groups: peripheral or central. Chronic pain that's peripheral starts outside the brain and spinal cord, in the peripheral nervous system — for example, in a damaged joint. Central pain is linked to damage in the brain or spine.

The peripheral nervous system connects your brain and spinal cord to other parts of your body. The nerves in this system take messages from your muscles and organs and send them to your brain.

## PERIPHERAL PAIN

There are several types of peripheral pain, as shown in the diagram on page 117. As you'll see, different types of arthritis — and other conditions you've read about — involve different types of pain, mainly under the umbrella of peripheral pain. The following sections give more information on the three types of pain that start in the peripheral nervous system.

***Noninflammatory pain*** This type of pain, also called localized pain, happens when at least one joint is damaged or altered. Osteoarthritis and other conditions that aren't caused by inflammation are examples.

***Inflammatory pain*** As you may have guessed by its name, inflammation in the body causes this type of joint pain. Rheumatoid arthritis and other conditions that cause pain and irritation are examples.

***Neuropathic pain*** Pain that's caused by one or more nerves is described as neuropathic. It happens when one or more nerves cause numbness, tingling or a burning feeling. Carpal tunnel syndrome is an example.

## CENTRAL PAIN

Central pain is different from these three types of pain, so it's unlike the pain of arthritis and other conditions you've read about already. That's because this kind of pain starts in the brain and spinal cord. Central pain is also known as central sensitization.

# PAIN TYPES: PERIPHERAL AND CENTRAL

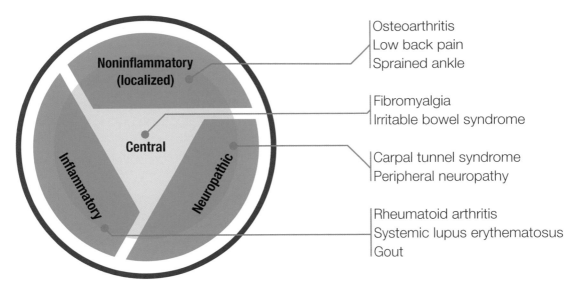

The cause of peripheral pain may be localized, inflammatory or neuropathic. Even when the source of pain is peripheral, each type of pain is modified in the brain and spinal cord, overlapping somewhat with central pain processing.

Here's how it works. Your body is covered in tiny sensor cells that monitor what you feel, taste, touch or smell. These sensor cells take the information they gather and send it to your brain.

When your brain gets these messages, it decides what to do about them. For example, if your brain gets the message that you're cold, it triggers shivering, and you may respond by grabbing a blanket or turning up the heat.

With central sensitization, the messages sent from these sensor cells to your brain get turned up, much like the volume on a radio. A slight chill may make you feel like you're freezing, for example. Lights may seem brighter, sounds may seem louder — and pain hurts more than it should. Even a light touch can hurt.

Mayo Clinic experts have found that central sensitization is linked to many symptoms and syndromes:

**Pain** Muscle or joint pain that isn't caused by inflammation is common.

**Fatigue** Another common symptom, fatigue is usually present all the time with central sensitization, and it doesn't get better after sleep. It may get worse with physical or mental activity. Fatigue is said to be chronic when it lasts for six months or more and isn't caused by another medical issue.

## CAN YOU HAVE BOTH TYPES OF PAIN?

Although pain is generally broken down into two types — pain that starts in the brain and spinal cord (central) and pain that starts outside of the brain and spinal cord (peripheral) — you can have both at the same time. In fact, as many as 2 out of 5 people with osteoarthritis, rheumatoid arthritis, and other joint diseases that cause pain and swelling in a joint have both types of pain.

This can make it hard to tell where the pain started. For example, if you've had arthritis but feel as though you hurt all over, are tired all the time and don't always have achy joints, you may have fibromyalgia.

An honest and thorough conversation about your symptoms can help your health care team uncover your true source of pain and treat it appropriately.

**Numbness or tingling** These sensations can appear with or without pain.

**Headaches** Both migraines and tension headaches can be symptoms of central sensitization. Tension headaches may cause pain and pressure in the head. Migraines can cause other symptoms, too, including nausea, vomiting, weakness, numbness, and feeling sensitive to light and sound.

**Sleep problems** Sleeping too much, being unable to sleep or not feeling refreshed after sleeping are all symptoms of central sensitization. Sleep apnea may need to be ruled out.

**Dizziness or lightheadedness** These feelings may happen all the time, or they may occur only upon sitting or standing too quickly.

**Weakness** A general sense of weakness can be a sign of central sensitization.

**Brain fog, memory issues and short attention span** Some people say they feel like their memory isn't as good as it used to be, or they have trouble paying attention.

**Sensitivities** The body may overreact to food, medication or changes in the environment. Sensitivities can increase in number and become more intense over time.

**Temporomandibular joint (TMJ) disorder** TMJ disorder involves pain in the jaw joint

## DO YOU HAVE CHRONIC WIDESPREAD PAIN?

If you've had pain in several different areas or all over for at least three months in a row, you may be experiencing chronic widespread pain due to central sensitization. Before making a diagnosis, your doctor will likely try to rule out other causes.

Your doctor may check to see if you have pain in your joints or in the soft tissues of your body. You may be asked to show where you feel pain and how long you've been feeling it. You may have a blood test and other tests that check your muscle strength and tone, reflexes, and coordination. Your doctor may also want to know if you're having other symptoms that could be causing your pain, such as fatigue or sleeplessness.

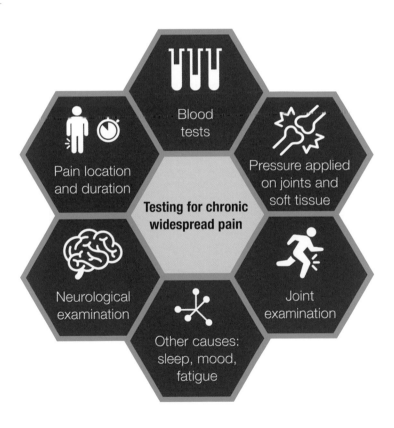

and the muscles that control your jaw. No injury can explain the pain.

**Irritable bowel syndrome** This condition affects the large intestine and often causes cramping, belly pain, bloating, gas, diarrhea and constipation.

**Interstitial cystitis** Pain and pressure in the bladder, pelvic pain, and the frequent urge to void are all symptoms of this disorder. It's linked to central sensitization when there's no tissue damage or infection to explain the symptoms.

**Chronic pelvic pain** This is also known as pain below the belly button. In women, it can happen with menstrual problems, so a doctor will usually rule out other causes of the pain first.

**Restless legs syndrome** Symptoms of this disorder can be mild or severe and tend to get worse at night. This disorder can lead to poor sleep and feeling tired during the day.

**Postural orthostatic tachycardia syndrome (POTS)** POTS is a condition that causes lightheadedness, fainting and a rapid increase in heart rate. This happens when a very low amount of blood goes to the heart after someone stands up after lying down. Symptoms are relieved by lying down.

**Fibromyalgia** This widespread pain disorder is commonly linked to central sensitization. Fibromyalgia affects the way the brain processes pain signals, causing even the slightest pain to hurt more. Aside from pain, fibromyalgia can cause fatigue and issues with sleep, memory and mood. Learn more about fibromyalgia below.

**Depression and anxiety** Depression and anxiety can lead to and be symptoms of central sensitization.

## FIBROMYALGIA: EXAMPLE OF CENTRAL PAIN

According to some estimates, nearly 1 in 5 people has a chronic widespread pain disorder, the most common of which is fibromyalgia. As you learned earlier in this chapter, fibromyalgia is a common syndrome linked to central sensitization.

As with other syndromes thought to be caused by central sensitization, pain isn't the only symptom of fibromyalgia. It also causes fatigue and issues with sleep and mood. Although there's no one way to describe what fibromyalgia feels like, some say they hurt all over, while others say they feel as if they always have the flu.

Fibromyalgia affects between 6 million and 12 million people in the United States. Between 80% and 90% are women. Researchers have learned that several factors may lead to fibromyalgia:

- Whiplash and other forms of physical trauma
- Sleep disorders

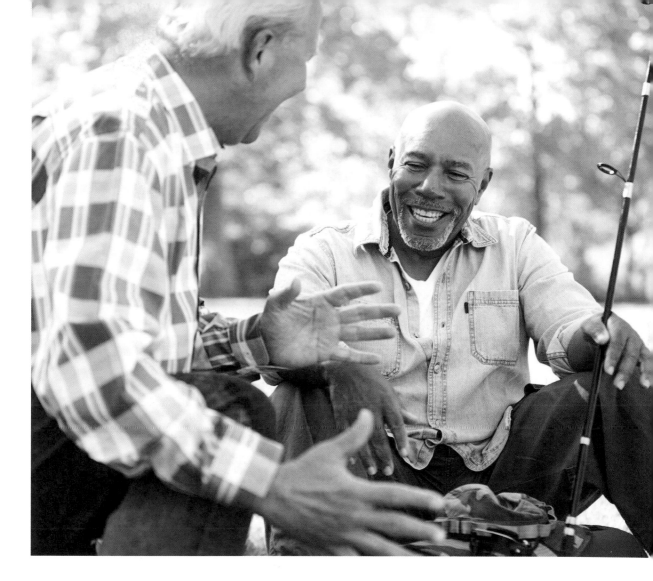

- Mood disorders
- Emotional trauma

## Signs and symptoms

The main symptom of fibromyalgia is chronic, widespread pain that persists for at least three months.

The pain may be a deep ache, a tingling sensation or soreness. It may vary depending on the time of day, your activity level, the weather, lack of sleep, and stress or anxiety. Most people feel some degree of muscle pain all the time. And the pain may move around all over the body.

Aside from pain, other signs and symptoms of fibromyalgia often include:

- Fatigue
- Stiffness

## FIBROMYALGIA VS. ARTHRITIS

Fibromyalgia has been confused with and linked to arthritis for many years. At one time, fibromyalgia was placed in the same category as rheumatoid arthritis. It was labeled as an autoimmune disorder. Although fibromyalgia and arthritis share pain as a symptom, they're two different disorders. Fibromyalgia differs from arthritis in that its pain isn't caused by swelling or damage to the joints. Instead, pain is largely due to the increased sensitivity of pain sensors, and it may hurt nearly anywhere. And unlike arthritis, fibromyalgia doesn't cause inflammation, just pain. It's not like tendinitis or bursitis.

However, some research shows that disorders such as rheumatoid arthritis may lead to fibromyalgia. Research also shows a possible link between the brain activity involved in pain processing in fibromyalgia and in osteoarthritis.

Even with these possible connections, it's important to keep in mind that fibromyalgia and arthritis are separate conditions with different causes. They're also managed differently. If you have symptoms that lead you to suspect that you have either condition, it's best to talk with your doctor.

- Sleep problems, such as trouble falling asleep, waking up during the night, or waking up unrefreshed or exhausted
- Pain in the jaw or face
- Digestive problems, including belly pain, bloating, constipation or diarrhea
- Numbness or tingling in the hands and feet
- Depression, anxiety or mood changes
- Sensitivity to weather and temperature changes
- Sensitivity to odors, noises, bright lights and touch

- Irritable bowel syndrome
- Headaches
- Not being able to think clearly
- Problems with attention and thinking quickly
- Pelvic pain and pressure
- Feeling the need to empty the bladder often or urgently
- Sensitivity to foods and medications

These signs and symptoms likely look familiar to you because they're all symptoms of central sensitization.

## Diagnosis and treatment

There's no standard lab test to show if someone has fibromyalgia. Instead, doctors will generally ask about your medical history, medications you take, and the symptoms you're having, what they're like and how long you've had them. You'll also likely have tests to rule out other causes for your symptoms.

Doctors used to look for tender points to tell if someone had fibromyalgia. Tender points are areas of the body that hurt or are sensitive to the touch when they're pressed. Although tender points are no longer part of today's fibromyalgia guidelines, some doctors still look for them in people who may have fibromyalgia. Researchers have found, though, that people with fibromyalgia don't always have tender points. Likewise, having tender points doesn't always mean that someone has fibromyalgia.

Instead of relying on tender points, today's fibromyalgia guidelines focus on a certain level of pain and other symptoms that have affected four out of five main parts of the body for at least three months.

Although fibromyalgia is chronic, it isn't life-threatening and doesn't get worse over time. It doesn't damage the body like arthritis can. With treatment, you can manage its symptoms.

While certain medications are approved by the U.S. Food and Drug Administration to treat symptoms of fibromyalgia, no one medication can relieve every symptom all of the time. And often, medication may not help at all or may even make you feel worse. Learn more about medications in Chapter 10.

Instead of relying on medications, doctors successfully treat fibromyalgia by focusing on overall well-being, including:

- Learning about fibromyalgia — in particular, that it is a real condition with a real cause and that it's treatable
- Getting regular physical activity that you increase little by little over time
- Pacing yourself by balancing periods of activity with periods of rest
- Moderating your activities so you're not doing too much — or doing nothing at all
- Taking steps to manage mood, including stress, anxiety and depression
- Setting a regular block of sleep time, so you're going to bed at the same time and waking up at the same time every day
- Following a healthy diet
- Reaching and maintaining a healthy weight
- Connecting with others

Special treatment programs that focus on all of these self-management steps — and more — can help. These types of programs are offered at Mayo Clinic campuses in Rochester, Minnesota, and Jacksonville, Florida.

# Evaluation for arthritis and other joint pain

Arthritis has many different signs and symptoms, causes, and outcomes. When you have a joint problem, identifying the cause and the best way to manage it may be a complex process.

Initially, your doctor will take a complete medical history and do a physical exam to sort out whether the joint problem is inflammatory or noninflammatory in nature. He or she will examine your tender joints and muscles and listen to your description of your symptoms. With a hands-on approach like this, a doctor can usually get a pretty good idea of what's going on inside your body in order to address the symptoms, make a diagnosis and decide treatment options.

Sometimes a doctor will need to run tests to confirm a diagnosis. Lab tests and imaging studies may also be needed to monitor dis-

ease progress, check medication effectiveness or determine if the drugs you're taking are causing harmful side effects. Most lab tests will require a simple blood draw. Other tests may need a sample of urine, joint fluid, or small pieces of skin or muscle tissue.

This chapter outlines the process of evaluating joint pain and the lab tests, imaging tests, procedures and specialty consultations you're likely to encounter. While lab tests and X-rays aren't needed for every form of arthritis, they are very important to confirm or rule out the presence of some diseases.

## LABORATORY TESTS

Lab tests are essential to the diagnostic and treatment process. The right tests, along with your doctor's observations and your honest feedback, can help you get the safest and most effective treatment for your disease.

Still, lab tests have their limitations. Some may show negative results even when a person has the disease being tested for (a false-negative). For example, many people with rheumatoid arthritis (RA) test negative for rheumatoid factor. Other tests may be positive in people who don't have a particular disease (a false-positive). Your doctor can talk with you about what the results of each test may mean.

## Anti-cyclic citrullinated peptide (anti-CCP) antibody

This test, like the test for rheumatoid factor (RF), checks for a particular antibody that is present in approximately 60% to 80% of people with rheumatoid arthritis. While most people with anti-CCP antibodies are also positive for rheumatoid factor, the RF antibody can occur in people with many other conditions besides rheumatoid arthritis. Thus, a positive anti-CCP antibody test is more specific to RA. The anti-CCP antibody may be present years before rheumatoid arthritis develops.

## Antinuclear antibody (ANA)

This tests detects antinuclear antibodies in your blood. A positive ANA test generally shows that your immune system is creating antibodies to attack your own tissue. ANA is commonly found in the blood of people

who have lupus, but it can also suggest the presence of polymyositis, scleroderma, Sjögren's syndrome, juvenile idiopathic arthritis or rheumatoid arthritis. It is also found in many people who are healthy, particularly people over age 65. Certain medications or infectious diseases may also lead to a positive ANA test.

When the test is negative, it helps to rule out certain connective tissue diseases. If the ANA test is positive, more-specific antibody tests may be ordered to check for underlying connective tissue disorders. The ANA test does not need to be repeated, as the result doesn't change with disease activity.

## C-reactive protein (CRP)

This test, like the sed rate (see next page), is a blood test that measures inflammation in your body. It measures a substance produced by the liver that increases with inflammation in the body. If you have an inflammatory type of arthritis, you may have this test periodically so that your doctor can monitor your inflammation levels.

## Creatinine test

This test is used to determine how well the kidneys are functioning. It measures the level of creatinine, a normal waste product of the muscles, in the blood. A high level of creatinine means that the kidneys are not working well enough to remove waste products from the body. This test is ordered to check for underlying kidney disease, which can occur with some types of arthritis. The test may also be used to monitor kidney function when people are on certain medications that can be toxic to the kidneys.

## Erythrocyte sedimentation rate (ESR)

This test is often called the "sed rate." It measures how fast red blood cells (erythrocytes) fall and settle, like sediment, in the bottom of a glass test tube over the course of an hour. Inflammation can cause the cells to clump together, and these dense clumps fall faster than other cells. So the higher the sed rate, the greater the amount of inflammation. Many different conditions can cause an elevated ESR, including infection, inflammation and cancer, as well as increasing age and pregnancy.

## Hematocrit (HCT) and hemoglobin (Hgb)

These tests measure the number and quality of your red blood cells. A low count of red blood cells (anemia) may suggest that your medications are causing gastrointestinal bleeding. Alternatively, an underlying disease may be the cause of the anemia.

## Human leukocyte antigen (HLA) typing

This test detects the presence of certain genes (genetic markers) in the blood. The genetic marker HLA-B27 is often present in people with ankylosing spondylitis or

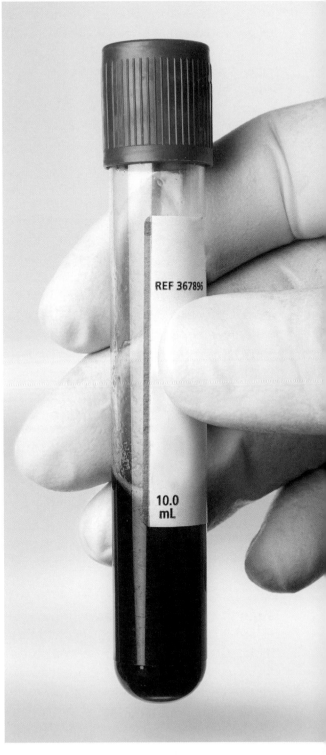

other spondyloarthropathies. About 6% of the general population has the HLA-B27 genetic marker, so having the gene doesn't mean someone has or will have one of the associated types of arthritis.

## Liver enzyme tests

These tests measure levels of liver enzymes in the blood, such as serum glutamic-oxaloacetic transaminase (SGOT), serum glutamic-pyruvic transaminase (SGPT) and alkaline phosphatase. They can help doctors determine if certain medications have caused damage to the liver. Liver enzymes can be elevated due to underlying liver disease or from medications that are toxic to the liver.

## Lyme serology

This test detects an immune response caused by the bacteria that cause Lyme disease. By confirming this immune response, the test can be used to diagnose Lyme disease, which can cause fatigue, stiffness and joint pain.

## Muscle enzyme tests

When muscles are damaged by inflammation in some rheumatic diseases, the muscles release enzymes, such as creatine phosphokinase (CPK) and aldolase. Blood tests can detect these enzymes and measure the amount of muscle damage. They can also see how well medication has reduced the inflammation that caused the muscle damage.

## Platelet count

Platelets are a substance in blood that helps the blood to clot. A low number of platelets is a concern because bleeding may be harder to stop. Medications, infections and certain diseases may lower the platelet count.

## Rheumatoid factor (RF)

This test measures the level of an antibody (rheumatoid factor) that can attack healthy tissue in your body. Rheumatoid factor acts against the blood component gamma globulin, mistaking it for a foreign invader. This test is often positive in people with rheumatoid arthritis. However, it can be seen in healthy people as well as those with other conditions, such as chronic infections, cancer or other inflammatory disorders. Because of this, your doctor may consider this test along with other test results in making a diagnosis.

In the early stages of rheumatoid arthritis, as few as 1 in 4 people tests positive for RF. Some people with rheumatoid arthritis have a negative RF throughout the course of the disease. In this case, the condition is called seronegative rheumatoid arthritis.

## Uric acid

Most people with gout will have an elevated uric acid level. Gout is a condition that occurs when excess uric acid crystallizes and forms deposits in the joints and other

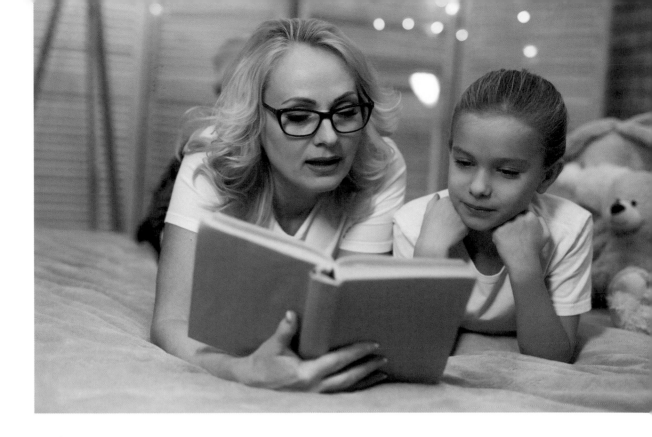

tissues, causing inflammation and severe pain. However, the uric acid level may be normal in 25% or more of people with gout. In addition, having an elevated uric acid level doesn't mean you have gout, as many people have elevated uric acid levels without any joint complaints. When gout is diagnosed, the treatment goal is to reduce the uric acid level to less than 6.0 milligrams per deciliter (mg/dL). Medications are often needed to reduce the uric acid level.

### White blood cell count

White blood cells help fight infection. A blood test showing a low number of white blood cells suggests that your body will have a harder time fighting an infection. You may have a low white blood cell count because of certain medications or an underlying disease.

## PROCEDURES

In addition to various tests, your doctor may request certain procedures to evaluate your joint symptoms. Some of the more common procedures are outlined here.

### Electromyography (EMG)

Electromyography measures the electrical activity of muscle fibers to detect the cause of nerve or muscle problems. This diagnostic procedure uses a needle and electrode stickers to measure activity within a muscle as well as signals traveling between two or more points. It may be ordered for further evaluation of people with nerve or muscle complaints such as numbness, tingling, weakness, or pain radiating down an arm or a leg.

### Joint fluid tests

If you have a swollen joint and the cause is unknown, withdrawing (aspirating) the fluid from the joint to have it analyzed in a lab may be helpful. This procedure is especially important if your doctor thinks the joint may be infected.

The doctor inserts a needle into a joint space and removes fluid into a syringe. The synovial fluid can be examined under a polarizing microscope to look for uric acid crystals, seen in gout, and calcium pyrophosphate crystals, seen in pseudogout. The fluid also can be sent to a lab to identify an infection. And the number of white blood cells in the synovial fluid sample helps your doctor determine whether the fluid is inflammatory or noninflammatory.

### Muscle biopsy

In some people, joint and muscle symptoms may include weakness and elevated muscle enzymes (CPK or aldolase). A muscle biopsy may be necessary to confirm the type of muscle disease. A surgeon can use a needle or make a small cut to take a sample of the muscle. The tissue can then be examined in a lab for signs of damage to the muscle fibers. Findings can confirm a diagnosis of muscle disease (polymyositis), inflammation of the blood vessel (vasculitis) or other conditions.

## Skin biopsy

If you're experiencing joint pain along with a rash, a skin biopsy may be ordered. A small sample of skin is taken and examined under a microscope. This can help doctors diagnose forms of arthritis that involve the skin, such as lupus, vasculitis and psoriatic arthritis.

## IMAGING (RADIOGRAPHIC) STUDIES

Often, imaging tests may be helpful in evaluating musculoskeletal complaints. Different imaging technologies create pictures in various ways, showing bones, joints and soft tissue with different levels of detail. Each technique can be useful in certain cases. For example, a simple X-ray may be all that's needed to confirm a diagnosis of osteoarthritis, while an MRI may be the best option in diagnosing a problem with a tendon or ligament.

## Arthrography

This X-ray procedure uses a dye that stands out against radiation (radiopaque dye). The dye is injected into a joint space before the X-ray is taken so that it will outline structures such as ligaments inside the joint. Arthrography can be used to view a torn ligament or fragmented cartilage in the joint, which would otherwise not show on a plain X-ray. However, magnetic resonance imaging (MRI) is now generally used in place of arthrography.

## Bone mineral density (BMD)

The most accurate way to evaluate bone density is with a bone mineral density test (dual energy X-ray absorptiometry). This test is needed when screening for or diagnosing osteoporosis or osteopenia, a less severe condition of low bone mass. A BMD test is also used to predict a person's risk of fracture, or to monitor the improvement during treatment for osteoporosis.

This test is quick and painless and involves very little radiation. X-rays of the lower spine and hip are used to measure how many grams of calcium and other bone minerals are packed into a segment of bone. Measurements of bone density at these sites are typically very accurate.

## Bone scan

Bone scanning is a type of nuclear imaging test that is highly sensitive to certain changes in bone. For the scan, a small amount of a radioactive substance is injected into a vein in your arm and is absorbed by any healing bone. It is then detected by a bone-scanning device, which creates an image of the bone that can be viewed on a computer screen.

A bone scan can be used to diagnose a fracture, particularly if a suspected fracture doesn't show on other tests, such as plain X-rays and CT or MRI. It may also be helpful to rule out a bone infection or a tumor that has spread from a cancer in another part of the body. However, while a bone scan can help reveal a problem in the bone, it may not show whether the problem is a fracture, tumor or infection.

## Computerized tomography (CT) and dual energy CT

Standard computerized tomography (CT) scanners use X-rays to take pictures of the body in cross-sectional "slices." This technology is best for imaging bone. Dual energy CT is a newer technology that combines the normal X-ray and also a second, less powerful X-ray to make the images. This helps show a wider range of materials on the image, such as calcium deposits appearing differently from bone. It gives advantages over standard CT for a wide range of tests and procedures. Dual energy CT can be helpful in diagnosing gout and assessing the amount of gout (uric acid crystals) present, especially when a joint aspiration can't be done.

A CT scan, like a conventional X-ray, exposes people to ionizing radiation. This form of radiation can potentially increase the risk of cancer or affect tissue in other ways. However, the risks with a CT scan are generally very low and usually far outweighed by the benefits of the test. Your doctor can talk with you about the risks of CT or other medical imaging.

## Magnetic resonance imaging (MRI)

Magnetic resonance imaging (MRI) creates highly detailed pictures and may be done to determine the extent and exact location of damage in the body. While CT scans use X-rays to create a "slice" image, an MRI uses a magnetic field and radio waves to take many high-resolution slices. It can combine them to create a 3D picture.

Like CT, MRI can be used to detect fractures that aren't visible on plain X-rays. MRI is especially valuable for imaging muscles, ligaments and tendons. MRI may be used if the cause of pain is thought to be a soft tissue problem — for example, rupture of a major ligament or tendon or damage to structures inside the knee joint. MRI can be more helpful than CT in detecting some abnormalities, such as small fractures or inflammation of the hip and pelvis.

MRI is more expensive than CT and takes more time — from 15 minutes to an hour or more. Some people may feel claustrophobic inside the MRI unit, which is typically a large tube open on both ends (see next page). An open-sided MRI can be used, but the image may not be as clear.

## X-rays

Plain (conventional) X-rays are typically the first imaging studies done when sorting out a musculoskeletal disorder. They are usually ordered to help evaluate painful, deformed or suspected abnormal areas of bone. Your doctor may diagnose fractures, tumors, injuries, infections and deformities from X-ray images.

X-rays can show changes that confirm a certain kind of arthritis. For example, in rheumatoid arthritis or other inflammatory arthritis, an X-ray will show that bone has worn away (eroded) in one or more joints. In osteoarthritis or other noninflammatory conditions, X-rays may show the joint space narrowing and bone spurs developing.

X-rays are most valuable for detecting breaks or changes in bone. Plain X-rays do not show soft tissues such as muscles, bursae, ligaments, tendons or nerves. More-specific imaging tests such as MRI or ultrasound may be needed to see those tissues.

## Ultrasonography

In recent years, ultrasound is being used more frequently to identify inflammation in and around joints and tears or inflammation of tendons. Ultrasonography is also used as a guide when a needle is inserted into a joint, for example, to inject medication or remove joint fluid. As an alternative to CT and MRI, ultrasound is less expensive. And unlike CT, it involves no exposure to radiation.

However, ultrasonography is not always available, and it requires highly skilled medical professionals to perform the scan and interpret it.

## SPECIALTY EVALUATIONS

If you see your medical provider for joint pain, the evaluation process is often complex. Depending on your symptoms, you may need to see doctors in several different subspecialty groups. Your doctor may refer you to the following medical specialties to help diagnose and manage your condition.

### Cardiology

A cardiologist specializes in heart conditions and often sees people with symptoms including shortness of breath, chest pain or dizzy spells. Sometimes a person without symptoms of heart trouble is referred to a cardiologist after a heart murmur is heard during a physical exam.

Your doctor may recommend that you see a cardiologist if you have inflammatory arthritis. The inflammation of this type of arthritis can affect the blood vessels, putting you at higher risk of heart disease.

## Dermatology

A dermatologist evaluates abnormalities of the skin, hair, nails and mucous membranes. You may need to see a dermatologist if you have certain joint conditions that occur with a rash. Sometimes, a dermatologist may need to take a sample of the rash for testing (a biopsy).

## Endocrinology

An endocrinologist is a clinician specially trained in conditions affecting the glands, including the pituitary, thyroid, adrenals, ovaries, testes and pancreas. If you have an inflammatory arthritis, you may need treatment with the corticosteroid prednisone, which can lead to diabetes and low bone mass (osteoporosis). You may need to see an endocrinologist to monitor those conditions. Rarely, the thyroid gland, adrenal glands and other glands can be involved with inflammatory conditions.

## Gastroenterology

A gastroenterologist is a physician with dedicated training in conditions of the gastrointestinal system — the esophagus, stomach, small intestine, colon, rectum, gallbladder and liver. People with inflammatory bowel disease (Crohn's disease and ulcerative colitis) may have an associated inflammatory arthritis, needing care for both conditions. Taking nonsteroidal anti-inflammatory drugs (NSAIDs) for arthritis pain also may cause esophagus or stomach issues. A gastroenterologist can help manage these side effects.

## Hematology

A hematologist is a specialist in blood disorders. A low red blood cell count (anemia), platelet disorders and white blood cell disorders are occasionally seen in people with arthritis as a result of the disease or as side effects of medications.

## Infectious disease

An infectious disease specialist focuses on diagnosing and managing infections. People with arthritis may see this type of specialist if they take immunosuppressive medications, which weaken the immune system and raise the risk of infection. Steroids, disease-modifying antirheumatic drugs (DMARDs), and biologics all weaken the immune system.

## Nephrology

A nephrologist evaluates and treats kidney disease. Various kidney diseases can be seen in people with certain types of arthritis. Many arthritis medications can affect the kidneys as well.

## Neurology

A neurologist specializes in nervous system disorders. These include problems in the brain and spinal cord (central nervous system) and peripheral nervous system. Several types of arthritis may affect the nerves. Imaging studies of the brain or spinal canal may be necessary. Nerve tests (electromyography) may be ordered for people who have symptoms of a nerve being pinched. Compression of a nerve can occur due to joint swelling or bone spurs from arthritis.

## Neurosurgery

A neurosurgeon specializes in the diagnosis and surgical treatment of nervous system disorders. If you have symptoms of a compressed nerve in your neck (cervical spine) or low back (lumbar spine) that don't respond to conservative therapy, you may need a neurosurgery consultation to discuss surgery as a treatment option.

## Ophthalmology

An ophthalmologist specializes in eye and vision abnormalities. People with inflammatory arthritis are at higher risk of inflammation of their eyes. Certain medications such as hydroxychloroquine (Plaquenil) also may affect the eyes, so if these medications are part of your treatment, you'll need regular eye examinations.

## Orthopedics

Orthopedic surgeons diagnose and manage musculoskeletal conditions. In most cases,

these problems are treated first with nonsurgical options such as medications, physical therapy and exercise. But if these treatments can't resolve the problem, surgery may be necessary. An orthopedic surgeon can review surgical treatment options with you.

## Physiatry (physical medicine and rehabilitation)

Physiatrists diagnose and treat a wide variety of medical conditions affecting the brain, spinal cord, nerves, bones, joints, ligaments, muscles and tendons. Also known as physical medicine and rehabilitation (PM&R), this specialty focuses on helping people to regain function.

People with arthritis may benefit from the expertise of PM&R specialists in guiding their rehabilitation to regain strength or movement needed for everyday activities. Physical and occupational therapy is an important treatment regimen for maintaining function in arthritic conditions.

## Psychiatry

A psychiatrist focuses on the diagnosis, treatment and prevention of mental, emotional and behavioral disorders. Many people with arthritis also have anxiety and depression symptoms due to their pain and decline in health, as well as related sources of stress such as financial costs. A psychiatrist can help manage these symptoms to improve overall health.

## Pulmonary medicine

A pulmonologist evaluates diseases of the lungs. Many forms of inflammatory arthritis can affect the lungs. Problems may include scarring or lumps (nodules) on the lung tissue, inflammation and buildup of fluid or mucus. In addition, some medications used to treat inflammatory arthritis, such as methotrexate, can affect the lungs. A pulmonologist may help diagnose issues with the lungs and guide treatment.

## Rheumatology

A rheumatologist specializes in the diagnosis and treatment of musculoskeletal diseases and systemic autoimmune conditions. Together these are known as rheumatic diseases. Rheumatic disease can affect the joints, muscles and bones, leading to pain, swelling and stiffness. Over time rheumatic diseases can cause abnormally shaped bones or joints. If you have arthritis, a rheumatologist is often the main doctor you'll see for your related symptoms after being referred by your primary care provider. The rheumatologist will coordinate care with other specialists if needed.

**PART 2**

# Treating arthritis

# Medications for arthritis

Just as there's a wide range of symptoms among people with different kinds of arthritis, a broad array of medications is available to help control these symptoms. It's important that you work with your doctor to find the best drug treatments for you.

Medications can help relieve pain, make joint movement easier and prevent further damage from inflammation. Some medications can be purchased over-the-counter at convenience stores, while others are powerful drugs that can only be obtained with a doctor's prescription. Some medications can be used to treat several kinds of arthritis, while others are used for a single type of arthritis.

Medications may help you feel better and allow you to lead a more active life. Like all drugs, though, arthritis medications can cause side effects, including dry mouth and upset stomach as well as an increased risk of infection, heart attack or stroke. The benefits of a particular drug must be weighed against its side effects. You and your doctor can discuss these risks in relation to your needs and circumstances.

For most people with arthritis, medications play a central role in their treatment plans, which may also include other therapies and lifestyle changes. In the past, rheumatoid arthritis and other forms of the disease were considered disabling and difficult to manage. But newer medications and combinations of treatments have greatly improved the overall well-being and outlook for many people with joint pain.

Because there are so many different types of medications to treat arthritis, and there may be different brand names of each, this chapter will refer to medications by their generic names for ease of reading. For the list of brand names, information on how a drug is given, and a summary of the benefits and risks for each, see the medication guide on page 147.

## DIFFERENT TREATMENT STRATEGIES

The treatment plan you and your doctor decide on will depend largely on the type of arthritis you have and the severity of your symptoms. Other important factors include your level of pain, how much your symptoms affect your daily life, and your personal preferences about medications and other therapies.

### Treating osteoarthritis and other noninflammatory arthritis

The main treatment goal for osteoarthritis or other noninflammatory arthritis is to manage the pain and inflammation and improve joint function.

Part of your treatment plan will include a healthy balance of exercise and rest. Exercise helps strengthen your joints and the muscles that support them, while rest can prevent pain and inflammation from getting worse.

If you're overweight, your doctor may also recommend weight loss to reduce stress on your joints.

Your treatment plan may include oral medications, particularly for pain relief. For mild to moderate pain, the pain reliever acetaminophen is often a first choice. Topical pain relievers in the form of creams, gels and ointments also can be rubbed onto painful joints.

For moderate to severe pain, or if you have signs of inflammation, you might take one of many medications that fall under the category of nonsteroidal anti-inflammatory drugs (NSAIDs).

If your joints are still painful in spite of using pain relievers, you may benefit from injections of medication directly into the joints. These medications may include corticosteroids or hyaluronic acid derivatives, which contain a substance similar to natural joint fluid. (For more on injections, see Chapter 14).

For pain that isn't controlled by other therapies, your doctor may recommend a short-term course of opioid medications. These are potent pain relievers. Their big drawback, as you may know from headlines in recent years, is that they can lead to dependency if used regularly over long periods of time. They can also make you drowsy.

If your symptoms are persistently severe, your doctor may refer you to an orthopedic surgeon to consult on surgeries that might help. (For more on surgical options, see Chapter 11.) Unfortunately, there is not a medication to stop the progression of osteoarthritis.

## Treating rheumatoid arthritis and other inflammatory arthritis

Treatment for rheumatoid arthritis has changed dramatically over the last several decades. The same is true for other inflammatory arthropathies, such as psoriatic arthritis and spondyloarthritis. Doctors used to start out with mild pain relievers and then progress to more powerful drugs if symptoms worsened — similar to the way osteoarthritis is treated. However, treatment for these types of arthritis is now more aggressive upfront.

Studies demonstrate that damage can occur in a joint within the first year or two of disease onset. Fortunately, there are now multiple treatment options to lessen or halt the inflammation that causes joint damage, and doctors will use the most effective medications available right away. Quick action stalls the inflammatory process in the early stages of the disease before serious damage to the joint can occur. This approach helps to prevent potentially lifelong symptoms or make them less severe.

***NSAIDs and steroids*** Doctors typically use NSAIDs to help reduce day-to-day pain in people with these conditions. They may also consider steroids, especially if someone has significant disability from the disease. Sometimes a steroid injection into the joint may offer significant benefit. Or your doctor may prescribe a low dose of an oral steroid as a "bridging therapy." The aim is to quickly reduce inflammation until the right medication, or combination of medications, is found to control the inflammation long term.

***Disease-modifying antirheumatic drugs (DMARDs)*** These synthetically produced drugs are the mainstay treatment for inflammatory arthritis. They work by slowing down or suppressing your immune system, which has been hijacked by the disease to increase inflammation in your joints. Early intervention with DMARDs can also improve your quality of life and life expectancy with the disease.

Many different DMARDs are available. Conventional DMARDs such as hydroxychloroquine, methotrexate, leflunomide or sulfasalazine are typically prescribed first. Each of these medications works differently and has its own unique set of side effects. The downside to all DMARDs is that they take time to work — usually three to six months. So a low dose of a steroid may be needed until the DMARD becomes effective.

Shots of a gold solution used to be prescribed but are no longer used, as DMARDs work better, faster and with fewer side effects. Other medications, such as the antibiotic minocycline, also may help to treat rheumatoid arthritis. Minocycline acts as an adjunct, or booster, to the DMARD, but it isn't effective enough to use by itself.

Studies have shown that, in certain situations, a combination of disease-modifying drugs (combination therapy) provides more benefits than taking just one — with no added side effects.

While you're taking these drugs, your doctor will monitor you for any signs of infection or disruption of organ function. You may have basic blood and urine tests. This is because DMARDs can inhibit your immune system and interfere with certain organs, such as your liver, lungs or kidneys.

***Biologics*** If a DMARD or combination of DMARDs doesn't effectively treat your symptoms, your doctor may recommend adding or switching to a newer category of medications called biologic DMARDs. They are also referred to as biologic agents or simply biologics. Like conventional DMARDs, they can relieve pain and stiffness and protect joints from damage by slowing or halting the inflammatory process. They differ from conventional DMARDs in that they're derived from living sources, such as cell cultures, while conventional DMARDs are made by way of a chemical process.

Biologic DMARDs are designed to work against specific targets. Some interfere with the action of immune substances called cytokines. Cytokines mobilize immune cells that fight off an infection or another perceived threat. With an autoimmune disease such as rheumatoid arthritis, where healthy cells are wrongly seen as threatening, cytokines contribute to the inflammatory reaction. (See diagram on page 143.) Biologics can stop or slow this response.

The largest group of biologics works against a cytokine called tumor necrosis factor-alpha (TNF-alpha). Others target a type of cytokine called an interleukin (IL). Specific targets include IL-1, IL-6, IL-17, IL-12/IL-23, and IL-23.

Some biologics disrupt the activation of certain T cells. These cells coordinate your body's immune response to invaders. Still other biologic medications work to deplete B cells, which produce antibodies that perpetuate the immune reaction. Antibodies are helpful when you're fighting an infection, but they're part of the problem in an autoimmune reaction.

The newest class of medications used for inflammatory arthritis is targeted DMARDs. These drugs interfere with specific signaling pathways, such as the Janus kinase pathway, inside immune cells.

Biologics are often used along with conventional DMARDs such as methotrexate. Some biologic medications are approved for the treatment of other inflammatory diseases, such as psoriatic arthritis, ankylosing spondylitis and inflammatory bowel disease. Biologics are either injected under the skin (subcutaneously), which can be done at home, or into a vein (intravenously), which is usu-

ally done at a doctor's office. The kinase inhibitors are small molecules and therefore can be taken by mouth (orally).

Biologics can weaken your body's ability to fight infection, so your doctor will want to make sure you don't already have an underlying infection, such as tuberculosis or pneumonia. Having another illness can put you at an increased risk of infection too. Existing infections should be treated before you receive a DMARD or biologic agent, since these medications can make the infection worse. It's also very important that you're up to date with vaccinations.

Because of the increased risk of serious infection, experts generally recommend against combining two or more biologic DMARDs.

## TNF, AN EXAMPLE OF CYTOKINES IN THE IMMUNE RESPONSE

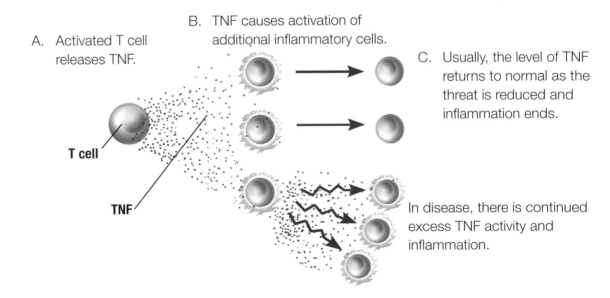

A. Activated T cell releases TNF.

B. TNF causes activation of additional inflammatory cells.

C. Usually, the level of TNF returns to normal as the threat is reduced and inflammation ends.

T cell

TNF

In disease, there is continued excess TNF activity and inflammation.

For some biologic medications, biosimilars can be substituted. A biosimilar is a biologic drug that is almost an identical copy of an original drug that is manufactured by a different company. Biosimilars can be produced when the original product's patent expires. In the United States, they still must be officially approved by the Food and Drug Administration (FDA).

If you've had an inflammatory arthritis for a long time, your doctor may focus less on disrupting the inflammatory process, which is likely to be less active at this point, and more on relieving pain and other symptoms.

## Treating gout

Gout is treated differently depending on where it is in its progression — during an attack of acute gout or in between attacks to prevent future attacks. When someone develops acute gout, one or more joints will have swelling, redness and warmth. A joint may need to be drained (aspirated) to confirm gouty crystals in the joint fluid.

Confirming these crystals is an important part of distinguishing gout from infections and other conditions.

An acute attack of gout can be treated with medications that reduce inflammation. Your doctor might prescribe NSAIDs unless you have a history of stomach issues, bleeding, kidney disease, using a blood thinner or other conditions. Steroids also can help and can be taken either by mouth or through a joint injection. Colchicine is another option. This drug can stop the inflammation from gout and help prevent attacks. However, it may cause nausea and diarrhea. Anakinra, an IL-1 inhibitor, may be used if you can't receive other treatments because of certain medical conditions or if other treatments haven't helped. It is typically reserved for people who are hospitalized with multiple conditions. Icing the area over the inflamed joint can be helpful too.

If you've been diagnosed with gout and you have more than two attacks a year, you'll need long-term treatment to lower the uric acid load in the body. The goal is to bring your uric acid level below 6.0 milligrams per deciliter (mg/dL), or in some severe cases, less than 5 mg/dL. Several medications may be used. For people who develop hard masses of uric acid crystals (tophi) the intravenous drug pegloticase may be helpful.

When you start a urate-lowering drug, there's a higher risk of a gout flare until the uric acid level stabilizes. Therefore, your doctor will likely place you on another medication such as an NSAID, low-dose steroid or colchicine for three to six months to prevent an attack.

The following different types of medications may be used to treat acute gout symptoms:

| Generic | Brand |
|---------|-------|
| NSAIDs: ibuprofen, naproxen, celecoxib, others | (multiple) |
| Steroids: prednisone, others | (multiple) |
| Colchicine | Colcrys, Gloperba, others |
| Anakinra | Kineret |

Some medications may reduce your risk of gout by limiting the amount of uric acid your body makes. This group, called xanthine oxidase inhibitors (XOIs), includes the drugs allopurinol and febuxostat.

| Generic | Brand |
|---------|-------|
| Allopurinol | Zyloprim |
| Febuxostat | Uloric |

Uricosuric and uricase medications also work in different ways to lower the amount of uric acid in the body. They help your body to remove more uric acid. These drugs include probenecid and pegloticase.

| Generic | Brand |
|---------|-------|
| Probenecid | (generic) |
| Pegloticase | Krystexxa |

Like all medications, each of these carries risks of certain complications. Before starting any of these drugs, it's best to talk with your doctor to make sure you understand the risks and any precautions you should take.

## Treating fibromyalgia

Fibromyalgia is a complex pain disorder, which is discussed more in Chapter 8. Typically, treatment of fibromyalgia includes improving sleep, reducing stress, and developing a slow and progressive exercise program. These steps can ease the pain and other symptoms.

Medications can be a helpful part of treatment. Various medications are used to help with sleep, stress and pain in people with fibromyalgia. Currently only three drugs are FDA approved for use in fibromyalgia. These include two antidepressants (duloxetine and milnacipran) and an anti-seizure drug (pregabalin).

However, depending on your symptoms and circumstances, your doctor might recommend off-label medications. These are drugs that haven't been approved by the FDA to treat fibromyalgia specifically, but may help relieve your symptoms. For instance, tricyclic antidepressants are frequently used to improve pain, fatigue and deep sleep.

The drugs currently approved by the FDA for treating fibromyalgia include:

| Generic | Brand |
| --- | --- |
| Duloxetine | Cymbalta |
| Milnacipran | Savella |
| Pregabalin | Lyrica |

These different types of medications work in different ways in the body, and each drug has its own risks and precautions. As always, talk with your doctor about your treatment options, the effects they may have and your needs. Making informed treatment decisions can help you to best manage your fibromyalgia.

## ARTHRITIS MEDICATION GUIDE

The following pages give more information about many of the most common medications used in treating arthritis. Still more may be available to you, as new research and drug innovation continue to change the landscape. If you have questions about medications or treatment, make sure to discuss them with your doctor.

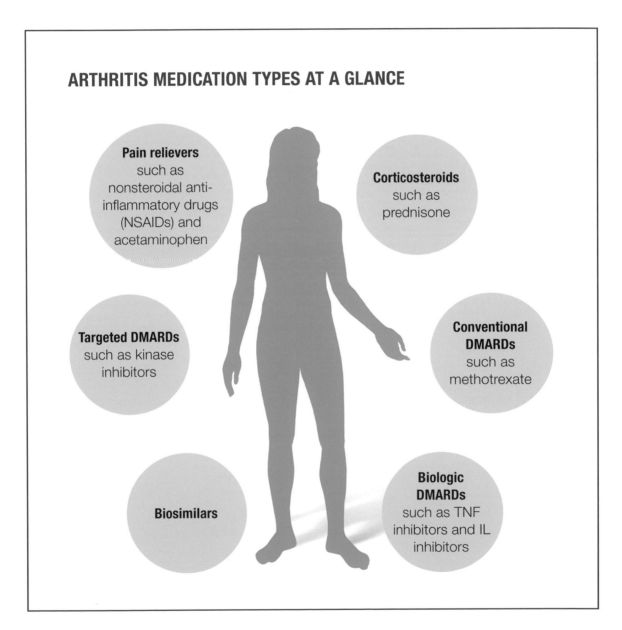

### ARTHRITIS MEDICATION TYPES AT A GLANCE

**Pain relievers** such as nonsteroidal anti-inflammatory drugs (NSAIDs) and acetaminophen

**Corticosteroids** such as prednisone

**Targeted DMARDs** such as kinase inhibitors

**Conventional DMARDs** such as methotrexate

**Biosimilars**

**Biologic DMARDs** such as TNF inhibitors and IL inhibitors

## PAIN RELIEVERS

When arthritis makes your joints hurt, you naturally want quick relief. A number of different types of pain relievers can help. Some are available over-the-counter (OTC), while others will need to be prescribed by your doctor.

A note of caution: These drugs can have serious side effects. With some, the risks include the potential for you to become dependent on or addicted to them.

Your body can also develop a tolerance to some pain relievers. So the longer you take them, the higher the dose you'll need to get the same relief.

In addition, by masking pain, these drugs may trick you into thinking that you can be more active than you should be, increasing the risk of additional damage or injury. Talk with your doctor about the risks of any medications you take.

### NSAIDs and aspirin

The medications in this group are effective pain relievers that also help ease stiffness and swelling caused by inflammation. Despite minor differences among different types of these drugs, they all work against inflammation in a similar way. They inhibit an enzyme called cyclooxygenase (COX), which is responsible for the production of prostaglandins. Prostaglandins are hormonelike chemicals that help send pain messages to your brain and are key to the inflammation process.

A larger dose of these drugs is required to reduce inflammation than is needed to relieve pain. If you have osteoarthritis, you may be able to take a smaller dose, because inflammation typically isn't severe and the pain may come and go. With rheumatoid arthritis or another inflammatory joint disease, however, you may need a larger dose to feel relief.

Many different types of these drugs are available. This group of medications includes over-the-counter medicines such as ibuprofen (Advil, Motrin IB) and aspirin, as well as other drugs available by prescription. Every person with arthritis is different, so the best choice of medication varies. What works for you may not work for a friend or relative.

Drugs in this group can cause an upset stomach, gastrointestinal bleeding, cardiovascular problems, and liver and kidney damage. Older people are at highest risk of complications. Because of the risk of side effects, your doctor will prescribe the lowest effective dose of these medications for the shortest time needed.

A subset of NSAIDs works by inhibiting only the cyclooxygenase-2 (COX-2) enzyme. COX-2 inhibitors relieve joint pain just as well as other NSAIDs yet cause fewer ulcers and less gastrointestinal bleeding. However, these may be more expensive and may increase your cardiovascular risks.

Based on your overall health — including your gastrointestinal and heart health — your doctor can help determine which type of medication in this group might provide the most benefits for you with the least risks.

| Generic | Brand |
|---------|-------|
| Diclofenac | Voltaren, Zorvolex, others |
| Diclofenac and misoprostol | Arthrotec |
| Ibuprofen | Advil, Motrin IB, others |
| Indomethacin | Indocin, Tivorbex |
| Meloxicam | Mobic, others |
| Naproxen | Aleve, Anaprox DS, Naprosyn, others |
| Piroxicam | Feldene |
| Sulindac | (generic) |
| Celecoxib (COX-2 inhibitor) | Celebrex |
| Aspirin | (multiple) |

*How they're usually given:*
• By mouth

*Benefits:*
• Provide mild to moderate pain relief
• Ease inflammation and joint stiffness

*Risks:*
• Upset stomach, abdominal pain, nausea
• Internal bleeding
• Heartburn, stomach ulcers
• Skin reactions
• Headache, dizziness, tiredness
• Ringing in the ears and hearing loss
• Constipation or diarrhea
• Kidney problems

*Precautions:*
• Use them with caution or consider other therapies if you have ulcers, gastrointestinal bleeding, asthma or cardiovascular disease. Talk to your doctor first.
• Don't take two or more different NSAIDs at the same time.
• Talk to your doctor about NSAID use in children, including over-the-counter brands.
• Risks, especially kidney and stomach problems, are increased if you're older than age 65.
• NSAID use with blood-thinning medications increases bleeding risk.
• Before any surgery or dental work, inform the surgeon or dentist of any of these medications you take.
• Consult your doctor before giving aspirin to children or teenagers. Aspirin use in children has been linked to Reye's syndrome.

# REDUCE YOUR RISK OF STOMACH PROBLEMS FROM NSAIDS

Nonsteroidal anti-inflammatory drugs can make life easier by helping control the pain and inflammation of arthritis. Unfortunately, they can also give you an upset stomach or even an ulcer.

Gastrointestinal bleeding is a potentially serious side effect of NSAIDs. In addition to suppressing prostaglandins associated with inflammation and pain, NSAIDs decrease production of a chemical that protects your stomach lining. This allows stomach acid to erode the lining and cause bleeding and ulcers.

Because bleeding and ulcers in the stomach can occur with no warning, it's important to get regular checkups. If you're taking NSAIDs regularly, your blood counts and liver enzymes should be checked periodically. Your doctor may also suggest that you take a medication, such as a proton pump inhibitor (PPI), to decrease some of the gastrointestinal side effects. PPIs are drugs that reduce the amount of stomach acid.

If you regularly take traditional NSAIDs, here are steps that may help you minimize the risk of stomach problems:

- Take NSAIDs with food and water or milk.
- Avoid alcohol, since this increases the risk of gastric bleeding.
- Take the lowest possible dose you can to reduce symptoms.
- Take your medication later in the day if possible. If you take an NSAID once a day, doing so in the afternoon or evening may be easier on your stomach.
- Don't take more NSAIDs than are prescribed or take them more often than are prescribed.
- Don't take other NSAIDs or medications containing NSAIDs, prescription or nonprescription, at the same time.
- Talk to your doctor or pharmacist about other medications you take that may interact with NSAIDs and increase your risk of stomach problems.

## Acetaminophen

Acetaminophen is a pain reliever used to treat common headaches, muscle aches, toothaches and sore throats. It is widely available over-the-counter and is often combined with other drugs in medications to treat multiple symptoms, such as for cold or flu relief. Acetaminophen works by interfering with how the body processes pain. Because the drug has a limited effect on inflammation, it's appropriate for arthritis that causes pain but little inflammation — as is often the case in osteoarthritis — and for people who are unable to take NSAIDs.

Many people with arthritis find that acetaminophen can ease their pain as well as an NSAID can. If you have mild pain from osteoarthritis, or other types of noninflammatory pain, your doctor may recommend acetaminophen as the first choice for pain relief. It is inexpensive and usually doesn't cause side effects as long as you don't take more than the recommended dose.

High doses of acetaminophen taken over a long period of time can lead to liver problems, especially if you consume alcohol daily or take other medicines containing acetaminophen.

| Generic | Brand |
|---------|-------|
| Acetaminophen | Tylenol, others |

*How it's usually given:*
- By mouth

*Benefits:*
- First choice for mild pain relief
- Works fast

*Risks:*
- High doses can lead to liver damage, especially if the medicine is consumed with alcohol or other medications.

*Precautions:*
- Check the labels of other medications you take to see if they contain acetaminophen.

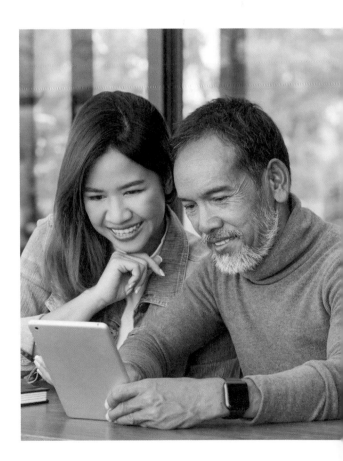

## Tramadol

If acetaminophen or an NSAID doesn't completely relieve your pain, your doctor may recommend a medication called tramadol. This drug is a less potent opioid that can be used alone or along with acetaminophen or an NSAID.

Studies show that taking tramadol can provide pain relief similar to other stronger opioids such as codeine. Tramadol may not make you as sleepy as codeine can, though it may increase the possibility of headaches.

| Generic | Brand |
|---------|-------|
| Tramadol | ConZip, Ultram |
| Tramadol with acetaminophen | Ultracet |

### How they're usually given:
- By mouth

### Benefits:
- Provide moderate to severe pain relief
- May cause less drowsiness than other opioids

### Risks:
- Drug abuse or dependency (especially when used for extended periods)
- Nausea, stomach pain
- Constipation or diarrhea
- Lightheadedness, dizziness
- Drowsiness

### Precautions:
- Avoid taking them with alcohol (including medicines containing alcohol).
- These medications can increase your risk of seizures.
- Serotonin syndrome may occur when using these medications with other medications (antidepressants, certain migraine drugs). Let your doctor know immediately if you experience agitation, hallucinations, irregular heartbeat or lack of coordination.
- Withdrawal symptoms can occur if these medications are stopped abruptly.
- Long-term use during pregnancy may result in neonatal withdrawal symptoms.
- These medications may increase suicidal thoughts.

## Opioids

Opioids are powerful pain relievers that block pain signals traveling to the brain. However, these drugs can be addictive and cause drowsiness. Because of this, they're prescribed mainly for a short duration and for intense pain. In certain cases, when other pain control methods aren't working or aren't an option, some doctors may prescribe an opioid medication to treat severe arthritis pain.

With increasing use of opioids in recent decades, cases of opioid abuse and drug dependency have become more common. If your doctor suggests an opioid as part of your treatment, make sure you understand the risks and how to take it safely.

| Generic | Brand |
|---|---|
| Codeine with acetaminophen | Tylenol No. 3, others |
| Fentanyl | Duragesic, others |
| Hydrocodone with or without acetaminophen | Norco, Vicodin, others |
| Hydromorphone | Dilaudid |
| Meperidine | Demerol |
| Morphine | (multiple) |
| Tapentadol | Nucynta |
| Oxycodone with or without acetaminophen | OxyContin, Percocet, others |

### How they're usually given:
- By mouth

### Benefits:
- Provide moderate to severe pain relief
- Work well for pain that hasn't responded to other therapies

### Risks:
- Drug abuse or dependency (especially when used for extended periods)
- Lightheadedness, dizziness
- Drowsiness
- Constipation
- Upset stomach, nausea

### Precautions:
- Breaking, chewing or crushing opioid medications that are extended release (ER), slow release (SR) or controlled release (CR) can lead to rapid and potentially fatal absorption of the drug.
- Avoid taking opioids with alcohol, including medicines containing alcohol.
- You can develop a tolerance to these medications, requiring larger doses to achieve the same amount of pain relief.
- Withdrawal symptoms can occur if these medications are stopped abruptly.
- Long-term use of opioids during pregnancy may result in neonatal withdrawal symptoms.

## Topical pain relievers

Topical pain medications are absorbed through your skin. The most common varieties are creams or gels that you rub onto the skin over your painful joints. Others come in the form of a spray or a patch that sticks to your skin. Some are available by prescription from your doctor, but others are available over-the-counter.

Because the ingredients are absorbed through the skin, topical preparations usually have fewer side effects compared with medications that are taken by mouth and absorbed through your bloodstream.

For adults over age 75 with osteoarthritis of the hands or knees, the American College of Rheumatology recommends topical NSAIDs instead of oral NSAIDs.

The active ingredients in topical pain medications may include:

**Capsaicin** Capsaicin (kap-SAY-ih-sin) creams inhibit a chemical that's important for sending pain messages. Capsaicin comes from chili peppers. For some people, the creams work well to relieve joint pain. But others dislike the burning or stinging sensation that can occur when they apply the cream. With continued use, the burning and stinging often lessens.

**Salicylates** Salicylates (suh-LIS-uh-lates) contain the pain-relieving substance found in aspirin. Although people with arthritis may use these creams, these products have not been studied specifically for their ability to relieve arthritis symptoms.

**Menthol** Menthol produces a sensation of hot or cold that may temporarily override your ability to feel arthritis pain. As with salicylate-based topicals, menthol-based preparations haven't been rigorously studied in a specific context of arthritis.

**NSAIDs** Some studies indicate that NSAID creams and gels may work as well as their oral counterparts. In the United States, the FDA has approved several versions of prescription gels and liquid drops containing the NSAID diclofenac to treat osteoarthritis in the hands, wrists, elbows, feet, ankles or knees. A topical patch containing diclofenac also is available.

**Lidocaine** In some situations, doctors may prescribe lidocaine patches for joint pain.

The patches are approved in the U.S. to treat a painful complication of shingles, but a doctor may also prescribe them for other forms of pain such as arthritis pain. This is called an off-label use. The lidocaine patches are placed on your skin over the painful joint for 12 hours at a time. The medication numbs the area.

When using topical pain relievers, be careful to wash your hands thoroughly after use, especially before you rub or touch your eyes. Don't use these pain relievers on broken or irritated skin or in combination with a heating pad, bandage, wrap or dressing.

If you're allergic to aspirin or you are taking an anticoagulant blood thinner, check with your doctor before using topical medications that contain salicylates.

| Generic | Brand |
|---|---|
| Capsaicin | Zostrix, others |
| Diclofenac (NSAID) | Voltaren gel, Pennsaid, others |
| Lidocaine | Lidoderm, Salonpas Lidocaine, others |
| Menthol | Bengay, Icy Hot, others |
| Salicylates | Aspercreme, others |

## GENERIC VS. BRAND NAME

Many drugs used to treat arthritis are available as both brand-name and generic medications. What's the difference?

A drug that's discovered or developed in a laboratory begins with a generic name selected by experts and governmental agencies. The company that developed the drug typically takes it to market with a brand name and sells it exclusively for a fixed period. When the patent rights on the drug expire, any other drug company can manufacture and sell the drug under its generic name or another brand name. In any case, the Food and Drug Administration still must approve the new versions before they can be sold.

Generic versions are available for many drugs on the market. For consumers, that's good news because generics often cost considerably less than their brand-name counterparts. Generic drugs have the same active ingredients, strength and method as the brand-name versions. They also carry the same risks and benefits.

Your doctor or pharmacist can determine whether you should use a brand-name medication or a generic version, based on your medical needs, the particular drug and its availability.

### How they're usually given:
- Topically, to your skin

### Benefits:
- Provide local pain relief

### Risks:
- Itching
- Stinging or burning sensation
- Rash

### Precautions:
- Avoid rubbing or touching your eyes after using the medication until you've thoroughly washed your hands.
- Don't rub the medication on broken or irritated skin.
- Check with your doctor before using topical medications that contain salicylates if you're allergic to aspirin or you are taking a blood thinner.
- Don't cover the medication with a bandage or wrap or use it in combination with a heating pad.

## CORTICOSTEROIDS

Corticosteroids are another group of medications used to fight inflammation caused by arthritis. Also called steroids or glucocorticoids, corticosteroids are artificial versions of a hormone called cortisol.

These drugs work by blocking your body's production of prostaglandins, hormonelike substances that cause inflammation. Corticosteroids also suppress the immune system to control inflammation.

Corticosteroids fight inflammation effectively and quickly. They ease symptoms of stiffness, pain and fatigue, and they reduce swelling, helping protect your joints and other affected areas. In the short term, corticosteroids can make you feel dramatically better.

Corticosteroids can be injected directly into a sore or inflamed joint. This allows the medication to go directly to the area needed without affecting the entire body. Relief can last for several months, and injections can be repeated in the future, although usually no more than two to four times a year.

Certain corticosteroids such as prednisone and other similar drugs can also be taken by mouth. They offer widespread relief of inflammation due to rheumatoid arthritis, usually in a matter of days.

However, taken in high doses over long periods of time, these drugs can have many side effects, including mood changes, weight gain, muscle weakness, loss of bone density, diabetes, cataracts, increased risk of infection and high blood pressure.

As a result, oral corticosteroids are generally reserved for treating acute symptoms or flare-ups. In rheumatoid arthritis, oral corticosteroids may be used to tide you over while you wait for other medications, such as a DMARD, to become fully effective. Once the DMARD kicks in, the corticosteroid can be slowly decreased and eventually discontinued.

| Generic | Brand |
|---|---|
| Betamethasone | Celestone Soluspan |
| Dexamethasone | (generic) |
| Methylpredniso-lone | Depo-Medrol, Medrol, Solu-Medrol |
| Prednisolone | Millipred, others |
| Prednisone | (generic) |
| Triamcinolone | Kenalog-10, others |

*How they're usually given:*
- By mouth, by injection into affected joint, or intravenously

*Benefits:*
- Provide fast relief for severe pain
- Ease inflammation
- Relieve flare-ups and sudden worsening of symptoms

*Risks:*
- Nausea
- Difficulty sleeping (insomnia)
- Increased appetite
- Anxiety and irritability
- Changes in mood
- Swelling of the hands, legs and feet
- Changes in vision
- Increased blood sugars
- Increased blood pressure
- Weight gain
- Osteoporosis

*Precautions:*
- Avoid live virus vaccines while taking corticosteroids.
- Corticosteroids may increase your risk of infections. Wash your hands frequently and avoid people who are ill.
- These medications should not be stopped abruptly if used for an extended period.

## CONVENTIONAL DISEASE-MODIFYING ANTIRHEUMATIC DRUGS (DMARDS)

If you have an inflammatory arthritis, such as rheumatoid arthritis, your doctor will likely recommend that you take one or more DMARDs — sooner rather than later.

All of these drugs work to slow or stop the inflammatory process that's characteristic of rheumatoid arthritis and other rheumatic diseases, such as psoriatic arthritis, ankylosing spondylitis and forms of juvenile arthritis. By halting the disease process, DMARDs help prevent further damage to your joints.

### Methotrexate

Methotrexate is one of the first DMARDs doctors turn to for established rheumatoid arthritis. It was originally used to treat cancer, but in lower doses it can treat rheumatic diseases. The drug relieves painful and swollen joints and prevents further joint damage. It inhibits an enzyme, interfering with cell division and slowing down the immune system. Side effects are typically manageable, and its cost is relatively inexpensive.

Methotrexate is often combined with other drugs, such as another DMARD. Using methotrexate as the cornerstone of combination therapy often results in better control of rheumatoid arthritis than can be achieved with methotrexate alone, with no increased side effects from combining medicines.

Methotrexate can be taken by mouth or by injection, typically as a single dose once a week. If taking it by mouth bothers your stomach, you might fare better with an injection. Taking regular doses of folic acid also can help minimize the side effects of nausea and gastrointestinal discomfort.

## DRUG INTERACTIONS

Many people use more than one medication. Unfortunately, the action of one drug can be altered by the action of another, either decreasing or increasing the desired effect or producing a potentially dangerous reaction. Even vitamins and herbal supplements can sometimes cause serious interactions with other drugs.

When taking medications for arthritis, be sure to tell your doctor about every drug you use, including nonprescription medications, vitamins, minerals, herbal supplements and alternative remedies.

Bring all current medications with you to a doctor visit. That way, the proper dosages can be determined for both prescription and nonprescription drugs you take. Your doctor or pharmacist also can create a schedule for taking your medications. This way, you can take the drugs you need to take, but minimize the chance of harmful interactions.

Liver damage is a rare but potential side effect of taking methotrexate. Before prescribing the drug, your doctor will likely have you tested for hepatitis B and C to make sure there's no existing liver inflammation. While taking the drug, it's important to limit alcohol consumption to avoid increasing your risk of liver injury.

Drugs such as methotrexate can also reduce the infection-fighting potency of your white blood cells, making you more vulnerable to infection. These drugs may lower the number of platelets in your blood, so you bruise or bleed more easily. They can also lower your red blood cell count, causing fatigue. Lung damage is another rare side effect.

At the low doses used for rheumatoid arthritis, these side effects are unlikely. But call your doctor immediately if you develop a fever or shortness of breath. Also tell your doctor if you experience unexplained bruising, fatigue or any other side effects.

If your doctor prescribes methotrexate, you'll need to have your blood tested regularly to help ensure that the drug doesn't produce unwanted changes in your liver and bone marrow. Visits with your doctor can help address any side effects quickly.

| Generic | Brand |
| --- | --- |
| Methotrexate | Trexall, Rasuvo, others |

### How it's usually given:
- By mouth or subcutaneous injection

### Benefits:
- Usually, the first choice in rheumatoid arthritis drug therapy

### Risks:
- Upset stomach or nausea
- Loss of appetite
- Mouth sores
- Serious infections
- Blood cell deficiencies, resulting in bleeding and bruising more easily than normal, fatigue or weakness

### Precautions:
- Methotrexate isn't recommended if you're pregnant, as it can harm the baby. If you hope to become pregnant, discuss potential alternatives with your doctor.
- Methotrexate may not be right for you if you have an existing infection, blood disorder, kidney, liver or lung disease, history of lymphoma, peptic ulcer, or ulcerative colitis.
- While taking this medication, you'll be monitored regularly for changes in your blood cell counts and kidney and liver functions.
- If you experience any reaction to the drug, contact your doctor right away.
- Don't drink alcohol when taking this medication.
- Discuss vaccination with your doctor before starting this medication.

## Leflunomide

If you need an alternative to methotrexate, your doctor may recommend leflunomide, an immunosuppressant that reduces pain, stiffness, inflammation and swelling. It may also slow or halt joint damage associated with rheumatoid arthritis.

Similar to other immunosuppressants, leflunomide inhibits certain substances — in this case, a type of enzyme — made by your immune system. It can be used alone or in combination with methotrexate to increase the benefits of DMARD therapy.

Leflunomide may cause a range of side effects, including nausea, diarrhea, skin rash, upset stomach, weight loss and hair loss. As with methotrexate, it can also increase your risk of liver damage and infection, so most of the same precautions apply. You'll undergo regular blood tests to monitor your red and white blood cell counts and platelet counts.

Your doctor will test your liver function before you begin taking the medication and will conduct regular tests from then on. If you already have a liver condition, you may not be able to take leflunomide. If you develop liver problems while taking the drug, your doctor may change the dosage or stop the medication altogether. Minimizing your alcohol intake can help reduce your risk of liver damage.

Avoid leflunomide if you're pregnant, breast-feeding or hoping to become pregnant. It can harm the developing fetus and may cause serious side effects in nursing infants. (Men hoping to become fathers may want to avoid this drug as well. Check with your doctor.)

This medication stays in your body for a long time. It can take many months to completely eliminate it from your system. If necessary, your doctor can prescribe a drug called cholestyramine to speed up the elimination of leflunomide from your body.

| Generic | Brand |
|---------|-------|
| Leflunomide | Arava |

### How it's usually given:
- By mouth

### Benefits:
- May be an alternative to methotrexate
- May be combined with methotrexate for rheumatoid arthritis that's hard to treat

### Risks:
- Diarrhea
- Nausea
- Rash
- Hair loss
- Hypertension

### Precautions:
- It's important to avoid pregnancy while on this medication and during the time the drug is being eliminated from your body.

- Leflunomide isn't recommended if you already have a liver disorder, as the medication can make it worse.
- Screening for infections such as tuberculosis and hepatitis B and C are recommended before starting the medication.
- While taking this medication, you'll be monitored regularly for changes in your blood cell counts and kidney and liver functions.
- If necessary, elimination of the drug from your body can be sped up by taking the drug cholestyramine. Without this procedure, it may take up to two years to clear the drug from your system.
- Discuss vaccination with your doctor before starting this medication.

## Sulfasalazine

If your rheumatoid arthritis symptoms are mild to moderate, your doctor may recommend sulfasalazine, a drug that's also used to treat inflammatory bowel disease. Research suggests that sulfasalazine may be more effective than the medication hydroxychloroquine at treating active inflammation. It's also useful in combination therapy.

Your doctor will likely order periodic blood tests to monitor the effect of this drug on your blood cells. Side effects are uncommon. Some people have stomach discomfort, which usually goes away after reducing the dose or switching to delayed-release tablets.

If you're allergic to sulfa or aspirin, sulfasalazine probably isn't for you, because it's derived from these ingredients. It could cause an allergic reaction, such as skin rash, wheezing, itching or fever.

| Generic | Brand |
|---------|-------|
| Sulfasalazine | Azulfidine |

**How it's usually given:**
- By mouth

**Benefits:**
- Effective for early, mild rheumatoid arthritis

**Risks:**
- Upset stomach
- Headache
- Rash
- Nausea, vomiting or loss of appetite

**Precautions:**
- Tell your doctor if you experience sore throat, fever, paleness, easy bruising, or a yellowish cast to the eyes or skin, as this may indicate a serious blood disorder.
- Caution is recommended with a serious blood disorder or liver or kidney disease.
- Urine or skin may change in color to mild yellowish orange.

## Hydroxychloroquine

Originally a treatment for malaria, hydroxychloroquine has also been found to be effective for rheumatoid arthritis — although how it works to reduce joint damage isn't clear. It takes about six months for this drug to become effective. If you have early, mild rheumatoid arthritis, your doctor may recommend starting out with hydroxychloroquine, reserving more potent DMARDs, such as methotrexate and leflunomide, for later if your symptoms get worse.

Hydroxychloroquine is a common choice for use in combination with other DMARDs or in combination with corticosteroids. Using it in this way can reduce the amount of steroids you need to take.

Hydroxychloroquine has few side effects, but at high doses it may increase the risk of damage to parts of the eyes, such as the retinas. The dose prescribed for rheumatic diseases generally isn't that high. Still, your doctor will probably want you to have an eye exam before starting the medication and regularly thereafter, to catch any changes.

Hydroxychloroquine is used to treat lupus and other rheumatic diseases, as well.

| Generic | Brand |
|---------|-------|
| Hydroxychloroquine | Plaquenil |

**How it's usually given:**
- By mouth

**Benefits:**
- Effective for early, mild rheumatoid arthritis and lupus

***Risks:***
- Upset stomach, nausea
- Rash
- Dizziness
- Headache
- Vision changes

***Precautions:***
- Before starting the medication, you will need a baseline eye exam. If you remain on this drug for more than five years, an annual eye exam is recommended thereafter to monitor for vision changes.
- Caution is recommended when liver disease or alcoholism is present.

## BIOLOGIC DMARDS

Biologics are recommended for early, severe rheumatoid arthritis or rheumatoid arthritis that hasn't responded to methotrexate or combination therapy. These targeted drugs can also be combined with DMARDs, NSAIDs and corticosteroids.

If you have an active infection, your doctor will want to treat the infection before starting you on a biologic medication. In addition, anyone taking these medications should be tested for tuberculosis to check for latent disease that could later become active.

### TNF inhibitors

Tumor necrosis factor (TNF) inhibitors appear to be as effective as the DMARD methotrexate in treating rheumatoid arthritis. For rheumatoid arthritis that doesn't respond well to either methotrexate or a TNF inhibitor, a combination of the two drugs may be more effective than using either drug alone.

When injected into the body, TNF blocking agents such as infliximab, adalimumab, certolizumab and golimumab attach to circulating TNF-alpha molecules (a type of cytokine) via an antibody. They neutralize the TNF-alpha molecules before the molecules can set off an immune reaction. Etanercept works by blocking the receptor that TNF attaches to.

Because TNF inhibitors can weaken the immune system, your risk of infection is increased, especially if you're also taking methotrexate or corticosteroids. Your doctor will monitor you for signs of infection. Let your doctor know if you have symptoms of infection, such as a fever, or if you aren't feeling well.

Some people have developed symptoms of disorders such as lupus or multiple sclerosis while taking TNF inhibitors. An increased risk of lymphoma, a type of cancer, has also been reported. However, studies suggest that this increase is a complication of rheumatoid arthritis rather than an effect of the biologic medication.

If you have congestive heart failure, your doctor may recommend against TNF inhibitors because they can worsen your heart function.

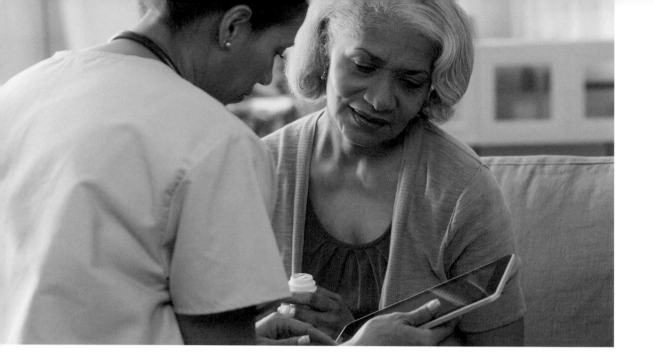

| Generic | Brand |
|---------|-------|
| Adalimumab | Humira |
| Certolizumab pegol | Cimzia |
| Etanercept | Enbrel |
| Golimumab | Simponi |
| Infliximab | Remicade |

### FDA-approved uses:
- Rheumatoid arthritis
- Psoriasis and psoriatic arthritis
- Ankylosing spondylitis
- Inflammatory bowel disease
- Juvenile idiopathic arthritis (JIA)
- Uveitis

### How they're usually given:
- Subcutaneous injection and intravenous (IV) infusions

### Benefits:
- They target TNF-alpha, an immune substance that plays a major role in the chronic inflammatory cascade that characterizes rheumatoid arthritis.

### Risks:
- Mild reaction at injection site (redness, pain, itching, swelling or bruising) or infusion reaction
- Headache
- Abdominal pain
- Upper respiratory tract infection
- Can cause a lupus-like reaction
- May exacerbate multiple sclerosis
- May increase risk of new or worsening heart failure

- May increase risk of serious infections
- May increase risk of nonmelanoma skin cancers
- May cause new or worsening psoriasis

***Precautions:***
- Prior to receiving a TNF inhibitor, you'll be screened for tuberculosis and hepatitis B and C. If necessary, an infection will be treated before you start therapy.
- Your doctor will monitor you closely for signs of infection while you're taking a TNF inhibitor. Call your doctor right away if you have a fever, don't feel well, or experience unexplained weight loss, excessive sweating, coughing or difficulty breathing.
- Vaccination with live vaccines isn't recommended while taking a TNF inhibitor.
- TNF inhibitors may not be appropriate if you have chronic or recurring infections or you have a history of heart failure.
- These medications may damage the protective coating that surrounds nerve fibers in the brain and spinal cord.
- Biologics can affect certain blood cells, so let your doctor know if you experience bleeding, bruising, fatigue or weakness more easily than normal while taking these medications.
- TNF inhibitors are likely safe during pregnancy and breastfeeding.

## Interleukin-1 inhibitors

IL-1 inhibitors are biologics that bind with cell receptors normally reserved for the cytokine interleukin-1. By taking the immune protein's spot on the receptor, IL-1 disrupts its activity. IL-1 inhibitors generally aren't as effective as the other biologics for treating rheumatoid arthritis. But they may be helpful with other autoimmune inflammatory conditions, such as systemic JIA and periodic fever syndromes.

In addition, IL-1 inhibition may be beneficial for some people with acute gouty arthritis.

| Generic | Brand |
| --- | --- |
| Anakinra | Kineret |
| Canakinumab | Ilaris |
| Rilonacept | Arcalyst |

***FDA-approved uses:***
- Rheumatoid arthritis
- Systemic JIA
- Periodic fever syndromes

***How they're usually given:***
- Subcutaneous injection

***Benefits:***
- Helps stall the disease process by targeting interleukin-1, another key player in the inflammatory cascade

***Risks:***
- Local reaction at injection site
- Diarrhea
- Flu-like reactions
- Increased risk of serious infection

**Precautions:**
- Your doctor will monitor your white blood cell and platelet counts while you're on these drugs.
- The medication can increase your risk of serious infections, including tuberculosis and bacterial, viral and fungal infections.
- Contact your doctor if you have a fever, don't feel well, or experience unexplained weight loss, excessive sweating, coughing or difficulty breathing. These could be signs of an infection.
- Receiving live virus vaccines isn't recommended while you're on these medicines.
- Risk of use during pregnancy and breastfeeding isn't known.

## Interleukin-6 inhibitors

The cytokine interleukin-6 is capable of activating T cells, B cells and other immune cells. IL-6 inhibitors work by blocking the cytokine from binding to cell receptors. This medication can be given by an infusion through your blood or by a subcutaneous injection.

| Generic | Brand |
|---------|-------|
| Sarilumab | Kevzara |
| Tocilizumab | Actemra |

**FDA-approved uses:**
- Rheumatoid arthritis
- JIA
- Giant cell arteritis

**How they're usually given:**
- Subcutaneous injection and IV infusion

**Benefits:**
- Targets interleukin-6, disrupting the inflammatory process

**Risks:**
- Common cold symptoms
- Local reaction at injection site
- Serious infections, including tuberculosis, bacterial sepsis and fungal infections
- Reactivation of dormant tuberculosis
- Allergic reaction, possibly severe (anaphylaxis)
- Tearing of the intestinal wall (bowel perforation), primarily if you have diverticulitis
- High cholesterol
- Blood cell deficiencies, resulting in bleeding and bruising more easily than normal, fatigue, or weakness
- Liver damage

**Precautions:**
- Prior to receiving an IL-6 inhibitor, you'll be screened for tuberculosis and hepatitis B and C. If necessary, an infection will be treated before you start therapy.
- Your doctor will monitor you closely for signs of infection while you're taking this drug. Call your doctor right away if you have a fever, don't feel well, or experience unexplained weight loss, excessive sweating, coughing or difficulty breathing.
- While taking this medication, you'll be monitored regularly for changes in your blood cell counts and liver function.
- Receiving live virus vaccines isn't recommended while you're on this medicine.

- IL-6 inhibitors may not be appropriate in patients with underlying liver problems or a history of diverticulosis.
- The risk of use during pregnancy and breastfeeding isn't known.

## Interleukin-17 inhibitors

IL-17 inhibitors target the cytokine interleukin-17. The IL-17 pathway has a role in psoriasis, psoriatic arthritis and ankylosing spondylitis.

| Generic | Brand |
| --- | --- |
| Ixekizumab | Taltz |
| Secukinumab | Cosentyx |

*FDA-approved uses:*
- Psoriasis and psoriatic arthritis
- Ankylosing spondylitis

*How they're usually given:*
- Subcutaneous injection

*Benefits:*
- Inhibits IL-17, a key cytokine in inflammation

*Risks:*
- Local reaction at injection site
- Diarrhea
- Headache
- Upper respiratory tract infection
- Candida infection

- May exacerbate inflammatory bowel disease activity
- Uveitis
- May worsen depression
- Low white blood cell count (neutropenia)
- May increase cholesterol

*Precautions:*
- You'll need to be screened for tuberculosis and hepatitis B and C. If necessary, an infection will be treated before you start therapy.
- Your doctor will monitor you closely for signs of infection while you're taking this drug. Call your doctor right away if you have a fever, don't feel well, or experience unexplained weight loss, excessive sweating, coughing or difficulty breathing.
- Receiving live virus vaccines isn't recommended while taking these medicines.
- IL-17 inhibitors may not be appropriate if you have chronic or recurring infections or a history of inflammatory bowel disease.
- Biologics can affect certain blood cells, so let your doctor know if you experience bleeding, bruising, fatigue or weakness more easily than usual.
- The risk of use during pregnancy and breast-feeding isn't known.

## IL-12/IL-23 inhibitors

The medication ustekinumab blocks both cytokines IL-12 and IL-23. It has been found to be effective in treating psoriasis and psoriatic arthritis. It can also be used to treat patients with Crohn's disease, one type of inflammatory bowel disease.

| Generic | Brand |
|---------|-------|
| Ustekinumab | Stelara |

**FDA-approved uses:**
- Psoriasis
- Psoriatic arthritis
- Crohn's disease

**How it's usually given:**
- Subcutaneous injection and IV infusion

**Benefits:**
- Blocks cytokines that aggravate psoriasis and psoriatic arthritis

**Risks:**
- Local reaction at injection site or infusion reaction
- Increased risk of infections
- Upper respiratory tract infections
- May increase risk of nonmelanoma skin cancers

**Precautions:**
- Prior to starting this medication, you'll be screened for tuberculosis and hepatitis B and C. If necessary, an infection will be treated before you start therapy.
- Your doctor will monitor you closely for signs of infection while you're taking this drug. Call your doctor right away if you have a fever, don't feel well, or experience unexplained weight loss, excessive sweating, coughing or difficulty breathing.
- Receiving live virus vaccines isn't recommended while you're on an IL-12/IL-23 inhibitor.

- This drug may not be appropriate for you if you have chronic or recurring infections.
- This medication may damage the protective coating that surrounds nerve fibers in the brain and spinal cord.
- Biologics can affect certain blood cells, so let your doctor know if you experience bleeding, bruising, fatigue or weakness more easily than usual.
- The risk of use during pregnancy and breast-feeding isn't known.

## IL-23 inhibitors

IL-23 inhibitors block this key cytokine found in the development of psoriasis and psoriatic arthritis.

| Generic | Brand |
|---------|-------|
| Guselkumab | Tremfya |
| Risankizumab | Skyrizi |
| Tildrakizumab | Ilumya |

**FDA-approved uses:**
- Psoriasis
- Psoriatic arthritis — in trials

**How they're usually given:**
- Subcutaneous injection

**Benefits:**
- Blocks the IL-23 cytokine, which is increased in psoriasis and psoriatic arthritis

**Risks:**

- Local reaction at injection site
- Increase risk of infections
- Upper respiratory tract infection
- Headache

**Precautions:**

- Prior to starting these medications, you'll be screened for tuberculosis and hepatitis B and C. If necessary, an infection will be treated before you start therapy.
- Your doctor will monitor you closely for signs of infection while you're taking this drug. Call your doctor right away if you have a fever, don't feel well, or experience unexplained weight loss, excessive sweating, coughing or difficulty breathing.
- Receiving live virus vaccines isn't recommended while you're on this drug.
- IL-23 inhibitors may not be appropriate for you if you have chronic or recurring infections.
- Biologics can affect certain blood cells, so let your doctor know if you experience bleeding, bruising, fatigue or weakness more easily than usual.
- The risk of use during pregnancy and breast-feeding isn't known.

## T cell inhibitors

The medication abatacept inhibits the action of T cells, which recognize invaders and trigger inflammation. The drug binds to the cells and blocks their signals. It's generally prescribed for people with moderate to severe rheumatoid arthritis that hasn't responded to other drugs.

Abatacept can slow damage to joints and improve physical function. It can be used with conventional DMARDs, but it shouldn't be taken with other cytokine inhibitors.

| Generic | Brand |
|---------|-------|
| Abatacept | Orencia |

**FDA-approved uses:**

- Rheumatoid arthritis
- Juvenile idiopathic arthritis
- Psoriatic arthritis

**How it's usually given:**

- Subcutaneous injection and IV infusions

**Benefits:**

- Inhibits activation of T cells, blocking the perpetuation of inflammation

**Risks:**

- Headache
- Dizziness
- Nausea
- Upper respiratory infection
- Increased risk of infection
- May aggravate chronic obstructive pulmonary disease

**Precautions:**

- Prior to receiving abatacept, you'll be screened for tuberculosis and hepatitis B and C and treated, if necessary.
- Your doctor will monitor you closely for signs of infection while you're taking this drug. Call your doctor right away if you have a fever, don't feel well, or experience unexplained weight loss, excessive sweating, coughing or difficulty breathing.
- Receiving live virus vaccines isn't recommended while you're taking this medication.
- Abatacept may not be appropriate if you have chronic or recurring infections or if you have a history of chronic obstructive pulmonary disease.
- The risk of use during pregnancy and breast-feeding isn't known.

## B cell inhibitors

B cells play an important role in sustaining the inflammation that's caused by rheumatoid arthritis. The drug rituximab is a genetically engineered protein that binds to B cells, causing them to self-destruct. Rituximab was first found to be effective in treating lymphoma, a type of cancer.

| Generic | Brand |
|---------|-------|
| Rituximab | Rituxan |

**FDA-approved uses:**

- Rheumatoid arthritis
- Vasculitis
- Lymphoma

**How it's usually given:**

- Intravenous infusion

**Benefits:**

- Targets and destroys immune system B cells
- Is usually reserved for severe disease that hasn't responded to other treatment
- Can be used in combination therapy with methotrexate

**Risks:**

- Infusion reactions
- Upper respiratory infection
- Urinary tract infection
- Fluid retention
- Rash, skin itching
- Nausea
- Diarrhea

**Precautions:**

- Prior to receiving rituximab, you'll be screened for tuberculosis and hepatitis B and C and treated, if necessary.
- The medication can cause side effects for 24 hours after receiving the infusion.
- To minimize its side effects, your doctor may give you a dose of a corticosteroids, acetaminophen or antihistamines.

- Receiving live virus vaccines isn't recommended while you're on this medication.
- This medication may damage the protective coating that surrounds nerve fibers in the brain and spinal cord.
- This drug lowers immunoglobulin levels.
- Your doctor will monitor you closely for signs of infection while you're taking this drug. Call your doctor right away if you have a fever, don't feel well, or experience unexplained weight loss, excessive sweating, coughing or difficulty breathing.
- A small number of people may develop antibodies to this medicine, but this effect is lessened when used with methotrexate.
- Avoid this drug during pregnancy, as it can affect the baby's developing immune system.

## TARGETED DMARDS

While conventional DMARDs restrict your immune system broadly, targeted DMARDs block specific pathways inside immune cells. Targeted DMARDs are small molecules that affect cell communication mechanisms such as kinase and phosphodiesterase pathways.

### Kinase inhibitors

Kinase inhibitors are not true biologic medications, as they aren't proteins. Rather, they're small molecules that block the action of the enzyme Janus kinase, which is important in activating the immune system. This category of medication is approved for treating moderate to severe rheumatoid arthritis that hasn't responded well to methotrexate. An advantage of these drugs is that they can be taken by mouth.

| Generic | Brand |
|---------|-------|
| Baricitinib | Olumiant |
| Tofacitinib | Xeljanz |
| Upadacitinib | Rinvoq |

**FDA-approved uses:**
- Rheumatoid arthritis
- Psoriatic arthritis
- Ulcerative colitis

**How they're usually given:**
- By mouth

**Benefits:**
- Inhibits the activation of Janus kinase (JAK), a protein kinase (enzyme) that contributes to inflammation
- Used in adults who have moderate to severe rheumatoid arthritis who haven't responded well to methotrexate

**Risks:**
- Upper respiratory tract infections
- Headache
- Diarrhea
- Inflammation of nose and upper throat
- Increased risk of serious infection
- Can increase cholesterol
- Increased risk of GI perforation if you have a history of diverticulitis

- Weight loss
- May increase hair growth
- Increased liver function on tests
- May increase the risk of nonmelanoma skin cancers
- May increase the risk of interstitial lung disease

*Precautions:*
- A kinase inhibitor can be used in combination with methotrexate or other nonbiologic DMARDS, but it shouldn't be used in combination with biologics or strong immunosuppressive drugs, such as azathioprine or cyclosporine.
- Before starting this drug, you'll need to be tested for a latent tuberculosis infection and treated if necessary. Even if you test negative, you should be monitored for active tuberculosis while on this medicine.
- While taking this medication, you'll be monitored regularly for changes in your blood cell counts, liver enzymes and blood cholesterol levels.
- This medication may not be appropriate for you if you have chronic or recurring infection or a history of diverticulosis.
- This drug may possibly increase your risk of a blood clot.
- If you develop kidney disease, you may need to reduce the dose of this medication.
- The risk of use during pregnancy and breast-feeding is unknown.

## Phosphodiesterase 4 (PDE4) inhibitor

The drug apremilast helps to stem inflammatory responses by blocking the enzyme phosphodiesterase 4 (PDE4). It's used to treat psoriatic arthritis when conventional DMARDs haven't been effective. It's easy to take by mouth, and unlike biologics, this drug doesn't weaken the immune system. If you have psoriatic arthritis and biologics are not an option for you, your doctor may suggest this medication.

| Generic | Brand |
|---|---|
| Apremilast | Otezla |

*FDA-approved uses:*
- Psoriasis
- Psoriatic arthritis

*How it's usually given:*
- By mouth

*Benefits:*
- No effect on liver
- Does not increase infection risk

*Risks:*
- Depression
- Weight loss
- Diarrhea
- Nausea
- Headache
- Upper respiratory tract infection

*Precautions:*
- The dosage may need to be decreased if you have or develop kidney disease.
- This drug is not recommended if you're interested in getting pregnant.

## BIOLOGIC MEDICATIONS AND INFECTIONS

The body's immune system is a well-regulated system. When bacteria, viruses and other invaders are discovered, white blood cells produce certain cytokines that induce inflammation (proinflammatory cytokines). These cytokines, including TNF, IL-1, IL-6, IL-12 and IL-23, mobilize the cells to engage and destroy the invaders. This temporarily causes inflammation.

Usually, after the infection is cleared up, your body stops making these excess cytokines. If you have rheumatoid arthritis, production doesn't decrease. As proinflammatory cytokines build up, more white blood cells collect in an area, causing inflammation, pain and tissue damage. Cytokine inhibitor medications work by blocking the action of the specific cytokine they target, thereby reducing inflammation.

Because of how they work, biologic agents also limit your ability to fight infections. In general, though, this risk isn't greater than that of some nonbiologic medications. Most people who develop a serious infection while taking a biologic medication are also taking other medications that suppress the immune system, such as methotrexate or a corticosteroid. The risk of serious infection also increases if you take a combination of cytokine inhibitors.

Before prescribing a biologic agent, your doctor may ask about any current or recurring infections you may have and may test you for tuberculosis and fungal infections. If you do develop an infection while taking a biologic agent, you may need to stop the treatment until the infection has been successfully treated.

It's not clear whether cytokine inhibitors can increase the risk of cancers such as lymphoma — people with rheumatoid arthritis have an increased risk of lymphoma even if they're not being treated with these medications. So far research hasn't shown a clear link between these drugs and an increased risk of cancer, but long-term studies are needed.

# Surgical treatments

If your joint pain from arthritis doesn't go away with other treatments, your doctor may recommend surgery to ease your symptoms. In certain cases, joint surgery can help you reach a more active and fulfilling life.

The primary goals of using surgery to treat arthritis are to relieve chronic pain, slow or prevent cartilage damage, and correct the joint's range of motion and stability. A surgical procedure aims to restore as much function to the joint as possible.

Some people choose surgery when they can no longer tolerate the pain and when other therapies they've tried, such as medications, exercise and weight loss, don't seem to help. Other people need surgery because arthritis interferes with their family life, work or ability to maintain a home.

Deciding to have joint surgery involves careful consideration and planning with your doctor. There are many different surgical procedures, and each one offers different benefits and risks.

Before deciding on a surgery, it's important to understand the possible outcomes and what each might mean for you. Is the surgery likely to completely resolve the pain? How long can you expect the improvement to last? How will the recovery time affect your routine? It's also important to be aware of any physical limitations that surgery may impose on the joint. For example, if you choose to go with a certain procedure, do you lose some flexibility in that joint or are some movements restricted?

The outcome of a surgery can be different for each person. It depends on a number of factors, including the strength of the bones, tendons and ligaments supporting your joints, your age, your weight, and your ability to participate in rehabilitation.

## COMMON TYPES OF JOINT SURGERY

Different types of surgical procedures are used to treat the joints affected by arthritis and make them more functional. A surgeon will recommend certain procedures in order to address your specific needs. Depending on your age and overall health, your form of arthritis, and your specific joint problems, one or more of the following procedures may be recommended.

### Debridement

Surgeons use this procedure to remove loose fragments of bone, cartilage or synovial membrane that cause joint pain, most often in the knees. The surgeon makes a small incision and inserts an arthroscope — a thin fiber-optic tube with a tiny camera. The camera lets the surgeon see inside the joint while other narrow tools cut or grind loose pieces as needed and suction out the fragments. The surgeon may make additional small incisions at different points around the joint to insert these instruments.

Debridement is often helpful to people in early stages of osteoarthritis. The loose fragments can create the sensation of your knee joint "catching" or "locking up." While removing the loose pieces won't reverse the arthritis, the procedure may help the joint move more smoothly and with less pain.

### Synovectomy

Synovectomy (sin-o-VEK-tuh-me) removes some of the synovial tissue lining an inflamed joint. It is used especially when rheumatoid arthritis is the cause of inflammation. Removing this tissue can reduce pain and swelling and delay or possibly prevent cartilage and bone destruction. Although it may provide pain relief, synovectomy is not a cure. Inflammation may recur as the synovium grows back over time.

Synovectomy is routinely performed on knees, fingers, wrists and elbows, before significant cartilage erosion or deformity occurs. Some specialists also perform synovectomy on the elbow. Synovectomy can be done arthroscopically or as open surgery. Arthroscopic surgery typically allows you to recover faster.

### Cartilage transplantation

This procedure is also known as autologous cartilage implantation (ACI). A small sample of cells is removed from the cartilage of the joint and cultivated in a lab. About six to eight weeks later, the lab-grown cartilage cells are inserted into a

## SELECTING A SURGEON

If your decision is to have surgery, your primary care doctor or rheumatologist can help refer you to an orthopedic surgeon. Orthopedic surgeons perform operations involving joints, muscles and bones. Typically, you want someone with extensive experience in joint procedures.

It's important to have confidence in the orthopedic surgeon you choose. Board-certified surgeons have met extensive requirements for training and experience. Some complete additional training and focus their practice on the treatment of specific joints. An experienced orthopedic surgeon should be able to answer questions about the options available to you, the risks and benefits associated with each, and what to expect during your recovery.

Questions you may ask the surgeon include:
- How often have you performed this kind of surgery in the past?
- What are short-term and long-term risks associated with this surgery?
- If the surgery involves implants, what type do you recommend?
- What kind of anesthesia will be used and what are the risks?
- Should I expect a lot of pain, and what measures can I use to relieve it?
- How long is the recovery process and what is involved?
- What outcome should I expect after this surgery?

Given the potential risks and costs associated with surgery, seeking a second opinion before proceeding may be a sensible option. Either you or your doctor can initiate the process of getting a second opinion. Don't be afraid to ask about it.

damaged joint as a tissue "scaffold" to help new cartilage grow.

Physicians use this procedure as a treatment for small areas of damaged cartilage — up to about 0.6 square inches. Transplantation for larger areas of damage has not yet been successful. Scientists are working to identify substances that will stimulate healthy cartilage growth (cartilage growth factors) to help advance this technique.

## ANATOMY OF AN ARTIFICIAL JOINT

When the gradual deterioration of a joint occurs due to arthritis, implanting an artificial joint can help eliminate pain and restore near-normal function. The implants are also called prostheses.

Artificial joints are made of various metals, ceramics or plastic-like materials called polymers. Surgeons choose the implants best suited to your needs from a wide selection of sizes, shapes and construction. At some medical centers, doctors may use computers to custom design the implant.

Traditionally, surgeons have secured joint implants to bones with a special cement. This method generally works well, but sometimes, the cement may eventually crack, causing the implant to loosen. If loosening occurs, you may need additional procedures to reattach or replace the implant.

Uncemented implants are used more commonly now, especially in hip surgery. These implants have a porous surface that the bone grows into, attaching itself. This may improve durability. But uncemented implants may also loosen. Rarely, the bone fails to attach itself to the implant and the implant becomes fixed with scar tissue.

Over time, artificial joints create debris from friction and wear. The tiny particles can cause inflammation that destroys bone or soft tissue in the joint and may ultimately contribute to loosening of the implant. Typically, you'll be asked to schedule regular follow-ups every few years to monitor your joint's condition.

## Osteotomy

During this procedure, a surgeon cuts and repositions bones near a damaged joint to help correct deformities caused by arthritis. These adjustments realign the joint and also help slow cartilage damage by distributing body weight more evenly across the joint. Osteotomy (os-tee-OT-uh-me) is most commonly used to correct curvature or bowing in the lower leg bones caused by osteoarthritis around the knee joint. It may be a good

The components of an artificial hip implant are shown above, assembled (left) and apart (right). The implant on the right is cementless, with a surface on the long stem to which bone attaches itself. Typically, younger, active people with good bone quality are the best candidates for cementless total hip arthroplasty. A cemented implant is preferred in people who have poor bone stock and in older people with low activity levels. Regardless of the type of implant, recent studies show that 85% to 90% of total hip replacements are still successful 15 years after surgery.

option for younger people wanting to avoid a joint replacement, particularly in the knee.

## Resection

Surgeons sometimes remove all or part of a damaged bone when diseased joints make movement painful. Called resection (resection arthroplasty), this procedure may be used in the feet to make walking easier. It's also done to reduce pain in the wrists and hands. It's less commonly used in larger joints such as hips or knees.

## Joint replacement

When arthritis severely damages a joint, your doctor may recommend replacing it with an artificial joint. This joint replacement procedure is called arthroplasty (AHR-throe-plas-tee).

For the procedure, the surgeon removes certain parts of the damaged joint and replaces them with an implant (prosthesis) made of high-density plastic, metal alloy or ceramic material. Most of the major ligaments and tendons are left in place and rebalanced so that the joint straightens and bends well, and is stable from side to side and front to back.

The hip and the knee are the most commonly replaced joints, but implants can also replace damaged bone and cartilage in other joints.

In some cases, the surgeon may choose to preserve more of the joint and replace only the most damaged part. In a knee joint, for example, damage may be limited to the inner or outer part of the knee or where the kneecap meets the thigh bone. Replacing only one part of the joint preserves more natural movement of the knee. A partial joint replacement may also allow for a faster recovery.

## Joint fusion

Also called arthrodesis (ahr-throe-DEE-sis), joint fusion is used most often to reduce pain and improve stability in the spine, wrist, ankle, and joints of the fingers and toes. During this procedure, surgeons remove a thin layer of tissue from the ends of two bones and bind them together, often using pins, rods or plates. Fresh bone cells then grow at the juncture, fusing the two bones. Once healed, the fused joint can bear weight but has no flexibility.

Joint fusion is typically used when total joint replacement isn't possible. This may be the case after an infection or a failed joint replacement with significant bone loss.

## Tendon and ligament repair

Surgeons can repair tendon tears to reduce pain, restore function and, in some cases, prevent tendon rupture. For example, you may need surgery if one of the tendons in the rotator cuff in your shoulder partially or fully tears. Other procedures can tighten or loosen tendons and ligaments. These are

## YOUR BODY'S JOINTS

Your body has several different types of joints. Together, they allow you to perform a variety of essential functions.

Fixed joints don't allow movement between bones. They absorb shock to help prevent the bones from breaking while also protecting the underlying tissue.

For example, fixed joints between the bony plates of your skull protect the sensitive brain tissue underneath. The sacroiliac joints connecting your spine and pelvis are another example.

Hinge joints work like the hinge in a doorway, allowing forward and backward movement (although there is slight motion in other directions). Your elbows, fingers, knees and toes contain hinge joints.

Pivot joints allow a rotating movement. The pivot joint in your neck allows your head to turn from side to side. Your elbow includes both hinge and pivot joints.

In ball-and-socket joints, the large round end of one bone fits snugly into a cup-shaped cavity of another bone. This allows movement in almost every direction, making swinging and rotation movements possible. Your shoulders and hips are ball-and-socket joints.

sometimes recommended to decrease pain, increase joint mobility or prepare a joint for total joint replacement. Surgeons may also perform procedures to relieve pressure on nerves that become pinched or irritated by tight ligaments.

## CHOOSING THE RIGHT PROCEDURE

Your joints vary greatly in size, shape, design and function. When you see a surgeon about procedures to treat your joint pain, he or she will consider these differences and tailor your treatment accordingly. This section explores how surgeons select procedures such as the ones described in the previous section to help relieve your arthritis symptoms in specific joints.

### Hands and wrists

The ability to grasp a spoon, turn a doorknob or button a shirt is something you may take for granted until arthritis starts affecting your hands or wrists. It's no secret that arthritis pain can make these movements difficult, if not impossible.

The primary goals of hand or wrist procedures are the same for all joint surgeries — to improve function and reduce pain. Some procedures can also improve the appearance of finger joints deformed by arthritis. But surgery is rarely recommended for cosmetic reasons alone — unless the arthritis is greatly hurting your self-image and social interactions.

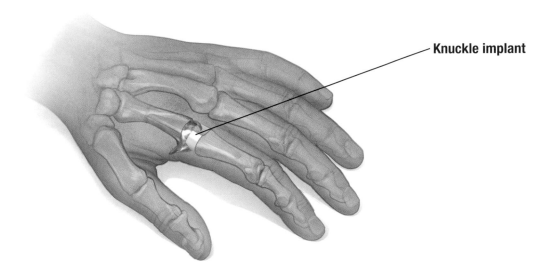

**Knuckle implant**

An artificial implant is shown in the knuckle of the index finger. The implant can reduce pain and restore motion in the knuckle joint and improve overall function of the hand.

***Tendon and ligament adjustments*** Sometimes, rheumatoid arthritis causes tears in the tendons of the hand and wrist, and an operation is performed to repair the damage and prevent rupture of these tendons. Other surgical procedures help tighten or loosen tendons and ligaments in the hand and wrist to decrease pain and increase your mobility and grip strength.

***Synovectomy or resection*** Removing inflamed tissue or damaged bone may help reduce pain in the wrists and fingers caused by rheumatoid arthritis.

***Joint fusion*** If you have severely damaged finger or wrist joints, fusing the joints together may relieve pain and improve stability. But fusing wrist joints also limits how you can move your hand.

***Joint replacement*** Hand and wrist joint replacements are performed less often than hip and knee replacements are. This is partly because the joints are small and require precise repair of ligaments and tendons.

The hand is a complex structure with many moving parts. Other surgical procedures, such as joint fusion and tendon adjustment, can usually have good results, so surgeons often use joint replacement for only the most severely damaged hand and wrist joints. Some surgeons reserve knuckle replacement for older adults who tend to use their hands less, allowing the artificial knuckles to last longer.

If you have joint replacement surgery on a hand or wrist, your hand will be placed in a splint for two to three weeks while your muscles and other soft tissues heal. After that, you'll have physical therapy to retrain the tissues. Post-surgical therapy is essential because there's so much soft tissue reconstruction involved in wrist or finger joint replacement.

## Elbows

If medications and daily exercise aren't providing enough relief from arthritis pain in your elbow, you may consider other options. Several surgical procedures can reduce pain and increase the range of motion, including complete surgical replacement of your elbow joint.

Elbow surgery is generally performed in one of two ways. Open surgery refers to working on the joint through an incision in the arm — the more traditional method. Open surgery on the elbow is widely available, and surgeons have been doing it for years.

The other option is arthroscopic surgery, done through small incisions. It has a lower risk of infection and leaves less scarring. But the procedure requires special expertise to move a tiny camera and surgical tools within your elbow. If the joint has deteriorated from arthritis, arthroscopic elbow surgery may not be an option. And because this is a relatively specialized procedure, it may not be available at all medical centers.

The specific surgical procedure that's right for you will depend on several factors, in-

cluding the type of arthritis you have and the condition of your elbow joint.

***Synovectomy or resection*** Removing inflamed tissue and, sometimes, damaged bone is usually the first choice of surgery for people in the early stages of rheumatoid arthritis. The procedure can help increase your elbow's range of motion and relieve pain. You and your doctor may consider synovectomy if you've tried medication and therapy for at least six months and you still have severe elbow pain.

The procedure can be open or done arthroscopically. Arthroscopic synovectomy is typically more thorough than the open option, because arthroscopy uses high-powered optics and small surgical instruments that allow your surgeon to access more of the joint.

The synovium in your joints eventually grows back, which means that elbow pain could return. But a synovectomy can delay the need for more-invasive surgical treatments, such as elbow replacement. Plus, medications can prevent the synovium from becoming inflamed again.

***Debridement*** For osteoarthritis, removing loose fragments is usually the first choice of surgery if medications and physical therapy fail to bring pain relief. Debridement can be performed either open or arthroscopically.

A more thorough form of debridement, known as osteocapsular arthroplasty, involves removing bone spurs, loose bone and cartilage, as well as performing a synovectomy and recontouring bones that have deteriorated due to arthritis. Osteocapsular arthroplasty can be an extremely successful procedure, relieving pain and improving range of motion. However, it's also relatively new and difficult to perform — so it may not be widely available.

**Interpositional arthroplasty** For this open-surgery procedure, your surgeon removes bone spurs or loose fragments from the elbow joint. He or she then separates your elbow and stitches a piece of skin tissue or tendon — usually taken from elsewhere in your body or from a donor — in place between the bones that make up the elbow joint. This tissue resurfaces the joint, keeping your bones from rubbing together to reduce pain.

This procedure is typically offered to younger or very active adults with severe arthritis of the elbow as a way to increase functionality and delay total joint replacement. Having total joint replacement carries limitations on activities and the amount of weight you can lift, which can be a difficult lifestyle change for some active people. However, neither surgery is a good fix for heavy laborers.

While interpositional arthroplasty may be the best choice for some people, pain relief and range of motion after the surgery can be unpredictable. Joint instability also is a significant risk. In addition, there's still a chance you may need to have replacement surgery later.

**Joint replacement** If your arthritis causes strong elbow pain that doesn't respond to medication and limits your daily activities, you might be considered for total elbow replacement (total elbow arthroplasty).

Replacing the entire joint is usually reserved for people with advanced arthritis that hasn't responded to nonsurgical treatments and less aggressive surgical options. It's generally done in adults age 60 and older, and isn't recommended for younger people unless other types of surgery have failed.

Replacing the diseased bone and tissue with an artificial joint can relieve pain and restore range of motion. During the procedure, your surgeon makes an incision in the back of the elbow and moves muscles and nerves out of the way. He or she then removes diseased parts of the bones, reshapes the remaining bones and places the prosthetic joint in place. Elbow implants are typically secured partly with cement and partly with bone regrowth into certain uncemented parts of the implant.

As with any surgery, elbow replacement carries the risk of infection and bleeding. Also, mechanical problems with the new elbow joint, such as loosening or breakage, are more likely to occur than in other joints because of the tremendous stress that the elbow typically undergoes with use. Damage to the nerves in your elbow also is possible as a result of the operation.

While elbow replacement can increase range of motion and reduce pain, you'll have limitations on the new joint. After surgery, you shouldn't lift more than 1 or 2 pounds regularly, and lifting up to 10 pounds can only be done occasionally. Heavier lifting could damage the new joint or the bones holding it in place. These restrictions remain for the life of your new joint.

## Shoulders

Doctors typically recommend daily exercise and medications as the first treatments for arthritis of the shoulder. However, if you've tried these options and you still have pain and limited motion, it may be time to consider surgery. Joint replacement is the most common surgical procedure for shoulder arthritis, but you and your doctor may consider other procedures.

***Synovectomy*** If you have rheumatoid arthritis and the bones in your shoulder joint aren't damaged, a synovectomy might be all that's needed to restore motion and reduce pain. A synovectomy can be done as either open or arthroscopic surgery.

While it's true that the synovium can grow back and become inflamed again, medica-

Humerus

Implant

Radius

Ulna

Total elbow replacement may be recommended if arthritis has severely damaged cartilage and bone (see inset). The components of the artificial joint are anchored with the help of long stems inserted into the humerus and ulna. Some implants permit movement in only one plane (hinge joint), while others permit rotation of the forearm (hinge and pivot joints), similar to a normal elbow joint.

tions can usually prevent that from happening. Most people with rheumatoid arthritis of the shoulder who have this procedure will have pain-free motion in the joint.

**Joint fusion** When bone or cartilage damage in your shoulder is extensive, more-aggressive surgery may be needed. Joint fusion can reduce pain and offer long-term stability. But because the fusion immobilizes your joint, the procedure significantly reduces your ability to use the shoulder.

Joint fusion is less common today than it once was. You may be a candidate for this procedure if damage from arthritis makes it impossible for the muscles and tendons in your shoulder to hold an artificial joint securely in place, or if you've lost cartilage due to an infection of the shoulder joint.

**Debridement** Osteocapsular arthroplasty is another surgical option for shoulder arthritis. During this arthroscopic procedure, your surgeon removes bone spurs and reshapes and smoothes the joint surfaces of the shoulder. This makes it easier for the bones in your shoulder to move without friction and pain.

**Joint replacement** Total shoulder replacement (arthroplasty) is the most common type of shoulder surgery for arthritis. It can increase the range of motion in your shoulder, making it easier to move your arm. It also improves strength and reduces pain in your shoulder.

During total shoulder replacement, your surgeon removes damaged parts of the bones that make up your shoulder joint, including the ball-shaped top of your upper arm bone (humerus) and the socket (glenoid cavity) of your shoulder blade. They're replaced with an artificial joint consisting of a metal ball and plastic socket. Your surgeon might also clean up the area around the joint by removing bone spurs and inflamed synovium.

Shoulder replacement involves a longer rehabilitation period than other types of joint replacement do. Learning to use your new joint and recovering its strength may take months, while regaining full function can take up to a year.

You'll need to diligently follow a prescribed set of exercises beginning the first day after surgery. Not sticking to the exercise regimen can lead to stiffness or instability in your new shoulder joint.

Shoulder replacement surgery is fairly safe and predictable, and most people are satisfied with their new shoulder joints. Like any surgery, though, it carries the risk of infection and bleeding, and complications can arise. A small number of artificial joints will eventually need to be replaced. The implant can loosen, requiring refitting. Sometimes, the shoulder becomes weak

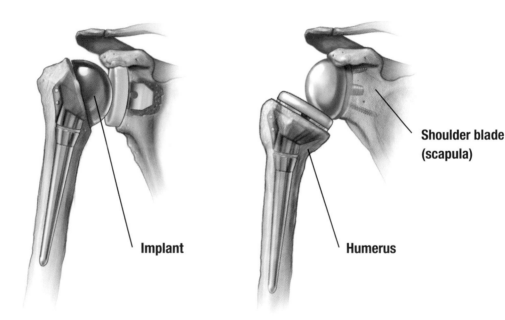

Implant

Humerus

Shoulder blade (scapula)

In total shoulder replacement (left), the ball component of the artificial joint is anchored to the humerus with the help of a long stem that's inserted into the bone, while the socket component is fixed to the shoulder blade. The implant replicates the structure and function of your natural shoulder joint. The implant design is reversed in reverse shoulder replacement (right). The ball component is fixed to the shoulder blade, and the socket component is attached to the humerus.

and unstable, which may require another surgery.

**Hemiarthroplasty** If the ball-shaped top of your humerus is damaged but the socket of your shoulder blade is still in good shape, your surgeon may recommend a version of joint replacement called hemiarthroplasty. In this procedure, only the ball is replaced. The socket remains, although your surgeon may smooth it out.

This procedure may also be considered if you have a tear in the muscles and tendons that support your shoulder (rotator cuff) in addition to arthritis. A rotator cuff tear may make it difficult for your shoulder muscles to firmly hold a prosthetic socket in place, which would lead to early loosening of the artificial joint.

If you're younger and want to use your shoulder more vigorously than is possible with total joint replacement, your surgeon may recommend resurfacing hemiarthroplasty, which affixes a synthetic surface cap to the ball part of the joint. This procedure provides pain relief — although perhaps with less predictable results than with a total replacement — and avoids years of wear and tear on an artificial joint. The possibility of a total shoulder replacement remains open for a later time.

**Reverse shoulder arthroplasty** As its name implies, reverse shoulder arthroplasty swaps the ball and socket parts of the typical shoulder implant. A reverse prosthesis is placed so that the ball portion is attached to the shoulder blade and the socket portion is attached to the upper arm bone.

This procedure is most appropriate for people who have shoulder arthritis along with extensive tears of muscles and tendons in the rotator cuff, severely limiting motion. It may also be the best choice if you have a failed previous shoulder joint replacement and a weak rotator cuff. The reverse technique compensates for a lack of strength and support from the rotator cuff. It allows another muscle of the shoulder to take over your shoulder's pulling function. This allows you to lift your arm again with relative ease.

Reverse shoulder arthroplasty is a newer procedure than traditional shoulder replacement. But for people who aren't otherwise good candidates for total shoulder arthroplasty, it has shown very promising results.

## Hips

The daily demands on your hips are impressive: bearing your weight, walking, climbing stairs, bending and twisting. It's no wonder the hips are commonly affected by arthritis. When weight loss, medications, reduced activity and use of a cane fail to provide relief, your doctor may recommend hip surgery.

**Osteotomy** This surgery, used to adjust and realign the bones of your hip joint, is occasionally used to help reduce hip pain, particularly in younger people with arthritis.

During this procedure, the surgeon makes a cut in the bone just below the joint to move healthier cartilage to the area that bears the most weight. This changes the joint alignment and helps evenly distribute your body weight. For some people, it brings pain relief and improved function of the hip joint. In best-case scenarios, osteotomy may delay the need for total hip replacement for 10 years or even longer.

***Joint fusion*** Although uncommon today, fusing the bones of an arthritic hip joint is another surgical option. Fusion of the hip joint is generally reserved for people who aren't good candidates for hip replacement, including younger people. During this procedure, your surgeon joins the round upper end of your thighbone (femur) and the socket in your pelvic bone (acetabulum), eliminating all motion. This surgery changes the mechanics of how you walk, but it can provide good relief from joint pain for many years.

***Joint replacement*** Hip replacement surgery (total hip arthroplasty) is by far the most successful surgical procedure for treating advanced arthritis of the hip. It's also one of the most common joint replacement

**Implant**

**Pelvis**

**Femur**

Severe osteoarthritis has destroyed cartilage and bone in the left hip. In total hip replacement, the surgeon replaces the head or "ball" of the thighbone (femur) with an implant consisting of a metal ball attached to a metal stem that is inserted into the femur (see inset). A socket implant is attached to your pelvic bone. The components may be cemented or uncemented, often depending on your bone quality.

surgeries, with more than 370,000 done annually in the United States.

The implants for an artificial hip joint come in many shapes, styles and materials. Your surgeon will decide which joint is best suited for you. The implants, which mimic the natural design of your hip, fit together and function like a normal joint. They are biocompatible — meaning they're designed to be accepted by your body — and made to resist corrosion, degradation and wear.

Some artificial hip joints are held in place with bone cement. More commonly, the new joint is uncemented and held in place by new bone growth into part of the prosthesis over time. No hard and fast rules dictate whether cemented or uncemented fixation should be used — it typically depends on the quality of the bone around the implant.

In general, uncemented fixation is used for people who have good bone quality. In certain cases, you may need to wait a few weeks for new bone growth to form before applying your full weight to the new joint. Cemented fixation is used for people with weakened health or weaker bones (such as from osteoporosis). A cemented joint can usually withstand your full weight immediately after surgery. For older adults, a doctor may use a hybrid form of joint fixation, in which the socket is placed uncemented while the stem is cemented.

During the procedure, your thighbone is separated from the socket on your pelvis.

Working between the large hip muscles, your surgeon removes damaged bone and tissue and leaves healthy bone intact. Next, an artificial socket is pressed into place on the pelvis. The top end of the thighbone is hollowed out so that the stem of the ball implant can be inserted. The ball and the socket join to form a new hip joint. Before closing the incision, your surgeon checks the alignment and stability of the new joint.

Hip replacement surgery is successful more than 90% of the time. It usually allows pain-free movement for many years after the procedure. Still, don't expect to do things that you couldn't do before surgery. High-impact activities, such as running and playing basketball, may not be possible after a hip replacement. But in time, you may be able to swim, play golf, walk or ride a bike comfortably.

Hip replacement surgery is generally safe, but complications — sometimes serious — may occur. Most can be treated successfully. Rare complications may include blood clots, dislocation, infection, fracture, loosening or breakage of the prosthesis, change in leg length or joint stiffening.

Hip replacement used to be an option primarily for older adults because implants would wear out. But improved technology has produced longer lasting artificial joints available for more active people, including young adults. However, active people face the possibility of more surgery to replace worn-out artificial joints if they don't reduce their activity after a hip replacement.

Repeated surgery, also called revision surgery, is more difficult and often isn't as successful as the original procedure.

A newer surgical approach to hip replacement is minimally invasive, avoiding the need to detach or cut through muscles to reach the joint. This surgery is similar to traditional hip replacement, but is performed with specially designed instruments inserted through one relatively small incision. It can still have the same complications, such as dislocated hips, bone fractures, and nerve and blood vessel injuries.

Because this technique is newer, there are a limited number of studies comparing outcomes with those of traditional hip replacement. Some studies have shown that people undergoing minimally invasive hip replacement may have a faster, easier recovery. Other research has shown no difference in long-term outcomes compared to the more traditional approaches. However, longer follow-up is still needed to evaluate the technique.

***Resurfacing*** In younger, more active people, some surgeons opt for a form of hip replacement that retains most of the ball of the hip joint, trimming only damaged portions and capping the ball with a smooth metal surface. The damaged socket on the pelvis is removed, just as with traditional hip replacement, and replaced with an artificial one.

An advantage of resurfacing is that the entire femoral head can be replaced at a later time, if necessary. This may be easier than correcting a total hip replacement if dislocation or implant failure occurs. One risk of hip resurfacing is that the femoral neck — the area just below the ball of the hip joint — might eventually fracture, requiring a full joint replacement.

## Knees

Surgery offers various options to relieve pain and restore mobility to an arthritic knee.

***Debridement*** This minimally invasive procedure is frequently used to remove cartilage tears or loose tissue fragments from

---

## EASING THE PAIN AFTER SURGERY

After joint replacement surgery, you may receive an anesthetic to numb the nerves surrounding the painful joint (peripheral nerve block). You'll get the medication through a catheter that's set up on the day of surgery and can remain in place for the first couple of days after surgery. It typically provides good pain relief. Some increase in pain is normal as the nerve block's effect gradually wears off.

Another option is to inject a combination of pain-relieving medications into the joint and surrounding tissues at the time of surgery. Both techniques reduce or eliminate the side effects from opioid pain medications normally used in such cases. They have also reduced the recovery time after surgery.

When the nerve block is stopped, you'll be given oral pain medication. The medication helps ease discomfort, but may not completely relieve the pain. Taking the medication before pain becomes significant is usually most helpful, so tell your doctor sooner rather than later if pain is increasing.

Express the level of pain you feel on a scale of 0 to 10, with 0 equal to no pain and 10 equal to the worst pain imaginable. Also tell your doctor if you have any other discomfort or suspect the pain medication is causing nausea or other symptoms. Cold packs can help reduce swelling and discomfort around the surgical incision.

around the knee joint. This may be a good option if you're young or middle-aged and the arthritis is a result of sports injuries. It's less effective for people with severe or long-term knee arthritis.

**Synovectomy** If the cartilage isn't significantly damaged, removing inflamed tissue from around the knee joint can decrease pain and swelling in people with rheumatoid arthritis. It doesn't appear to slow the progress of arthritis. But in younger people, synovectomy may delay the need for total joint replacement.

Because the knee is a relatively large joint, surgeons typically perform the procedure with arthroscopy. This allows the surgeon to view inside the joint and remove diseased tissue with small instruments. An arthroscopic procedure requires a much smaller incision than a conventional operation does, so recovery is usually quicker.

**Osteotomy** Doctors sometimes recommend surgery to realign the bone (osteotomy). This is done to slow cartilage damage in the knee and relieve pain.

Trimming and repositioning the leg bones allows your body weight to be more evenly distributed across the knee joint, taking pressure off the arthritic area and moving it to intact cartilage. It also corrects curvature or bowing in the lower leg bones caused by osteoarthritis. Surgeons typically recommend this procedure for younger, more active people with damage mostly on one side of the knee.

**Joint fusion** Permanently fusing the parts of the knee together is an option for people who aren't candidates for knee replacement surgery — perhaps because of age, activity level or weight, or if an artificial knee becomes infected and can't be saved. Although fusion limits knee motion, it allows your leg to bear weight without pain.

**Joint replacement** Knee replacement surgery (total knee arthroplasty) can help relieve pain and restore function in severely diseased knee joints. More than 600,000 knee replacement surgeries are performed in the United States each year. Your doctor can choose from a wide variety of implant designs that take into account your age, size, activity level and overall health.

Most replacement procedures attempt to replicate your knee's natural ability to roll and glide as it bends. Although most people who undergo knee replacement are between the ages of 50 and 80, surgeons occasionally replace the knees of people who are younger. The active lifestyles of younger people may cause greater wear on an artificial knee, requiring it to be replaced in the future.

During the surgery, your surgeon cuts away damaged bone and cartilage from the lower thighbone (femur), the upper portion of the lower leg bone (tibia) and the kneecap. Your knee is kept in a bent position so that all surfaces of the joint are fully exposed.

After making an incision, the muscles, kneecap and connective tissues are moved aside, and the damaged bone and cartilage are cut away. The ligaments are realigned to hold the joint together after the prosthesis is in place. Leg bones also may be realigned.

Your surgeon smoothes the bones' rough edges and carefully measures the cut to ensure a good fit for your new prosthesis. The artificial joint is then put in place. Most implants are affixed with bone cement. Others are held in place by new bone growth. Before closing the incision, the surgeon will bend and rotate the new joint, testing and balancing it to ensure proper function.

Although you probably won't forget that you have an artificial knee — for example, your range of motion with a knee implant may never completely return to normal or you might hear clicking sounds when you walk — about 90% of people who have total knee replacement experience significant pain relief, improved mobility and better overall quality of life.

During the first weeks after surgery, physical activity will typically include a graduated walking program — first indoors, then outdoors — and knee strengthening exercises that you learn from a physical therapist. You may also be advised to slowly resume other normal household activities, including walking up and down stairs.

Femur

Tibia

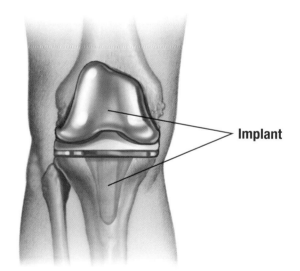

Implant

In total knee replacement, diseased bone and cartilage is removed from the end of the femur and a U-shaped component is attached. A T-shaped component is attached to the tibia, firmly anchored in the bone. The top of the T provides a resting place for the femoral component. A plastic spacer inserted between the two components functions as artificial cartilage by creating a smooth gliding surface. Some joints include another small component — a circular piece of plastic that attaches to your kneecap to replace damaged cartilage.

Three to six weeks after surgery — depending on your doctor's assessment — you can typically resume most normal daily activities, such as shopping and light housekeeping. You can usually start driving in four to six weeks if you can bend your knee far enough to sit in a car and you have enough muscle control to properly operate the brakes and accelerator. As early as six weeks after surgery, you may start to notice the improvement in your knee, compared with how it felt before the joint replacement.

Being active after joint replacement is important for keeping your new artificial joint working smoothly. After recovery, you can enjoy low-impact activities such as walking, moderate hiking, swimming, golf and recreational biking. Some surgeons recommend avoiding high-impact activities such as running or jogging, contact or jumping sports, high-impact aerobics, skiing, and tennis. Also avoid repetitive lifting of objects over 50 pounds. The stress these activities place on the knee may increase the risk of artificial joint failure.

***Partial knee replacement*** The knee joint includes three parts (compartments): the inside (medial) compartment, the outside (lateral) compartment, and the patellofemoral compartment, where the kneecap meets your femur. If arthritis has affected only one part of your knee, your doctor may suggest an implant to replace just the damaged part. This is known as a unicompartmental knee arthroplasty. This procedure is less extensive than total replacement and usually allows for faster recovery. A partial replace-

ment may also feel and move more like your natural knee.

To determine whether you're a candidate for the partial procedure, your surgeon must be certain that other parts of the joint are undamaged. Usually this can be determined by X-rays or MRI scans, but in some cases, your doctor may not make the decision until the time of surgery.

***Minimally invasive surgery*** In recent years, some surgeons have offered a procedure using a smaller incision. This may reduce trauma to muscles and tendons and result in a faster recovery and less scarring. Some early research suggested that overall

A partial knee replacement may be a good option for you if arthritis has affected only part of your knee joint. This surgery preserves the joint's healthy bone and tissues. Here, only the inside (medial) compartment of the knee joint was removed and replaced.

limb alignment may suffer when knee surgery is performed through smaller incisions, leading to complications. More research is still needed to know whether the procedure is as safe and effective as the conventional procedure in the long term.

## Ankles and feet

The joints in your ankles and feet, like those in your hips and knees, help carry the weight of your body. Various procedures are used to relieve pain and stabilize these joints. Bone resection in the feet — for example, the removal of bunions, bone spurs or other bony growths — can make walking and standing less painful.

***Debridement or osteotomy*** Removing cartilage and bone spurs (debridement) or surgically realigning the bone (osteotomy) can provide temporary relief from pain. These procedures may delay the need for more extensive surgery, perhaps for several years. They are most often performed arthroscopically. However, they can also be done as open surgery.

***Synovectomy*** For people with rheumatoid arthritis in the front of the foot, removing the inflamed synovial tissue in early stages of the disease may be able to provide pain relief before the cartilage becomes badly eroded. After the procedure, your doctor will likely recommend taking certain drugs to help control disease activity and reduce inflammation in your foot. (See Chapter 10 for more on medications.)

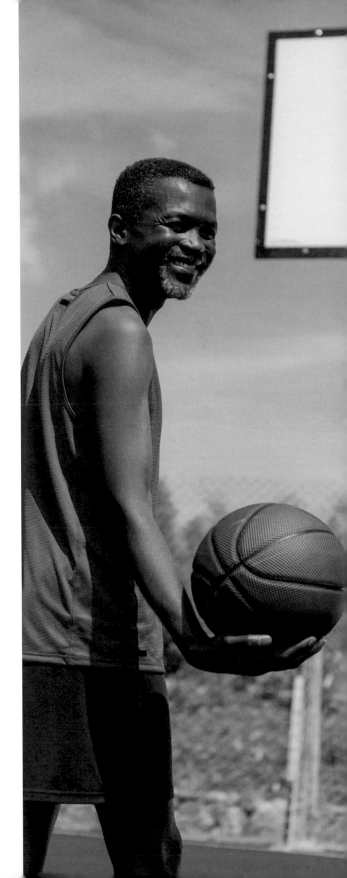

## WHAT ABOUT ARTHRITIS INVOLVING MULTIPLE JOINTS?

If you'll need more than one surgery to treat arthritis pain, you and your doctor can discuss which procedure should be performed first.

Surgery on the hips, knees, ankles and feet is usually done before surgery on the upper body joints. That's because using crutches after surgery on the lower extremities puts a lot of stress on the upper body.

When multiple lower body surgeries are required, hip surgery is typically performed before knee surgery to get the best possible knee alignment and pain relief. Ankle and foot surgeries are usually done before hip or knee replacement to provide stability for hip or knee rehabilitation.

When more than one surgery is needed on upper body joints, the order is controversial. Often, the more symptomatic joint is done first, but it's best to discuss options with your surgeon.

*Joint fusion* If your symptoms are severe, the surgeon may recommend fusing the bones in your foot or ankle to improve stability and reduce pain, particularly if the condition has changed the shape of the joint (caused deformity). Joint fusion is a standard treatment for arthritis of the ankle, although it can lead to changes in gait. It may also eventually cause arthritic changes in other joints of the foot. The procedure may be a good option if you're younger and you want to resume more-strenuous activities.

*Joint replacement* Ankle joint and foot joint replacements are newer and evolving

procedures that aren't widely used, partly because they lack a strong record of success. Early ankle implants often had complications, such as loosening, infection and persistent pain after the procedure.

Newer implant designs have reduced some of the problems and can provide good relief. And because implants allow the joint to move, unlike a joint fusion, they don't risk causing arthritis in other parts of the foot. But more research is still needed to know how these newer ankle replacements perform over time and who the best candidates are. If an artificial joint fails, it may be difficult to find a different treatment that can be successful.

## THINGS TO KNOW BEFORE SURGERY

Once your surgery is planned, you and your surgeon will determine when you can be admitted to the hospital. It's also good to arrange ahead of time for meals and other assistance to help you cope with changes in your activity level during recovery (see "Plan ahead for recovery" on pages 200–201).

Before surgery, your doctor will want to know your medical history and do a physical exam. People with arthritis need special considerations before surgery because of certain risks related to the disease:

*Cardiovascular risk* People with arthritis have a greater risk of heart disease. Your doctor may recommend a preoperative cardiac stress test to check whether you're at risk of a heart attack or other heart problems during or after surgery.

*Anesthesia concerns* Your doctor will discuss the risks of anesthesia with you before surgery. Arthritis in the neck (cervical spine) or jaw (temporomandibular joint) may increase the risk of problems with your airway while under anesthesia. If you have severe shifting (subluxation) of the cervical spine, the risk of a spinal cord injury is higher. In addition, having limited range of motion in your joints may make positioning your body for surgery difficult. X-rays may be needed before the surgery to assess these concerns.

*Infection risk* While taking your medical history and doing a physical exam, your doctor will assess your risk of infection. You may be checked for dental cavities; open, crater-like wounds especially around the feet (skin ulcerations); and signs or symptoms of a urinary tract infection. Your nutrition level also may be assessed since you're more likely to develop an infection if you're malnourished. As prevention, your doctor may have you take preoperative antibiotics.

*Disease activity and medication use* Before you have elective surgery, your rheumatologist should evaluate your level of disease activity and identify major organ involvement that may impact the surgery. Ideally, you should have surgery during periods when the disease is well controlled and you have a successful medication regimen. Your doctor will review your medications with you and explain any changes that may need to occur before, during and after surgery. He or she will consider the risks and benefits of changing any drug or dosage in your particular situation.

- *Steroids* Some corticosteroids may increase the risk of surgical site infections, skin tearing, fracture, gastrointestinal hemorrhage or ulcer. Most physicians will taper the steroid dose to the lowest dose possible prior to surgery to reduce these risks. One study found that among people who had hip or knee replacements, those taking more than 15 milligrams of prednisone daily had a twentyfold increase in risk of postoperative infection.
- *NSAIDs* These medications are typically stopped about a week before surgery to

## PLAN AHEAD FOR RECOVERY

Expect your recovery from surgery to take some time. It may be several months before you can resume all of your normal activities. To make things easier on yourself, plan for your return home after surgery before you go to the hospital:

- Talk with your doctor about how long you can expect to stay in the hospital after surgery. Some people now go home the same day after total hip or knee replacement surgery. Most people stay one or two nights, while some may need to stay longer. Certain other surgeries are outpatient procedures, meaning most people can plan to go home the same day.
- The best option after you've been discharged is to go directly home. Another option is to go to a loved one's home. Ask someone to accompany you as you leave the hospital, as you may not be able to drive right away.
- Ask someone — family member, friend or neighbor — to assist you for the first week or two at home. Or you may arrange for a temporary caregiver from a home health care agency or a short stay at a step-down care facility during this time. You shouldn't be alone for more than three or four hours at a time during this period.
- Your caregiver must be able to help you with activities around the house, such as getting dressed, using the bathroom, preparing meals and doing laundry.
- Leave your home clean and tidy before you go to surgery so that you won't need to clean much during your recovery.
- Move throw rugs, cords and other tripping hazards and clutter out of walkways.
- If possible, rearrange your bedroom with extra space around the bed to allow room to get in and out while using a walker or crutches. If your bedroom is up or down a flight of stairs, you may need to have your bed temporarily moved to a room on the main level of your home.

minimize the risk of bleeding. Acetaminophen (Tylenol, others) can usually be substituted for pain control, if necessary.

- ***Disease-modifying antirheumatic drugs (DMARDs)*** In the past, DMARDs such as methotrexate were often stopped before surgery. Doctors feared they might increase the risk of infection. But newer research suggests that in most cases, you can safely continue taking these medications leading up to a joint surgery. If you have a high risk of infection — say, due to

- Be sure to get instructions on how best to lie down and sit up in bed (see the illustration on page 349).
- Consider installing safety bars or a secure handrail in your shower or bath and arrange for a toilet-seat riser with arms if you have a low toilet. Try using a stable bench or chair in your shower.
- Make sure the handrails along your stairways are secure.
- Rearrange your kitchen so that you can easily reach utensils, tableware and food without bending, stretching or lifting.
- Stock up on food supplies. Prepare some meals in advance and freeze them to use after you return home.
- Set up one location as a "recovery center" where you'll spend most of your time. Make sure to have a sturdy armchair with a firm seat cushion and back — not a recliner. Gather the things you might want to have within easy reach: remote controls, telephone or cellphone, laptop computer or tablet, chargers, books, music player, tissues, medicine, and a pitcher of water.
- Ask your mail carrier to deliver to your door, if possible.
- If you wish, request a visit from your clergy person or spiritual adviser while you recover.
- Consider placing a clean plastic trash bag on the car seat to make it easier to turn and adjust your body once you're seated in the vehicle.
- If you're interested in getting assistance from a home health care agency or public health nurse while you recover from surgery, arrange it beforehand. Your doctor may be able to help you with referrals and arrangements.

uncontrolled diabetes or serious lung or liver disease — or a weakened immune system, your doctors may recommend skipping a few doses of the DMARD before and after surgery. Some doctors still recommend stopping medications such as leflunomide, sulfasalazine and azathioprine for a brief time before surgery.

- ***Biologics*** These medications are still not as well studied regarding the safety of taking them over the time of your surgery. Because of this, your doctor may ask you to stop taking them at least one cycle before the procedure to minimize the risk of infection. Your doctor may want to balance the risk of an infection or wound complication against the risk of a disease flare-up if you stop taking your medications. If you do discontinue a medication, you can usually start it again one or two weeks after surgery.

## Potential risks and complications

Joint surgeries can greatly improve your quality of life. Still, every surgery carries a risk of complications. Your medical team will monitor you closely during and after surgery to reduce the chance of infection, a blood clot in the lung, blood loss or a heart attack. Other rare complications may include having a nerve or blood vessel injured, a joint dislocation, bone loss, and even death.

*Infection* The location of an artificial joint implant is susceptible to infection, even in the long term. Bacteria can travel through your bloodstream and infect the site years after the procedure. Let your doctor know immediately if you notice warning signs such as a fever over 100 F, shaking, chills, drainage, and increasing redness, tenderness, swelling and pain around the artificial joint.

If you take a course of antibiotics and they fail to clear up the infection, you will likely need surgery to remove the infected joint and replace it with a new joint.

To reduce the risk of implant infection, your doctor may recommend antibiotics each time you have certain dental procedures, such as tooth extraction or periodontal work, as well as urological procedures and bowel surgery. Bacteria may also enter your bloodstream through cuts, scrapes and skin ulcers.

*Blood clots* Dangerous blood clots may form in a vein of the leg (deep vein thrombosis) or lung (pulmonary embolus) after surgery. Doctors commonly prescribe blood thinners, especially after hip and knee replacement, to help reduce the risk of developing a clot. During your hospital stay, you'll be encouraged to move your foot and ankle, which increases blood flow to your leg muscles and helps prevent swelling and blood clots. You may also need to wear support hose or compression boots to further protect against swelling and clotting.

*Blood loss* Joint surgeries may require a blood transfusion. The vast majority of people who receive transfusions have no adverse reactions. The use of a person's own blood (autologous transfusion), while popular in the past, is now rarely used. Analysis of people who used their own blood versus donated blood shows no difference in terms of side effects or reactions.

Certain methods now commonly used can lower the likelihood that you'll need a blood transfusion. These include medications given during surgery and blood collection devices used during the procedure that quickly infuse lost blood back to you. The method used will depend on the results of blood tests taken before your surgery and the anticipated blood loss.

***Loosening of artificial joints*** Implants may loosen, dislocate or wear out. However, improved designs and surgical techniques have helped replacement joints to last longer. Rarely, certain movements or an injury can dislocate an implanted artificial hip joint.

## Hospital stay

The length of your hospital stay after surgery will depend on many factors, including the type of joint operation you've had, your age and overall health. It also depends on whether you experience any complications after surgery.

After the procedure, the surgical care team will monitor your vital signs, alertness, and pain or comfort level and adjust your medications accordingly. Your doctor may prescribe an antibiotic to prevent infection and a blood thinner (anticoagulant) medication to reduce the risk of developing blood clots.

Procedures that use only small incisions and local anesthesia, such as arthroscopic debridement or synovectomy, frequently do not require an overnight stay in the hospital.

Physical therapy begins almost immediately after most joint procedures. Even though you might need assistance at first, you can expect to be up and out of your hospital bed several times daily. A physical therapist will help you practice the best ways to dress, sit down in a chair, get out of bed, use the toilet

## DISEASE-SPECIFIC ISSUES

Some forms of arthritis involve greater risk of certain complications during or after surgery. These include:

- *Sjögren's syndrome.* This condition causes dry eyes and mouth. During surgery, the care team may use lubricating gel and artificial tears to keep the corneas from becoming dry and scratched.
- *Rheumatoid arthritis.* People with rheumatoid arthritis have an increased risk of neck (cervical spine) and jaw problems. Special cervical spine X-rays may be necessary before surgery, and the anesthesiologist may need to use a flexible tube for intubation. In addition, people with rheumatoid arthritis may have low white blood cell counts and have an increased risk of infection, especially if they are taking arthritis medication that weakens the immune system.
- *Juvenile idiopathic arthritis (JIA).* Children with JIA who have surgery may have disturbances in their bone growth afterward. Joint replacement surgery is usually delayed until their bones are done growing. Intubation — for help with breathing during surgery — may be difficult in children who have disease activity in the cervical spine and jaw.
- *Ankylosing spondylitis.* People with this form of arthritis have an increased risk of heart disease and problems with the aortic valve. They also are at risk of lung disease, and changes in the upper back can affect their breathing motion. Positioning and intubation for surgery also may be difficult. After surgery, the disease may cause extra bone to form at the surgical site. This can cause pain and limit motion.

- *Psoriatic arthritis.* The risk of a skin flare may be higher at the time of surgery, due to stopping medication and the stress of the procedure.
- *Connective tissue diseases (lupus, scleroderma).* These diseases may affect multiple organs and can increase the risk of infection, blood clots and anemia, as well as heart, kidney and lung disease.

and climb stairs. Remarkably, most people leave the hospital within two to three days after total joint replacement — if not sooner.

## Rehabilitation

Exercise and rest are both important elements of recovery from joint surgery. It's absolutely essential that you follow the activity guidelines that your surgeon or physical therapist prescribes.

If you don't do the exercises, you can end up with a stiff, painful joint. But appropriate rest also is important. If you have rheumatoid arthritis in other joints, putting extra stress on them during the recovery period, while you're protecting the operated joint, may cause a flare-up.

Physical therapists can help you learn the proper way to move and protect a new or altered joint. Exercise can improve joint motion, strengthen the muscles around your joint, reduce pain and improve mobility. You may need to learn how to use assistive devices such as a walker, cane or crutches for support while the surgical site heals.

Occupational therapists can help you become more independent in daily activities. They may work with you on getting dressed, preparing food and bathing. They can also help you learn to use assistive devices such as dressing aids, grab bars, raised toilet seats and bath benches. The goal of rehabilitation is for you to become as independent as possible in your daily living.

Depending on your age, physical condition and home situation, your surgeon may recommend a short stay in a skilled nursing facility or rehabilitation center to allow you to focus fully on recovery before returning home.

## Recovery at home

To recover more quickly, you'll likely need to continue doing the recommended exercises at home. Your doctor and physical therapist can help you determine when you'll be able to resume your favorite activities. They can also identify positions or movements to avoid that may damage your joint.

If your surgery involved any joint below your waist (a weight-bearing joint), you'll probably need to use a walker, cane or crutches for a time after returning home. If you have difficulty getting around, your doctor may recommend in-home visits by a physical or occupational therapist.

Joint infection may still be a risk after you leave the hospital. Make sure to contact your doctor if you develop a fever, if your incision opens, or if you notice an increase of pain, tenderness, swelling, redness, warmth or fluid draining near the surgical site. Also watch for signs of circulation problems, such as increased swelling, pain or tenderness in your limbs.

During the first few weeks at home after getting a new weight-bearing joint, you'll typically have a graduated walking program. You'll start slowly and then build activity as you become more fit and accustomed to the artificial joint. You'll also continue strengthening exercises. You may be advised to slowly resume other normal household activities, including walking up and down stairs.

Three to eight weeks after a joint replacement — depending on the procedure you had and on your doctor's assessment — you generally can resume most normal daily activities, such as shopping and light housekeeping. Driving is generally possible in four to eight weeks after hip or knee replacement. You'll need to be able to bend the knee far enough to sit in a car and have enough muscle control to operate the brakes and accelerator.

## NEW LEASE ON LIFE

Full recovery from a joint operation may take only a few weeks for certain tendon, ligament or cartilage procedures. Some types of joint fusion, osteotomy or joint replacements can require several months to a year of recovery before your bones fully heal and you regain maximum strength, stability and mobility.

Many people have less pain and swelling, as well as easier movement, in just days after the procedure. Your age, overall physical health and commitment to rehabilitation can all play a role in how quickly you recover. Follow-up visits with your doctor also are important.

Although recovering from joint surgery takes time, the outcome gives many people a new lease on life. Many years after surgery, most recipients of an artificial hip or knee are still able to move around comfortably. You may need to permanently avoid vigorous, high-impact activities, even after successful joint replacement and dedicated rehabilitation and care. Nevertheless, if you and your doctor decide it's time, joint surgery can lead you toward an active, fulfilling future.

# Pain management

Sharp. Throbbing. Nagging. Stiff. Burning. Achy. Agonizing. There may be millions of ways to talk about arthritis pain — one for each person who has arthritis.

No matter how you describe the sensation, joint pain can keep you from doing the things you would like to do. Treatment can help fix what's making your joint hurt. But meanwhile, you may have to deal with the discomfort.

Pain is influenced by many factors, including your activity level, your physical condition, the amount of swelling in your joints, your tolerance of pain and your state of mind.

Your approach to treating pain may be as individualistic as the symptoms that you're experiencing. The use of medications to re-duce inflammation and relieve pain is a major element of most treatment plans (see Chapter 10). Some approaches focus on building a lifestyle that minimizes pain. You can learn better posture and body mechanics and use special devices that help with daily tasks (see Chapter 18).

You can also work at strengthening your muscles, tendons and ligaments to stabilize your damaged joints (see Chapter 15). In addition, losing weight may lessen the stress on joints (see Chapter 16). And building a positive attitude that helps keep pain in perspective can be valuable as well (see Chapter 17).

In many ways, this entire book is about the defining characteristic of arthritis — pain. There are many ways to understand it and to deal with it.

This chapter focuses on common approaches to pain management. The first section explains simple treatments for short-term (acute) pain. Many of these can be performed at home. The second section discusses professional treatment of pain aside from medications.

## TREATING ACUTE PAIN

Acute arthritis pain comes on quickly and lasts a short time, but it completely disrupts your day. It's severe pain that prevents you from working in the kitchen, typing on a keyboard or climbing a flight of stairs.

You can use either cold or heat to help relieve pain, but it may be a matter of trial and error to find which temperature — or combination — works best. Before using cold or heat, make sure your skin is dry and free of cuts and sores. Use a towel to protect the skin from direct contact with cold or heat, especially in areas where bone is close to the skin surface.

### Cold

Cold is especially good for pain from arthritis flare-ups, as well as overuse injuries. Cold has a numbing effect on the painful area, dulling the sensation. It decreases muscle spasms and may reduce swelling and inflammation. Applying cold is typically recommended in the initial days of a flare-up. However, don't use cold if you have poor circulation or numbness in your skin.

*Ice packs* You can pick up ice packs at many drugstores, department stores and pharma-

---

### HOT AND COLD PACKS

A reusable gel-filled pack is perhaps the safest, most convenient commercially available product for applying either heat or cold to an affected joint. It's inexpensive and is found in most pharmacies.

You typically heat the pack in hot water or a microwave oven or chill the pack in a freezer. The heat or cold dissipates as the pack is used, so it's generally safe to apply it for 20 to 30 minutes at a time. You can also use it to treat minor muscle sprains and strains and minor tendinitis. Be sure to follow the product manufacturer's instructions.

cies. Instant ice packs may be helpful if you don't have easy access to freezer gel packs. They're simple to use — squeezing the pack will activate its contents.

Before using an ice pack, make sure to wrap it in a thin towel so the cold surface isn't directly against your skin. This will also help the pack stay cold longer.

You may apply cold several times a day for 15 to 20 minutes at a time. Regularly check that skin color is normal where you apply it. Losing color in your skin may mean you're starting to get frostbite. Stop immediately if this happens.

*Helpful hint:* To make your own ice pack, combine ⅓ cup of rubbing alcohol with ⅔ cup of water. Seal the mixture inside a freezer bag. Put this bag inside another freezer bag, seal it and chill the pack in a freezer. It's ready to use when it's slushy. You can refreeze the contents after use. A bag of frozen vegetables, such as corn or peas, also can work. Just take care not to eat the frozen vegetables if they have been defrosted and frozen again.

**Ice massage** This method also applies cold to your skin. Wrap an ice cube or small ice block in cloth and hold it comfortably in your hand. Use a circular motion to move the ice in and around your painful joint for five to seven minutes. Apply mild pressure and remember to keep the ice moving when it's in direct contact with your skin.

Remember to watch for color changes in your skin. If you notice your skin losing its underlying natural tone, stop immediately. If your skin becomes numb during the massage, stop the treatment.

*Helpful hint:* Make an ice block by freezing water in a paper cup. Peel back part of the cup to expose enough ice for a massage. Wrap the sides of the cup in a towel to protect your hands.

## Heat

Heat helps relax muscles and soothes painful joints. It also encourages blood flow to the affected area. Heat is especially good for easing stiffness and getting muscles limber.

If you have poor circulation or numbness in the area, don't apply high heat — you won't know if you're getting burned. In addition, don't apply heat after acute trauma or over an area that is swollen. It could increase the swelling and pain even more.

***Hot packs and heating pads*** Lay a towel or cloth over the painful area. Lay a hot pack on top of the towels. Cover the pack with another layer or two of towels to keep it hot. Add or remove towels above or below to vary the heat. You may add extra layers over your skin in spots where bones sit close to the skin. Apply the heat for 20 to 30 minutes.

Check your skin every 15 minutes. If you see red and white blotches, stop treatment immediately. Continuing to heat the area could cause a burn or blister.

## DESCRIBING PAIN

It's not hard to recognize pain when you experience it. It's more difficult to describe what you're feeling to your doctor. And yet the details you provide at a medical visit may be extremely valuable in diagnosing and treating a condition, such as arthritis, or in helping you manage its symptoms.

In fact, it's hard to be objective when you're describing pain. Your personal experience of pain is influenced, in part, by your physical and emotional health and your mood, all of which may change from day to day. Pain tolerance varies greatly, and the pain that you may try to brush off as "nothing" one day may feel unbearable on another day.

Your doctor may use a numerical rating scale, which allows you to verbally rate pain on a scale of 0 to 10, with 0 representing no pain and 10 representing the worst pain imaginable. When you're talking to your doctor, the following questions also may help you describe your symptoms better:

- Where is the pain located? Does it remain in that place or does it tend to spread to other areas?
- When and how did the pain start? Were you doing any activities at the time that you normally don't do? Did you have any illness before the pain started?
- Is the pain continuous or intermittent? If intermittent, how long does the discomfort last?
- Does the pain feel mild, moderate or severe?
- What is the quality of the pain? For example, does it feel throbbing, dull, sharp or burning?
- Are there associated symptoms? For example, is there weakness, headache, or numbness and tingling along with pain?
- Does the pain change when you do certain activities or movements? Does it affect your ability to perform simple tasks?
- Does the pain keep you from sleeping or does it awaken you from sleep?
- Have you tried anything to manage the pain?

To protect your skin from burning, don't lie on a hot pack or heating pad or apply pressure during treatment.

*Helpful hint:* Make your own heat pack by placing a wet washcloth in a freezer bag and heating it in the microwave for one minute. Wrap the hot pack in a towel and place it near the affected joint. You can also fill a cotton tube sock with rice or another grain (other than popcorn), knot the open end, and warm it in the microwave.

**Baths, showers and hot tubs** One of the easiest, most effective ways to apply heat to a painful joint is to take a 15-minute hot shower or bath. A standard bathtub can be just as effective as a hot tub.

In a very warm bath or shower, remember to use extra caution — and the grab bars — when entering or leaving the stall. You could become lightheaded or even faint, causing a fall.

*Helpful hint:* Sticking clothes in the dryer for a few minutes before dressing can help erase morning stiffness. Or turn on an electric blanket for a few minutes before getting out of bed.

**Heat lamps** You can also warm a painful joint using an infrared heat lamp with a reflector heat bulb, or clamp lamps or incubator lights equipped with low-cost incandescent bulbs. Incandescent lights release most of their energy as heat, significantly increasing blood circulation in the affected area.

Position the heat source approximately 18 to 20 inches from your skin. Then apply the heat for 20 to 30 minutes. You can decrease the intensity of the heat by moving the lamp farther away. Direct the lamp at the skin from the side rather than from above.

*Helpful hint:* Use an alarm clock or timer while you're using the heat lamp to make sure the heat doesn't stay on too long. Or ask someone to wake you if you think you might fall asleep.

## Contrast baths

Contrast baths are helpful to many people with rheumatoid arthritis or osteoarthritis of the hands and feet. Alternating between warm and cold water may provide more relief than a hot or cold bath alone.

Start with two large pans. Fill one pan with warm water (approximately 97 to 104 F) and the other one with cool water (approximately 55 to 61 F). Place your joint in the warm water first for 10 minutes and then in the cold water for one minute. Cycle back to the warm water for four minutes and then to the cold for one minute.

Repeat this process for half an hour. Always end with your hands or feet in the warm water. If pans aren't available, twin sinks work just as well for soaking your hands.

*Helpful hint:* Because you're immersing your skin directly into the baths, use water that is warm, not hot, and cool, not icy.

## PROFESSIONAL HELP FOR PAIN

Various health care professionals may bring a broad range of experience and expertise to your pain management team. Your family physician or rheumatologist may prescribe medication to help control your discomfort, along with exercises and other therapies. But your treatment may also include seeing a physical therapist, occupational therapist, physiatrist, psychiatrist, psychologist and perhaps even a specialist of integrative medicine, such as an acupuncturist. These professionals may use different methods and techniques to help you manage pain.

### Devices to control pain

Orthotics is a medical specialty dealing with supportive devices for the body. The devices may control the function of a joint, assist or restrict its movement, and reduce pressure on the joint. Many products including insoles, splints and braces can be used to help relieve arthritis pain.

***Foot orthotics*** If you've lost foot or ankle support due to the deterioration of a joint, most often from rheumatoid arthritis, it can lead to strain on the associated knee or hip. Foot orthotic devices, including heel cups, arch supports and molded boots, can help stabilize arthritic joints, thus reducing stress on other joints and helping relieve pain.

***Shoe insoles*** Special insoles placed inside your shoes may provide pain relief due to osteoarthritis of the knee. The doctor may recommend a medial-wedge insole or a lateral-wedge insole, depending on how it alters knee function. When using insoles, it's important to wear appropriate footwear with cushioning that properly supports your weight-bearing joints and your back.

***Knee braces*** Braces are used on the lower limbs to decrease weight-bearing pressure and provide stability. Knee braces are helpful to some individuals with osteoarthritis. They may help reduce pain and increase knee mobility.

### Therapies to control pain

Professionals may prescribe the following to help you reduce or manage pain. Some of these fall under the heading of integrative medicine. A full discussion of various integrative medicine treatments used for treating arthritis pain can be found in Chapter 13.

***Physical exercise*** Exercise is perhaps your best defense against pain. Your doctor may have you work with a physical therapist to develop an exercise program that maximizes your range of motion. It can also strengthen the muscles around your painful joints. Exercise is discussed in more detail in Chapter 15.

**Massage** Massage can improve blood circulation, help you relax, and reduce pain and swelling. Some therapists are specially trained in massage techniques for people with arthritis.

During massage, heed the warnings of pain. If you're giving yourself a massage or a family member is massaging you, remember to stop the moment it starts to hurt. If the joint itself is swollen or painful, avoid massaging it and instead massage adjacent muscles.

Try warming or cooling the area before massage. Use a lotion or massage oil to help hands glide smoothly over the skin.

*Helpful hint:* If you're using massage oil or lotion on the affected area, wash it off before heat treatment to avoid burns.

**Specialized heat treatments** Unlike more simplified home heat treatments, a physical therapist may use specialized techniques or equipment to provide pain relief.

One of these treatments may involve soaking sore joints, particularly hands, in a warm paraffin bath. With instruction from the therapist, you may be able to use warm paraffin at home.

For deeper penetration, the therapist may use ultrasound or shortwave diathermy, which applies an electromagnetic current at higher frequencies to generate heat. This procedure requires careful monitoring because it may worsen some forms of arthritis.

**Steroid injections** Steroid medications are prescribed to reduce pain and inflammation in joints. Your doctor may inject cortisone directly into an acutely inflamed joint — for example, a knee, a hip or an ankle — to ease discomfort. For more information on joint injections, see Chapter 14.

**Nerve block** Your doctor may use an anesthetic injection to deaden the nerves in a targeted area of your body that's painful, interrupting pain signals to the brain. The relief is temporary, but treatment provides a welcome respite from chronic arthritic pain.

**Transcutaneous electrical nerve stimulation (TENS)** This therapy is used to treat targeted areas of your body that are painful. Electrodes placed on your skin near the painful areas deliver mild, painless electric pulses to nearby nerve pathways. The strength of the pulses may be adjusted as needed to control pain.

TENS is thought to work in several ways. The stimulation may overpower pain signals in nerve pathways, reducing the pain messages that reach your brain. TENS treatment may also trigger a release of endorphins — chemicals in your body with painkilling effects similar to those of morphine.

TENS generally works best for acute pain from a pinched nerve. Studies show that TENS has mixed results in treating chronic pain, but it does give relief for some people with arthritis. Most often, TENS is used in combination with exercise and other pain treatments.

Similar to TENS, a treatment called percutaneous electrical nerve stimulation (PENS) delivers electric pulses to the nerve pathways. But instead of delivering the current through electrodes, PENS uses needles that penetrate your skin to just below the surface. These needles are very thin, like those used in acupuncture. Most people feel some sensation, but not pain, when the needles are inserted.

## Behavioral approaches to control pain

Positive thinking can be vital to coping with chronic pain. Being positive doesn't mean you're trying to ignore the hurt. It means that you approach your condition in a positive, productive manner, looking for ways to make the best happen, not the worst.

However, you may reach a point at which you need extra support to cope with arthritis symptoms. That's when professionals may be able to help you.

***Cognitive behavioral therapy*** With cognitive behavioral therapy, you work with a counselor in a structured way to become more aware of inaccurate or negative thinking. The therapy allows you to view challenging situations clearly and respond to them in more-effective ways.

The goals for treating arthritis will likely include identifying and modifying your negative reactions to pain. And you'll learn how to change behavior in ways that help you better manage life despite the pain.

Cognitive behavioral therapy is generally focused on specific problems and uses a goal-oriented approach. It requires you to be more aware of your thoughts, emotions and beliefs about your condition. It also helps you recognize habits in everyday life that may be contributing to the problem.

## Related treatments

In addition to behavioral approaches to managing pain, you may learn other ways to build support.

***Biofeedback*** Your body has automatic, involuntary reactions to stress and pain: changes in muscle tension, skin temperature, blood pressure and heart rate. The goals of biofeedback are to teach you to recognize these reactions and learn to modify them.

During a session with a therapist, you're attached to monitors that track your physiologic systems — heart, respiration, muscle tension, skin temperature and brain activity. The therapist, with the help of this output, can teach you to control involuntary reactions that trigger the stress symptoms.

***Relaxation training*** You can learn to relax your body and mind with a variety of techniques, including progressive muscle relaxation, deep breathing, guided imagery and meditation. Some of these techniques are described in greater detail in Chapter 13.

With the help of an instructor, you can learn how to take short breaks, whenever you're feeling overwhelmed by stress or pain, to concentrate and relax. Eventually, you learn to relax on your own, without taking cues from someone else.

The ideal location for relaxation is a quiet room where you can rest comfortably on a bed, in a reclining chair or even on the floor. You should feel at ease, not cramped or confined.

You may enjoy audiovisual resources to help you focus, for example, playing a soft recording of ocean waves or forest sounds. Soft lighting that's easy on the eyes is often preferable.

The goal of a relaxation strategy is to reduce tension buildup in your body. You can employ the strategy throughout the day, whenever you feel stress or pain building up. In this way, you may prevent the tension from getting worse and successfully complete activities in your daily life.

***Chronic pain centers*** If your arthritis pain is severe, your doctor may recommend visiting a chronic pain center. In this setting, you may undergo outpatient treatment from a team of pain specialists. The program may last from several days to several weeks.

The center may be useful if you're not getting any respite from chronic pain and the pain treatments you're using, such as medications, injections and surgery, don't seem to affect it. An interdisciplinary approach to pain relief at these centers is essential because it's unlikely that any one technique will work to control pain.

The professionals can help treat pain and associated conditions such as depression. They may also help you deal with potential consequences of arthritis, such as family disruption and loss of income.

# Integrative medicine

Conventional medicine has much to offer in helping you manage your arthritis. But standard arthritis medicines may not "cure" arthritis or completely control your symptoms. You may still have good days and not-so-good days.

In addition, some conventional arthritis treatments carry the risk of unwanted and even serious side effects, especially after long-term use. For these reasons and others, many people with arthritis turn to integrative medicine.

Integrative medicine is the practice of using proven complementary treatments alongside conventional treatments. Integrative treatments don't replace conventional medicine. Instead, they complement existing treatments with the goal of improving outcomes. You may know these treatments by other names, such as complementary and alternative medicine.

More than a third of adults in the United States use some kind of integrative medicine as part of their health care. Supplements, meditation, chiropractic care, yoga and massage are all examples.

Pain is a powerful motivator in the hunt for new treatments that may provide relief. In fact, research shows that chronic pain is the top reason people try integrative medicine. Integrative therapies can effectively treat many types of pain, including back pain, neck pain, and arthritis and joint pain.

This chapter will help you learn about integrative therapies that may enhance your treatment plan. You'll find background information as well as tips on using these treatments wisely. Use the information here to guide you when you talk with your arthritis team about options for your care.

## CHOOSING AN INTEGRATIVE THERAPY

One of the key differences between integrative therapies and conventional medicine is testing. Conventional medicine, particularly in the United States, is designed around clinical trials that rigorously test the medicines on thousands of people.

When a medicine or therapy is approved by the Food and Drug Administration, it means that regulators are fairly certain that the drug is safe and effective for most people who are meant to take it and who take it as instructed.

Many integrative therapies — such as massage therapy, herbal supplements and meditation — have been used for a thousand years or more. But these therapies didn't start out in a lab or go through a study. Instead, they were found by trial and error. They're still used today because many people find them helpful.

This means scientists are playing catch-up in their efforts to test many of these therapies on a large scale. Researchers are still learning how they work and making sure they're truly safe and effective. Evidence is still emerging, so it's important to use common sense when considering integrative therapies.

### Discuss your options

Many people who use integrative therapies often don't talk about them with their doctor. They assume their doctor either won't be interested or will be opposed to the treatments. But not telling your doctor about all of the therapies you're using, traditional or nontraditional, can be dangerous.

For example, just because an integrative therapy is said to be "natural" doesn't mean it's safe to use. Some dietary supplements and herbs touted as being natural can cause problems with the conventional medications you may be taking.

If you're thinking about trying an integrative therapy, talk about it with your doctor first. Many doctors see the value of integrative practices and can help you blend them into your treatment plan. Your doctor may not know enough about a particular therapy to endorse it, but he or she may be able to show you studies on its risks and benefits or give you resources that can help you evaluate your options.

Regardless of what your doctor thinks about integrative medicine, it's important that he or she knows what you're doing. That allows you to get the best possible care and avoid dangerous interactions.

### Assess the risks and benefits

Some integrative therapies pose very little risk while offering wonderful benefits. For

## WHAT'S IN A NAME?

The terms used to describe health care methods that fall outside of mainstream medicine have shifted over the last several decades.

In the early 1990s, many of these methods were labeled as "unconventional" or "alternative." Later, they were referred to as complementary and alternative medicine (CAM), an umbrella term that's still used today. It includes a diverse range of systems, practices and products that aren't typically part of conventional practice.

There's an important distinction to be made:
- Complementary therapies are treatments used in conjunction with conventional medicine. For example, you may practice tai chi along with taking standard pain medication to relieve pain.
- Alternative therapies are used in place of conventional medicine. An example of this is seeing a homeopath or naturopath instead of your regular doctor.

Among the general public, this distinction isn't always clear. Many people use the term "alternative medicine" as a catchall phrase for all health practices that aren't typically part of mainstream medicine.

Today, medicine has shifted in focus toward prevention and whole-body wellness, and doctors are integrating unconventional therapies into their practices. Therapies that were once called alternative or complementary may now be described as integrative. As the term suggests, integrative medicine refers to using natural or holistic practices as a complement to conventional medicine. Integrative therapies are used alongside conventional medicine to optimize health through nutrition, exercise, stress management and social connection.

This is done by combining the best of today's high-tech tests and procedures with the best of nontraditional practice. This approach can help soothe stress, reduce pain and anxiety, maintain strength and flexibility, and promote a sense of well-being.

## WHAT MAKES A GOOD STUDY?

When doing research on treatments for arthritis, here are two types of studies you may find.

*Randomized controlled trial.* A randomized controlled trial is basic to most medical research. It's designed to evaluate a new medication or other form of treatment. In this type of study, participants are usually divided into two groups. One group gets the treatment being studied. The other group is the control group. People in the control group get standard treatment, no treatment or an inactive substance called a placebo. Participants are placed in these groups randomly. This helps ensure all of the groups will be similar.

*Double-blind studies.* In this type of trial, neither the researchers nor the participants know who's getting the active treatment and who's getting the inactive treatment, or placebo. With this approach, the results are objective. Still, because people can vary so much, many doctors prefer to see whether the results of later trials can confirm the results of a particular study. Often, only then are a study's results considered to be conclusive.

example, meditation and relaxed breathing are unlikely to cause harm. They're easy to learn, you can do them anywhere at any time, and they can help you to relax and reduce stress.

On the flip side, buying an herbal supplement that's touted as an arthritis cure may be risky. Supplements are complex mixtures of compounds found in nature. While there are many reputable supplement manufacturers in the United States, dietary supplements in general aren't regulated with the same strict oversight as are prescription drugs. Your product may have varying or unknown amounts of the active ingredient.

Even though stronger regulations have been in place in the United States since 2010, herbal products of poor or unreliable quality can still reach store shelves. This may cause your doctor to be skeptical about taking them. Keep in mind that any potential benefits may be offset by the risks. So think critically, and use reputable sources and providers.

## Finding a provider

When you're looking for someone who practices the type of integrative therapy you're interested in, choose someone in the same way you would choose a new doctor. Look at his or her qualifications and experience. Ask for a referral from a trusted health care professional or a friend or family member who has had the treatment you're considering. Many universities and teaching hospitals, including Mayo Clinic, now have integrative health programs that offer a holistic, evidence-based approach to health care.

If you're evaluating a licensed practitioner, check with your local and state medical boards for information on credentials and whether any complaints have been filed against the individual.

You can also contact well-established professional organizations, such as the American Academy of Medical Acupuncture, for the names of certified practitioners in your area. Keep in mind, though, that for many integrative therapies, there are no licensure or certification standards.

## Consider treatment cost

The integrative treatment you're considering may not be covered by your health insurance plan. Check with your insurance company first. If you have to pay for it out of pocket, find out how much it will cost. If possible, get it in writing before you start treatment.

## Keep your mind open and objective

Look at integrative therapies objectively. Stay open to possibilities, but take a close look at any treatment you're considering.

# FORMS OF INTEGRATIVE THERAPY

Many different forms of integrative medicine can ease symptoms and help you cope with arthritis. Each type of therapy may work in a different way to improve your physical and emotional health and your quality of life.

This section outlines five common types of integrative medicine:
- Mind-body medicine
- Herbs and other dietary supplements
- Energy therapies
- Hands-on therapies
- Alternative medical and healing systems

In each section, you'll learn about therapies that are used the most and have shown to be the most helpful.

# MIND-BODY MEDICINE

People have long believed that your state of mind can influence your physical body and your health. More recently, research using imaging techniques such as functional MRI have confirmed this. Mind-body techniques that promote relaxation can be helpful for people with arthritis. They can help ease tension, which may also help reduce pain and improve physical functioning. Mind-body techniques usually get the green light for use from doctors.

You can learn to do most of these techniques yourself. Many are inexpensive or free. To get the full benefit, practice them regularly.

## Aromatherapy

This ancient form of healing uses essential oils from flowers, herbs and trees to promote health and well-being. Practitioners believe that when these oils are massaged into the skin or inhaled, they help treat symptoms, including arthritis pain and inflammation. Originally popular in Europe, aromatherapy is increasingly being used in the United States. Aromatherapy treatments are found in stores that sell natural health products.

More study is needed to say for sure if the plant oils used in aromatherapy are of benefit to health and well-being. Limited research has been done on the use of aromatherapy for arthritis.

## Biofeedback

Biofeedback teaches you how to control your body's responses to arthritis pain. During a biofeedback session, a trained therapist applies electrodes and electronic sensors to your body. The sensors monitor your physical response to stress — including your heart rate, breathing patterns, body temperature and muscle activity. The sensors then feed the information back to you via sound and visual cues.

With this feedback, you can learn how to control your body's responses and enter into a relaxed state that helps you cope with arthritis pain. Once you learn how to control the responses in your doctor's office, you can learn to control them on your own at home, without the help of a therapist or technology.

You can get biofeedback treatments in physical therapy clinics, medical centers and hospitals. To find a qualified biofeedback therapist, ask your doctor for a recommendation. The Biofeedback Certification International Alliance is another resource for finding a biofeedback therapist.

There are also self-directed, computer-guided biofeedback programs currently on the market that may help you learn basic breathing and meditation exercises for stress management.

## Guided imagery

Imagery is a thought process that invokes the senses — you use it to see in your mind's eye. Guided imagery, also called visualization, has been used by different cultures throughout the ages as a healing tool.

With guided imagery, you close your eyes to the outside world and create a soothing mental picture that helps your mind to promote healing. In your mind's eye, for example, you might see yourself lying on a beach on a warm summer day listening to gentle waves lapping on the shore.

When you imagine the beach, your brain is activated almost as if you were actually feeling the sand on your toes. The message your brain receives is relayed to other parts of your body that control your heart rate and blood pressure. With repeated practice, your relaxed state during guided imagery may help relieve pain, fatigue and other symptoms. In turn, this may reduce your need for medications.

## Hypnosis

Hypnosis is often portrayed humorously on TV and in films, but it can be an effective health treatment. Hypnosis induces a state of deep relaxation that helps you concentrate and makes you more open to the power of suggestion.

For instance, if you're open to a suggestion to relax, you may respond less to the world around you. You can use hypnosis to help manage pain — or at least shift your attention away from it. Several studies have found that hypnosis can be useful in pain management, although they haven't focused specifically on its use with arthritis. And research shows that hypnotism works better for some adults than others.

Scientists don't understand exactly how hypnosis works. It appears to alter brain wave patterns in much the same way that other relaxation techniques do. It seems to influence nerve impulses, hormones and chemicals that affect how your brain communicates with your body.

## Meditation

Meditation has been around for thousands of years. It can help you enter into a deep, restful state that reduces your body's stress response.

There are many paths to meditation. In general, when you're meditating, you're paying attention to the present moment, not on past

## GET STARTED WITH RELAXATION TECHNIQUES

You can master simple relaxation techniques with a little practice. Use this approach whenever you feel increasing stress, pain or muscle tension.

*Relaxed breathing.* Stress or pain typically causes rapid, shallow breathing. This kind of breathing helps your body respond to stress by boosting your heart rate and causing you to sweat. By controlling your breathing, the effects of stress will become less intense, and you'll be able to keep the effects of stress from spiraling out of control.

Here's how to use relaxed breathing in times of stress:
- *Inhale.* With your mouth closed and your shoulders relaxed, inhale deeply by slowly pushing your stomach out as you count to six. Allow the air to fill your diaphragm, the muscle under your rib cage.
- *Exhale.* Release the air through your mouth as you slowly count to six.
- *Repeat.* Complete this cycle three to five times.

*Progressive muscle relaxation.* The goal of progressive muscle relaxation is to reduce muscle tension. First, find a quiet place where you'll be free from interruption. Loosen tight clothing and remove your glasses or contacts if you'd like. Find a comfortable position — seated or lying down.

Starting with your feet and working up through your body to your neck and head, tense each muscle group for at least five seconds and then relax the muscles for up to 30 seconds. Repeat before moving to the next muscle group. Areas to concentrate on include your feet, legs, stomach, back, chest, hands, arms, shoulders, neck and face. Each session should last about 10 minutes.

As you learn to relax, you'll start to notice when stress causes your muscles to tense up. You'll also start to notice other physical changes that stress causes in your body. Knowing how stress makes you feel will help you make a conscious effort to relax whenever you feel stress building. And remember, relaxation is a skill. As with any skill, you'll get better with practice.

concerns or future anxieties. You focus on your breathing or on a mantra — a simple sound or phrase repeated over and over.

During meditation, you suspend the flow of emotions and thoughts that normally fill your mind. This helps you achieve a deep mental calmness and state of relaxation. It may also help you control how you respond to challenging and stressful situations.

Today, many people meditate for spiritual reasons, but meditation may have health benefits, too. Meditating regularly can slow your brain waves, boost your mood and decrease your muscle tension, blood pressure and heart rate. It can also lessen your body's response to the chemicals it produces when you're stressed by pain.

Meditation is often practiced on its own. Some people start with simply sitting quietly and paying attention to their breathing. Meditation can be combined with other therapies, such as yoga and tai chi. You can even meditate while walking or jogging.

### Yoga and tai chi

Yoga and tai chi are efficient, low-impact activities that can help you maintain both physical fitness and mental clarity. With regular practice, you can gradually increase your strength and flexibility while enhancing the connection of your mind, body and spirit.

Yoga combines breathing exercises, physical postures, meditation and other techniques that originated in India more than 5,000 years ago.

There are many different styles of yoga. Hatha is one of the most common forms. It involves different body postures that are held for various lengths of time and done in a sequence.

In the United States, yoga has become increasingly popular as a fitness activity. Don't be intimidated, though, if what comes to mind are "power yoga" or "hot yoga" classes featuring strength-intensive moves. Many forms of yoga can benefit your strength and flexibility with gentler movements. In a class, you also can ask the instructor to suggest modified poses to accommodate joint pain or a limited range of motion.

Tai chi is an ancient Chinese tradition that combines rhythmic movements, breathing techniques and focused attention. A self-paced series of postures are performed in a slow, graceful manner. Each body position flows into the next as one continuous movement.

Yoga and tai chi may improve quality of life and relieve pain from osteoarthritis. In part, these practices help by improving how well you move and enhancing your strength, flexibility and balance. Studies have shown that tai chi can improve range of motion in people with rheumatoid arthritis. Both yoga and tai chi promote relaxation and help reduce stress, which often goes hand in hand with chronic pain.

Some postures may strain your lower back and joints, so be careful. Don't push to perform a pose that feels uncomfortable. It's best to work with a yoga and tai chi instructor who knows about your health condition and can help you make adjustments if needed.

## HERBS AND OTHER DIETARY SUPPLEMENTS

Herbs and dietary supplements make up the broadest category of integrative therapies. This category encompasses a range of ingredients found in nature, including herbs, vitamins, minerals, amino acids, animal extracts and enzymes.

Herbs and dietary supplements are the most commonly used form of integrative medicine in the United States. About 1 in 5 adults uses some type of natural product.

Herbal treatments have been in use for thousands of years. Many of today's conventional medicines — including digoxin, which is used for congestive heart failure, and quinine, used for malaria, were once considered folk medicines. Scientists continue to discover new medicines derived from plants and herbs.

Many herbal preparations are marketed as alternative pain relievers and inflammation fighters for arthritis. As experts learn more about how to treat pain and other symptoms of arthritis, researchers are also working to improve evidence-based knowledge about these herbal treatments.

But it's hard to apply traditional scientific research to dietary supplements. Many products are complex mixtures of natural ingredients that often can't be tested in the same manner as conventional medications, in which one compound is tested for one disease. Different brands of the same herb may have varying amounts of the active ingredient in them.

In addition, research hasn't established guidelines around how much of a supplement to take and what side effects supplements may cause. So it's important to talk to your doctor before taking any herbs or dietary supplements.

## Best bets

If you're interested in adding an integrative medicine supplement to your arthritis treatment, you may want to look to the following products. While everyone responds differently to treatments, research has shown these to be generally safe and sometimes helpful.

***Glucosamine and chondroitin*** Glucosamine and chondroitin are natural compounds found in cartilage — the tough, pliable tissue that cushions joints. Glucosamine supplements are made from the outer skeletons of shellfish. Chondroitin supplements are made from sources such as shark cartilage. The two compounds are often used together. Taken separately or together, these supplements are the second most used of all natural products, second only to fish oil.

There have been dozens of clinical trials on glucosamine for osteoarthritis — most often for osteoarthritis of the knee. Unfortunately, these studies have yielded mixed results.

In a two-year study from the National Institutes of Health known as the Glucosamine/ Chondroitin Arthritis Intervention Trial (GAIT), glucosamine and chondroitin were used to treat more than 1,500 people with osteoarthritis of the knee. Results suggested that glucosamine sulfate, when used with chondroitin, helped a small group of people with moderate to severe knee pain. But the researchers couldn't say for sure if it was helpful for overall pain relief.

More research is also needed to say how effective these supplements are in treating rheumatoid arthritis. Early research suggests that glucosamine and chondroitin may lessen pain, but they don't seem to lessen inflammation or help with painful and swollen joints.

Glucosamine and chondroitin appear to be safe, with few side effects. However, if you're allergic to shellfish, you should avoid them. And be cautious if you take a blood thinner, such as warfarin, because glucosamine may increase the risk of bleeding.

Like many supplements, glucosamine can take longer than most prescription drugs to be effective. So you may want to use a supplement for four to six weeks or longer before deciding if it is helpful or not. Keep track of your pain levels and the side effects to see if the treatment is working for you.

## A NOTE ON DIET

You may have read about specific diets that help with arthritis symptoms. Some of them involve removing wheat, bacon, pork, milk, rye, beef or coffee from your diet. But there's no proof that these strategies help relieve symptoms.

Likewise, no one diet has been proved to help arthritis symptoms. However, some research suggests that following a Mediterranean diet may help. It has been touted as anti-inflammatory and focuses on eating whole grains, fruits and vegetables, and limiting saturated fats, sodium and processed foods. Regardless of what diet you follow, healthy-eating principles can help. See Chapter 16 for more guidance on healthful eating and arthritis.

Gout is the one type of arthritis that does require a specific diet, because certain foods can contribute to the excess uric acid in the body. See pages 302–303 for more details on eating to help manage gout symptoms.

Glucosamine may take up to eight weeks before it becomes most effective.

**Gamma-linolenic acid** Gamma-linolenic acid (GLA) is an omega-6 fatty acid. It's necessary for good health, but it isn't produced in the body. Your body obtains GLA from the breakdown of certain foods during digestion. GLA supplements are typically made from the seeds of the borage plant, black currant plant and evening primrose.

Once in your body, GLA is converted into compounds with anti-inflammatory properties. There's some proof that it may moderately reduce pain, joint tenderness and morning stiffness from rheumatoid arthritis.

Borage seed oil is available in liquid or capsule form, as are oils made from black currant seeds and the evening primrose plant. These oils may cause mild stomach upset.

**SAMe** S-adenosyl-L-methionine (SAMe) is a dietary supplement that has gained attention as a treatment for osteoarthritis. It's a man-made version of a compound that occurs naturally in the body. Pronounced "sam-E," this supplement is thought to repair, stimulate growth and increase the thickness of cartilage. In Europe, SAMe is available as a prescription medication for arthritis and depression.

SAMe has been studied in a number of clinical trials. It appears to relieve pain from osteoarthritis as well as NSAIDs do, but with fewer side effects. And it can improve how well your joints work. You may need to take SAMe for more than a month before you see significant relief from your symptoms.

Side effects are uncommon and may include minor nausea or stomach upset. SAMe may lessen the effects of a drug used to treat Parkinson's disease. It may also interact with drugs and supplements used to increase levels of serotonin in the body, such as antidepressants. SAMe may also worsen symptoms of mania in people with bipolar disorder.

**Fish oil** Cold-water fish such as salmon, mackerel, herring, sardines and trout are high in polyunsaturated fats called omega-3 fatty acids. These fatty acids play an important role in many bodily functions and can help reduce inflammation. Eating at least two servings of fish a week has many health benefits.

For people with arthritis, taking a supplement of the oil derived from fatty fish may also be helpful. Fish oils are high in two specific fatty acids — eicosapentaenoic acid (EPA) and docosahexaenoic acid (DHA) — that play a role in the anti-inflammatory process.

Fish oil has been shown to improve pain, tender joints, morning stiffness and other symptoms in people with rheumatoid arthritis. In addition, fish oil supplements may protect against developing heart disease, which is more likely in people with rheumatoid arthritis.

Fish oil supplements may also allow some people with rheumatoid arthritis to reduce their use of anti-inflammatory drugs. Taking a low dose of fish oil daily may also improve pain and function for people with osteoarthritis.

Fish oil is sold as a supplement in liquid, capsule or pill form. Side effects are usually mild and may include a fishy aftertaste, bad-smelling sweat, headache, heartburn, nausea and diarrhea. Fish oil supplements may cause problems with drugs that affect how the blood clots.

**Ginger** Ginger is an aromatic spice from Asia. The product you buy in the grocery store is the underground stem of the plant. It's also available as a powder, tablet, extract, tincture and oil.

Some studies have found that ginger can modestly reduce pain associated with arthritis. Researchers believe that compounds in ginger have anti-inflammatory effects. Research is ongoing.

In low doses, ginger causes few side effects. In some people, it may cause mild stomach discomfort, heartburn, diarrhea and gas. It may interact with blood thinners, and people with gallstone disease should use ginger with caution.

**Vitamins** Vitamin C, vitamin E and beta carotene, which contain antioxidants, have been studied as possible treatments of arthritis because they may help prevent cell damage that leads to joint pain and further progression of the disease. Dietary sources include fruits and vegetables, which are important parts of a healthy diet in general. Should you take vitamin supplements as well? More studies are needed to answer this question.

So far, some research indicates that vitamin C may make it less likely that your osteoarthritis will get worse. Taking vitamin E along with standard care for rheumatoid arthritis seems to help with pain, but not inflammation. Vitamin E doesn't seem to help with the pain and stiffness of osteoarthritis.

Vitamin D, best known for its bone-protecting properties, is sometimes taken to treat and prevent arthritis. Some research shows that boosting vitamin D may lower your risk of developing rheumatoid arthritis, but taking vitamin D supplements doesn't seem to reduce pain from this type of arthritis. Some research shows that vitamin D may help with pain and function in people who have osteoarthritis and don't get enough of the vitamin in their diets.

Vitamin B-3 is made up of niacin and niacinamide. Preliminary studies suggest that niacinamide — found in meat, fish, milk, eggs, green vegetables and cereals — may be useful in treating osteoarthritis. But more research is needed before a recommendation can be made about taking vitamin B-3 supplements.

***Avocado-soybean unsaponifiables*** This supplement is a mixture of avocado and soybean oils. It's widely used in Europe to treat knee and hip osteoarthritis. It acts as an anti-inflammatory, and some studies have shown it can slow or even prevent joint damage. Some research shows that it may improve pain and help you move more easily, but more research is needed.

***Capsaicin*** This topical cream made from chili peppers is widely used for pain relief. The product is generally considered safe for use but can cause unpleasant effects such as a burning sensation on the skin. Some experts recommend this cream for hand osteoarthritis but not for some cases of osteoarthritis of the knee.

***Turmeric*** Turmeric contains the chemical curcumin, a yellow pigment that makes for a popular fabric dye. It's a popular spice in Indian and Asian dishes. Studies suggest that its anti-inflammatory qualities may help treat osteoarthritis. Specifically, turmeric may reduce pain and make it easier to move. It may also help lessen joint swelling and morning stiffness in rheumatoid arthritis.

When it's taken by mouth or applied to the skin, it's generally considered safe. Because turmeric may slow blood clotting, it should be avoided if you take blood thinners.

**Devil's claw** Devil's claw is widely marketed as a remedy for osteoarthritis. It's been used extensively in Europe, and more and more proof shows it can lessen arthritis pain.

The plant may have some anti-inflammatory, pain-relieving and antioxidant properties. Studies have shown that it reduces pain from osteoarthritis, especially hip and knee pain. Unfortunately, it doesn't appear that devil's claw can help with symptoms of rheumatoid arthritis.

Side effects appear to be minimal. The most common side effects include diarrhea and stomach upset. It may also cause problems with drugs used to treat and prevent blood clots and some medications used to treat high blood pressure.

## More evidence needed

A number of other herbs and supplements on the market may also have therapeutic effects. But more research is needed to better understand how the possible benefits balance any risks.

**Marijuana** Now that a number of states have legalized marijuana for medical use, doctors are often asked about using it. It may be available in the form of a pill, oil, oral solution and spray, or whole plant material. Studies show that marijuana may help treat symptoms of a variety of conditions, including chronic pain. However, there's limited evidence for this use, particularly for pain from rheumatic disease.

Some evidence suggests that a specific mouth spray containing a certain marijuana extract may help with sleep and morning pain in rheumatoid arthritis. It doesn't seem to help joint stiffness in the morning or make pain less intense, though.

Safety concerns and side effects are two more reasons that marijuana generally isn't recommended for treating pain. Side effects of medical marijuana can include dizziness, slower reaction times, increased heart rate and, in rare cases, psychosis. It has additional risks when used with other medications.

Experts in rheumatology and pain management offer this advice for using medical marijuana to treat arthritis symptoms:

- Don't smoke it. Inhaling it through a vaporizer or ingesting it have fewer health risks.
- Know the levels of active ingredients and choose an application with low tetrahydrocannabinol (THC) content, up to 9 %, and high cannabidiol (CBD) content.
- Start with a low dose.
- Don't drive or operate heavy machinery for 24 hours after taking it. It can impair reaction time.
- Avoid cannabis if you're under 25 years old, as the brain is still maturing until this age. Marijuana can negatively affect brain development.

## RISK OF DRUG INTERACTIONS WITH CBD

Cannabidiol (CBD) is one of the components of marijuana, known for having anti-inflammatory effects without psychoactive or "high" effects. CBD oil is on the rise as an integrative therapy for a number of conditions, including arthritis.

But because of the ways that certain medications and CBD work in the body, they may interact if you use both. This could make each less effective or increase the risk of adverse effects.

The following medications may interact with CBD:
- Certain antidepressants including amitriptyline, citalopram (Celexa), fluoxetine (Prozac), mirtazapine (Remeron), paroxetine (Paxil) and sertraline (Zoloft)
- Gabapentin (Neurontin)
- Some NSAIDs including celecoxib (Celebrex) and naproxen (Naprosyn)
- Steroids including prednisone, prednisolone and hydrocortisone
- Pregabalin (Lyrica)
- Tofacitinib (Xeljanz)
- Tramadol (Ultram)

Some other arthritis medications appear less likely to interact with CBD. These include certain conventional DMARDs such as hydroxychloroquine, methotrexate and sulfasalazine, and biologic DMARDs such as abatacept, adalimumab, anakinra, baricitinib, etanercept, infliximab, rituximab and tocilizumab.

Research in this area is still early and ongoing. In addition, some emerging reports show higher liver enzyme levels after CBD use. Talk with your doctor about the risks of using CBD or other marijuana components as part of your treatment.

- Consider using medical marijuana only when your symptoms flare, and follow up with your doctor regularly to monitor its effects.

***Bovine cartilage*** Cartilage that comes from cow tissue is thought to have anti-inflammatory effects. Some researchers think it can spur growth of new cartilage in people with osteoarthritis. Injections of bovine cartilage given under the skin seem to help ease symptoms of both osteoarthritis and rheumatoid arthritis.

**Cat's claw** Cat's claw is made from a woody vine from the tropical rainforests of Central and South America. Its name comes from hooked thorns that run along the vine's surface. The herb comes in tablet or capsule form and is sold as tea.

Cat's claw inhibits two substances that trigger inflammation. For osteoarthritis, this supplement may relieve knee pain. For rheumatoid arthritis, it may have a modest effect on reducing joint pain and swelling.

More study on the benefits and risks of cat's claw is needed. The supplement may lower your blood pressure, so if you take drugs to lower high blood pressure, talk to your doctor before taking cat's claw.

**Dimethyl sulfoxide (DMSO) and methylsulfonylmethane (MSM)** These related supplements are used for many conditions, including osteoarthritis. Some research shows that used alone or with glucosamine, MSM may lessen symptoms of pain and swelling and improve how well joints work. But not enough research has been done to say if these supplements are helpful for osteoarthritis.

**Selenium** Some studies suggest that selenium, a trace mineral with antioxidant properties, may decrease joint pain and inflammation. Other research, however, has failed to show a benefit. More research is needed.

**Willow bark** Willow bark contains salicin, an ingredient similar to the active ingredient in aspirin. Yet, there's no strong evidence that willow bark can help treat osteoporosis or rheumatoid arthritis. This supplement should not be taken with blood thinners.

## ENERGY THERAPIES

Energy therapies center on the belief that illness results from a blockage or disturbance of the free flow of energy through your body. According to this theory, rebalancing your energy fields can restore health and allow healing to occur. Of all the energy-based therapies, the most well-known and well-studied is acupuncture.

**Acupuncture** Originating in China more than 2,500 years ago, acupuncture is one of the oldest forms of medicine in the world. The system is based on a belief that the body contains a vital life energy that runs along pathways within the body. Imbalances in energy flow are thought to cause illness.

The energy pathways, called meridians, are accessible at approximately 400 different locations, or points, on the body. Practitioners of acupuncture attempt to rebalance energy flow by inserting extremely fine needles into these points.

During a typical acupuncture session, the practitioner inserts disposable, sterilized stainless steel needles into the skin. He or she may manipulate the needles manually or by electrical stimulation or heat.

A typical acupuncture visit may last from 15 to 60 minutes. Therapy usually involves a series of weekly or biweekly treatments. It's common to have several treatments, which can get expensive if acupuncture isn't covered by your insurance.

Scientists don't fully understand how or why acupuncture works. It's possible that it may work, in part, by stimulating your body's painkilling chemicals, called endorphins. When performed properly by a trained practitioner, it has proved to be safe and effective for various pain-related conditions, including low back pain, headaches and fibromyalgia.

In a study on acupuncture for osteoarthritis of the knee, people were randomly assigned to get one of three treatments: acupuncture, sham acupuncture or a self-help program. People receiving acupuncture saw a significant decrease in pain and were able to move more easily compared with people in the other groups.

Researchers suggest that acupuncture can complement standard care for knee osteoarthritis. Other studies on the use of acupuncture for arthritis have varied in quality, but most have shown some benefit.

Acupuncture may be particularly appealing to people who can't tolerate side effects from long-term use of nonsteroidal anti-inflammatory drugs (NSAIDs), as well as those with moderate to severe pain who don't want or can't undergo surgery.

**Dry needling** Dry needling is a type of acupuncture used by physical therapists for intra-muscular stimulation. It's also known as trigger point therapy. A needle is inserted directly into tender areas, or trigger points, to try to break up scar tissue and calcifications. The idea behind dry needling is that irritating the surface of the bone may increase muscle relaxation and stimulate faster healing. However, it's not clear how it works, and more study of its use for arthritis is needed. In contrast to acupuncture, dry needling is strictly based on Western medicine principles and research.

**Magnetic therapy** Many people wear magnets based on the idea that they can help reduce arthritis pain. Static magnets are placed in shoe insoles, headbands and bracelets. They aren't very strong. Electromagnets, on the other hand, are made to be magnetic with the help of electrical current. Devices with these types of magnets are used for health purposes, but it's not clear if they can relieve the pain of rheumatoid arthritis or osteoarthritis much, if at all. Magnets can disrupt implantable defibrillators and pacemakers and shouldn't be used during pregnancy.

**Copper bracelets** Some people have worn copper bracelets to ease arthritis pain. The practice is based on the thought that your body may not be getting enough copper from your diet, so you might absorb some

from the bracelet. However, researchers who have studied their use for both osteoarthritis and rheumatoid arthritis have found they bring no relief.

## HANDS-ON THERAPIES

Also called manual therapies, this popular group of treatments involves the movement or manipulation of one or more parts of the body. These therapies may relax the tissues surrounding joints, improving blood circulation and joint mobility.

### Chiropractic manipulation

A chiropractor may gently manipulate your soft tissues to stop muscle spasms and relieve tenderness. Chiropractors focus on the relationship between structure and function of joints. If the structure of a joint is not right, then it can't work as it was designed. The American College of Rheumatology supports chiropractic therapy for low back pain. However, not much research has looked at chiropractic care specifically for arthritis. It is not recommended in people with active joint swelling.

### Massage

You might think of a massage as a luxury limited to exotic spas and upscale health clubs. But massage can be an excellent way to ease arthritis pain and stiffness. During a massage, a therapist uses his or her fingers,

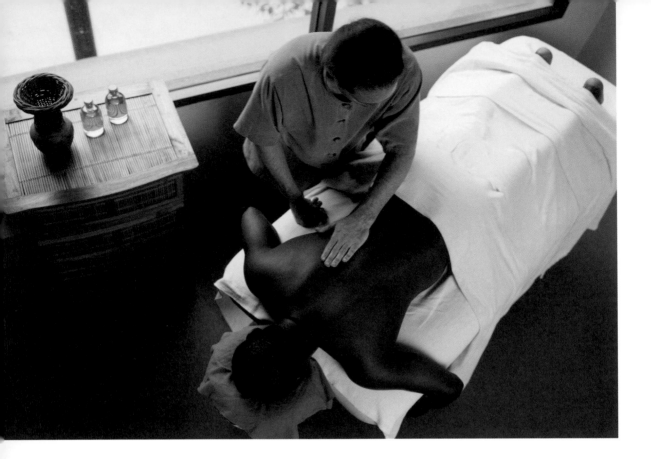

hands, and fists to knead, stroke and manipulate your body's soft tissues — skin, muscles and tendons. There are many types of massage; it's done in health clubs, salons, massage studios and hospitals. According to one small study, massage helped lessen pain and increase grip strength in people with rheumatoid arthritis in the arms and shoulders. It may also help people with osteoarthritis in the knee.

Massage can help loosen tight muscles, improve flexibility and reduce stress. Studies show that it can temporarily relieve pain. But if you have painful, swollen joints from rheumatoid arthritis, massaging the area di-

rectly may worsen your pain. Any pain that's more than just a momentary discomfort could mean something is wrong. If you feel uncomfortable, speak up.

## Prolotherapy

Prolotherapy is a natural therapy that reduces pain by relying on the body's ability to repair itself. A local irritant, such as a dextrose solution, is injected into the soft tissue of a painful joint. The goal is to cause an inflammatory response that kick-starts the body's healing response. This, in turn, strengthens and repairs damaged tissues.

Prolotherapy has been used in many parts of the body; the back, knees, shoulders, and other joints and ligaments are all examples. Several shots at the site of the injury are usually needed for it to be helpful. Medical professionals who support using prolotherapy believe that it may help with some chronic musculoskeletal injuries, but how well it works overall is still questioned. Irritation at the site of the injections may occur.

## ALTERNATIVE MEDICAL AND HEALING SYSTEMS

These complete medical systems are distinct from traditional Western medicine. They typically emphasize the whole person — mind, body and spirit — in treating and preventing disease. The systems are based on customs that may date back thousands of years. Traditional Asian, American Indian, African, Tibetan and South American practices fall into this category.

These approaches are based on beliefs that the mind and body have a powerful connection, and that the body has the power to heal itself. Alternative systems are individualized; no two people with similar symptoms get the same treatment. For example, you may take a different amount of herbs than someone else.

### Ayurveda

Ayurveda dates back thousands of years to ancient India. The aim of ayurvedic medicine is to promote health rather than fight disease. This is done through an emphasis on harmony in body, mind and spirit. Treatment may include fasting, breathing exercises, massage, herbs, meditation and yoga.

Few scientific studies have examined the use of ayurveda in treating arthritis. The research that has been done has focused on the use of herbal medicine, not other aspects of ayurveda. Some studies have shown that various herbal mixtures may help with osteoarthritis and rheumatoid arthritis. Ayurvedic herbs may help reduce pain and stiffness, but better-designed research is needed to confirm these findings.

### Homeopathy

Homeopathy was developed in Germany in the late 18th century. Today, it's practiced around the globe. Homeopathy is based on two principles — the law of similars and the law of infinitesimals.

The law of similars maintains that a disease can be cured with a substance that produces similar symptoms in healthy people. According to the law of infinitesimals, the substances used to treat disease are most effective when they're highly diluted to the point that none of the original substance remains. Most homeopathic treatments are highly diluted forms of natural substances, such as plants and minerals.

Some researchers have tried to learn how homeopathic medicines might work. Since the active ingredients in the preparations are so diluted, most scientists are skeptical about how well they work. A few studies have focused on the use of homeopathy for arthritis. Some indicate that these treatments may improve pain, stiffness, grip strength and other symptoms of rheumatoid arthritis. But for osteoarthritis, no studies have found it to be any more effective than conventional treatment.

Because homeopathic medicine mainly involves diluted substances, the risk to your health is likely to be minimal. A bigger concern may be the time and money you spend on something that may not work, while forgoing proven conventional treatment.

## EVALUATING INTEGRATIVE THERAPIES

It's easy to become frustrated by the limitations of conventional medicine on treating arthritis. What's the point of using it if it's not going to cure you, right? You may believe that trying an unproven treatment is better than doing nothing at all.

In fact, you may encounter wonderful opportunities to improve your health with integrative therapies. Unfortunately, their practice also attracts a few unscrupulous or fraudulent businesses and practitioners who are ready to prey on people desperate for a cure at any cost.

So, it's important to protect yourself. If you opt to try an integrative approach, your

safest bet is to separate the help from the hype. But finding out how effective and safe a therapy is can be hard because many haven't been studied as extensively as mainstream medicine has.

Conventional medicine practiced by most doctors is grounded in scientific method, which relies on experimentation and established research practices. Before a new therapy is widely accepted, scientists typically publish study results in established journals that are reviewed by experts who aren't associated with the study or sale of the product.

Throughout the process, researchers attempt to identify the health benefits and risks of the therapy. They also try to sort effective treatments from the ineffective ones that are enhanced by the placebo effect. The placebo effect happens when someone feels better simply because he or she is receiving treatment of any kind, whether it's a sugar pill or a real medication.

The cyclic nature of rheumatoid arthritis can make it hard to say how effective a treatment is. Because flares and remissions can occur suddenly and for no clear reason, you may be tempted to think that the treatment you just tried is what's making you feel better. This type of "coincidental cure" can be misleading and make a treatment appear more effective than it actually is.

The symptoms in osteoarthritis also may vary for reasons that are unclear. Changes may occur after a joint is used more strenuously than usual. Or you may see no recognizable cause at all. All of these normal variations make it hard to say whether any therapy is actually working.

With this in mind, it's important to look carefully at a therapy before you try it. Here are some steps to take as you get started:

- **Gather information.** Find out what's known about the safety and effectiveness of any integrative therapy you're considering. Check scientific studies to determine the advantages and disadvantages, risks, side effects, expected results, and length of treatment. The National Center for Complementary and Integrative Health (*https://nccih.nih.gov*) is an excellent resource that's updated regularly.
- **Consider the source.** When looking for facts, rely on reputable sources, such as well-known medical schools or health care institutions, government agencies, and professional associations or organizations, such as the Arthritis Foundation.
- **Use the internet wisely.** When using the internet for research, look for a site featuring an editorial board or medical advisory board involved with developing its information. Check the dates posted on the site. Outdated information can be wrong and dangerous. Look for a site that regularly reviews and updates its information.
- **Know when to be suspicious.** Think twice about any product or practitioner who promises cures, makes claims that sound too good to be true or encourages you to give up conventional treatments. Be wary of terms such as quick cure, mir-

acle cure, new discovery or secret formula. If a cure for arthritis or another disease had been discovered, it would be widely reported and prescribed. Also be suspicious of claims that a product cures a wide range of unrelated diseases, for example, cancer, arthritis and AIDS.

In general, when it comes to using a nontraditional practice, try to steer a middle course between uncritical acceptance and outright rejection of the therapy. Stay open to various treatments but evaluate them carefully.

The list of what's considered integrative is ever changing. Every day, new approaches to health care emerge and what were once fringe therapies become part of mainstream practice. Indeed, many hospitals, doctors and health insurers are integrating a variety of nontraditional treatments into their services — with good reason.

Talk to your doctor about the best natural therapies and your treatment plan. If he or she is uncomfortable with these practices, ask for a referral to a pharmacist or specialist who can help.

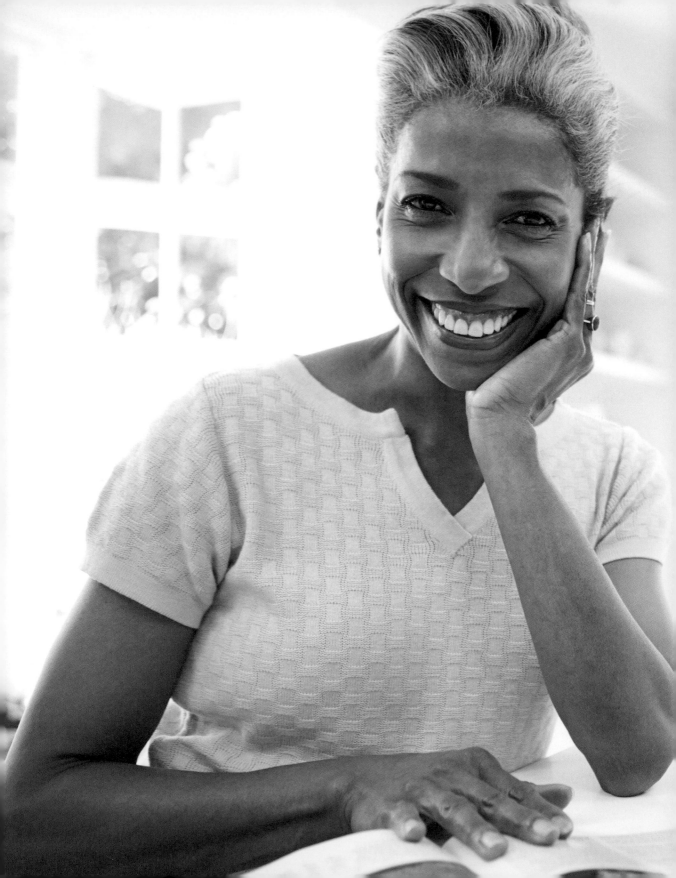

# Injections

When arthritis causes persistent joint pain, sometimes medications and other methods of pain management aren't enough to bring relief. What if other treatments haven't helped enough, but surgery still isn't recommended for your circumstances? Joint injections may be another option.

Injecting different substances into the joints can treat arthritis pain in a number of ways. Corticosteroid shots may be able to bring quick and targeted pain relief. Other types of injections can help replace natural lubrication in a joint or work to boost your body's own ability to heal damaged tissues. Researchers are continuing to explore newer treatments such as stem cell therapy to see how these may help provide joint relief.

This chapter will explore several types of joint injections your doctor may recommend.

## CORTICOSTEROIDS

Corticosteroid shots are injections that may help relieve pain and inflammation in a specific area of your body. These shots use a synthetic form of cortisone, a hormone naturally made in your body. Cortisone decreases inflammation by blocking inflammatory molecules.

Cortisone shots are most commonly injected into joints such as the ankle, elbow, hip, knee, shoulder, spine and wrist. Even the small joints in your hands and feet may benefit. The injections usually contain the corticosteroid medication and a local anesthetic. Often, you can receive a cortisone shot at your doctor's office.

Cortisone shots may be most effective in treating inflammatory arthritis, such as rheumatoid arthritis. They can also be part of treatment for other conditions. These injections may effectively treat bursitis, plantar fasciitis, tendinitis, trigger points, ganglion cysts and carpal tunnel syndrome, as well as gout and other types of inflammatory arthritis. People with pain from osteoarthritis and back and neck pain may benefit from cortisone shots too.

As with any medication, cortisone shots carry a risk of certain complications. These are somewhat different from the side effects of corticosteroids taken by mouth, because the medication is concentrated in one area instead of circulating throughout your body. The risk increases with larger doses and repeated use. Side effects can include:

- Joint infection
- Nerve damage
- Thinning of skin and soft tissue around the injection site
- Temporary flare of pain and inflammation in the joint
- Tendon weakening or rupture
- Thinning of nearby bone (osteoporosis)
- Whitening or lightening of the skin around the injection site
- Death of nearby bone (osteonecrosis)
- Temporary increase in blood sugar

There's concern that repeated cortisone shots might cause the cartilage within a joint to deteriorate. So doctors typically limit the number of cortisone shots into a joint. In general, you shouldn't get cortisone injections more often than every 12 weeks and usually not more than three or four times a year.

## Receiving the shot

If you take blood thinners, you might need to stop taking them for several days before your cortisone shot to reduce the risk of bleeding or bruising. This is usually recommended with spine injections. Some dietary supplements also have a blood-thinning effect, which may increase your risk of bruising. Ask your doctor what medications and supplements you should avoid before your cortisone shot.

When you go in for the shot, your doctor might ask you to change into a gown. You'll then be positioned so that your doctor can easily insert the needle. The area around the injection site is cleaned. Your doctor might also apply an anesthetic spray to numb the area where the needle will be inserted. In some cases, your doctor might use ultra-

Medicine injected

Sacroiliac joint

A cortisone shot in the sacroiliac joint may help relieve pain and inflammation in the low back and pelvis.

sound or a type of X-ray called fluoroscopy to watch the needle's progress inside your body — to make sure it's placed in the right spot.

You'll likely feel some pressure when the needle is inserted. Let your doctor know if you have a lot of discomfort. The medication is then released into the injection site. Typically, an anesthetic in the cortisone shot provides immediate pain relief, while a corticosteroid medication relieves pain and inflammation over time.

Some people have redness and a feeling of warmth in the chest and face after getting a cortisone shot. The shot also might temporarily increase blood sugar levels in people who have diabetes. If you take insulin, you'll need to pay close attention to your blood sugars for the first few days after your shot.

Your doctor might ask that you take certain steps after the shot to minimize the risk of complications, including:
- Protect the injection area for a day or two. For instance, if you received a cortisone shot in your shoulder, avoid heavy lifting. If you received a cortisone shot in your knee, stay off your feet when you can.
- Apply ice to the injection site as needed to relieve pain. Don't use heating pads.
- Watch for signs of infection, including increasing pain, redness and swelling that lasts more than 48 hours.
- It may be recommended not to use a bathtub, hot tub or whirlpool for two days. It's OK to take a shower.

Results of cortisone shots typically depend on the reason for treatment. Cortisone shots commonly cause a temporary flare in pain and inflammation for up to 48 hours after the injection. After that, your pain and inflammation in the affected joint should decrease, and the relief can last up to several months.

## HYALURONIC ACID

Hyaluronic acid (hyaluronan) is a natural substance found in normal joint fluid. It works by acting like a lubricant and shock absorber and helps the joint work properly. In people with osteoarthritis, natural hyaluronic acid molecules in the joints break down and their lubricating effect is reduced. This can result in more rapid wearing down of the joints.

Scientists have discovered other sources for hyaluronan — most commonly, the red combs of roosters. They have discovered ways to extract and purify hyaluronan into a gel for clinical use. Animal-free products also are available. Treatment with this type of shot is commonly referred to as viscosupplementation. So far, the Food and Drug Adminstration (FDA) has approved hyaluronan injections only for osteoarthritis of the knee.

By injecting this compound into a knee joint affected by arthritis, this shot may help restore more-normal lubrication of the joint. For many people it can improve mobility and reduce pain, although its effect is usually modest. The injection may work by helping your body to produce more hyaluronic acid and preserve cells in your cartilage. It may also help reduce pain signals and limit your body's inflammatory response. However, more research is needed to prove whether it actually slows progression of the disease.

This type of injection may be recommended for people with osteoarthritis who don't get relief from physical therapy and pain medications. It may also be a good option for people who can't take nonsteroidal anti-inflammatory drugs (NSAIDs) or other pain relievers. Usually, people might receive hyaluronic acid injections after trying a steroid shot first.

### Receiving the shot

Hyaluronic acid is usually given in a series of injections. You'll receive one a week for three to five weeks. You'll see your doctor for each one to make sure the injection is given safely and in the right location, as with cortisone shots. And similarly, it's best to avoid putting heavy stress on your knee for a day or two after the shot.

It may take several weeks to notice relief from symptoms. While cortisone shots work faster, relief from hyaluronic acid injections may last longer — up to six months or more.

As with any joint injection, there's a small risk of infection with this treatment. Occasionally, you may have muscle pain, stiffness or swelling in the joint for a day or two. If these symptoms persist, you should con-

tact your doctor. But the risk of side effects is low, even with multiple courses of treatment. For many people, hyaluronic acid shots can safely provide better joint function and more manageable pain that may help delay knee surgery for months or years.

## WHAT IS REGENERATIVE MEDICINE?

Regenerative medicine deals with the process of engineering or replacing human cells and tissues to help your body function normally. There is growing interest in regenerative medicine, such as stem cell therapy, for people with arthritis and other musculoskeletal issues.

Your body has the ability to heal itself from certain injuries or conditions. For example, think about a paper cut. Within a day or so, most people get a scab at the site of the cut. That scab is the body working to heal the skin and the tissue beneath it. Regenerative medicine relies on the body's ability to heal itself. The goal is to replace or restore human cells, tissues or organs that aren't functioning or healthy. Over time, your injured tissue will work normally again.

Regenerative medicine is still a relatively new type of treatment with ongoing research. So far it has been used to treat a variety of musculoskeletal injuries and conditions, such as Achilles tendinitis, rotator cuff injuries and tennis elbow. Muscle and ligament sprains, plantar fasciitis, degenerative disk disease and arthritis have also been treated

## IS REGENERATIVE MEDICINE THE RIGHT TREATMENT FOR YOU?

Regenerative medicine is a promising area of research and treatment for a wide range of conditions. But it's important to understand that regenerative medicine therapy doesn't work for everyone with joint pain. It's often one of the last treatments tried.

Some studies have shown that regenerative medicine may be helpful for musculoskeletal and spine conditions. However, the FDA has not yet approved regenerative medicine as a treatment for these uses. In addition, these therapies have possible side effects and complications. Talk to your doctor or a regenerative medicine specialist if you have questions.

You'll also want to talk with your doctor about any medications you're already taking and how they may affect regenerative therapy. Corticosteroids can interfere with platelet and stem cell function. They also can affect how well you heal, so you may need to stop taking them several weeks before a stem cell procedure. You may need to stop blood-thinning medications and NSAIDs, as well.

Finally, these treatments usually aren't covered by insurance plans, and they can be very expensive. If you have questions about the cost and how to pay for this, ask a member of your care team.

by these experimental therapies. Studies are continuing to explore how different types of regenerative medicine may help people with arthritis pain.

Two regenerative therapies are used more commonly to treat joint pain: platelet-rich plasma (PRP) and stem cells from bone marrow aspirate concentrate (BMAC). These innovative procedures are minimally invasive, use local anesthesia and don't require a hospital stay.

## PLATELET-RICH PLASMA (PRP) THERAPY

In recent years, there has been some enthusiasm that injecting whole blood, or more specifically, the plasma (the liquid component of your blood), into painful tissues may help with healing and reduce pain. This treatment aims to take advantage of the blood's natural healing properties to repair damaged cartilage, tendons, ligaments, muscles or even bone. Plasma includes platelets, proteins and growth factors. Although not well understood, these growth factors may increase blood flow, provide healing and decrease inflammation.

### How does PRP work?

When you're bleeding, your body quickly sends platelets to the injured area. Platelets act like "first responder" cells. They form a clot to help stop the bleeding. Platelets also help create a foundation for new tissue to grow. In addition, they release growth factors and other proteins. These proteins attract stem cells and other cells to the area. Each of these cells is needed to help the area heal.

When PRP is injected into a diseased or injured area affected by arthritis, it acts like glue. The platelets bind the damaged tissue together. The PRP also releases growth factors, which stimulate your body's healing. Multiple studies are evaluating PRP injections into painful areas of the body as a way to treat different musculoskeletal conditions such as tendon injuries, plantar fasciitis and osteoarthritis.

## How is PRP made?

Blood has different components, including:
- Red blood cells: cells that carry oxygen to the body
- White blood cells: cells that work to fight infection
- Platelets: cells that help blood to clot and help the body heal from injury
- Plasma: the colorless, fluid part of blood

The first step in creating PRP is to draw blood from a vein and place it into a machine called a centrifuge. This spins the blood, separating the platelets from the other blood cells in about 20 to 30 minutes.

The PRP layer is then injected into the site of arthritis, tendon degeneration or ligament tears to allow your body to regenerate tissue.

**Platelet-rich plasma (PRP) is separated from blood for use**

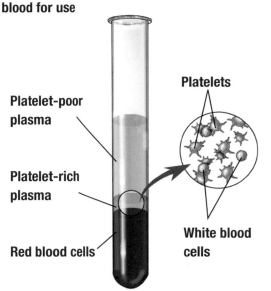

Platelets

Platelet-poor plasma

Platelet-rich plasma

Red blood cells

White blood cells

## Is it effective?

PRP therapy acts very differently from cortisone injections, which simply decrease inflammation and have no healing capabilities. If PRP is successful, it generally results in long-lasting relief. This is because it helps the damaged or worn-out tissue start to regenerate.

Recent research studies have looked at this treatment, with mixed results. Some people have reduced pain with PRP injections in conditions such as tennis elbow, rotator cuff disease and osteoarthritis. Studies suggest that PRP may provide similar or better relief than hyaluronic acid shots, and PRP therapy may have a longer lasting effect. But not all PRP is created equal. There are different preparation and delivery techniques, which can lead to different results.

The FDA hasn't officially endorsed PRP as a treatment for musculoskeletal conditions. But doctors are able to provide this treatment off-label for people who've exhausted other options. Still, more high-quality, controlled clinical studies are needed to determine the best candidates and the most effective techniques before this may become a more common therapy for joint pain.

## STEM CELL THERAPY

Stem cells are the basic building blocks of all human tissue. In the body, they can divide and form more stems cells. Stem cells may become specialized cells with a more specific function, such as blood cells, red cells, heart muscle cells or bone cells. No other cell in the body has the natural ability to generate new cell types. The thought is that these cells can communicate valuable information about tissue growth and healing to other cells in the body.

In regenerative medicine, researchers and doctors are studying whether stem cells may be used to generate healthy cells and replace diseased cells. If stem cells can be guided to become specific cells that regenerate and repair diseased cells in people, this process could help a wide range of diseases.

Stem cells are powerful cells. They can:
• Copy (replicate) themselves
• Ooze (secrete) anti-inflammatory proteins
• Turn into different types of cells, such as cartilage, bone and tendon

When you are sick or injured, stem cells help tissue heal and regenerate. They also help control any nearby inflammation. Your bone marrow — the tissue inside your bones — has stem cells and many other cells that help in healing. Blood cells are made in bone marrow. Cells found in bone marrow can be used to treat damaged tissue, improve function and help control pain.

Stem cells are obtained from a concentrated form of bone marrow called bone marrow aspirate concentrate (BMAC). Compared with typical bone marrow, BMAC has more regenerative cells, including stem cells. It also has platelets and growth factors like those found in PRP. BMAC has been injected into injured joints, tendons, ligaments, muscles, intervertebral disks and other areas.

### How is BMAC made?

Bone marrow is most commonly taken from the back of your pelvic bone. While you lie on your side or your stomach, a member of your health care team will locate your pelvic bone with help of an ultrasound machine or an instrument called a fluoroscope. Your skin will be cleaned, and you'll receive an anesthetic to numb the tissue down to the bone. A special needle is guided into the bone, and the marrow is withdrawn.

The bone marrow is placed in the centrifuge. Spinning the marrow removes much of the fluid and unwanted components. It concentrates the bone marrow cells. The result is BMAC.

**Removing bone marrow from pelvis**

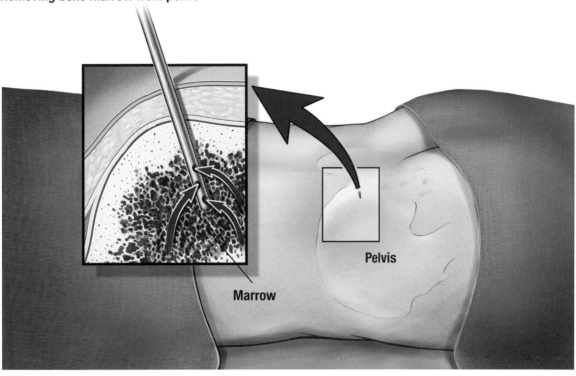

Pelvis

Marrow

This process usually takes about 30 to 60 minutes. The time depends on how much marrow was drawn from your bone.

Your doctor will then use ultrasound or fluoroscopy to identify the part of your joint to receive the stem cells, and the BMAC is injected into the target area. Altogether, it takes about two hours to make and inject BMAC.

## Promising, but not yet proved

Unfortunately, the excitement surrounding emerging stem cell therapy has led some patients and health care providers to overlook the lack of scientific evidence to support its use at this time. Stem cell therapies currently used outside clinical studies do not contain pure stem cells. Instead, they are a mix of a variety of cells, of which only a very small percentage are stem cells. It is possible that many of these treatments do not contain enough stem cells to help.

In addition, many stem cell therapies are now marketed directly to patients. To meet the growing interest, some clinics offer these injections without proper assurance of the contents or quality. Some forms of mislabeled stem cell therapies do not contain any living stem cells. Such practices are cause for concern. While the risks with joint injections are low, misleading treatments used in other parts of the body may actually cause harm to people looking for relief. They can also delay the scientific progress needed to turn stem cell therapies into cures.

What the research into stem cells and arthritis shows is that there are opportunities for stem cell treatment to be used as injection therapy. It may be used alone or in addition to joint surgery procedures. Successful stem cell therapies thus far have resulted mostly in pain relief and improvement in function or quality of life. Only a few limited early studies have demonstrated improvement in new cartilage or bone formation needed to cure arthritis. Exactly how that cartilage regrowth occurs, or even how pain relief is achieved, is still unknown. That means if you have a stem cell procedure, it will be used to treat only the symptoms of arthritis. This therapy can't yet cure the disease entirely.

As with other types of regenerative medicine, stem cell treatment for arthritis also isn't covered by most insurance companies. You'll likely pay out-of-pocket for it, which can be expensive.

Stem cell therapy for joint pain appears to be a fairly safe treatment option. If evidence of its effectiveness continues to grow, it may possibly be used more widely for arthritis in the future. Meanwhile, until the scientific evidence provides proof of its promise, it remains an experimental option that you and your doctor might discuss if you haven't been able to manage your joint pain with other treatments.

**PART 3**

# Living with arthritis

# Staying active

Your joints are stiff, swollen and achy. Sometimes it hurts when you stand, get up from a chair or climb stairs. Won't exercise just aggravate these symptoms and make you feel worse?

In fact, it's just the opposite. The idea that you should rest your joints when you have arthritis is outdated. Today, it's clear that movement is good medicine for osteoarthritis, rheumatoid arthritis and many other types of rheumatic disease. Physical activity is not only safe — it can also reduce pain and stiffness while improving your overall health, mood and quality of life.

In addition, physical activity can help fend off the natural loss of joint strength and range of motion that comes with arthritis. Being active helps you perform everyday tasks and maintain your independence.

There's no reason not to be as physically active as your abilities and symptoms allow. Exercising at least 30 minutes on most days of the week is recommended.

If that's far more activity than you're used to, you're not alone. Many people don't meet this benchmark — with or without arthritis. But studies show that people affected by arthritis are typically less active than people without joint conditions.

The best plan for arthritis includes aerobic activity, as well as muscle-strengthening exercises, flexibility exercises and balance exercises. If you're already doing some of these things, keep it up. Or, if that sounds overwhelming, just start slowly — every bit helps. Use the tips in this chapter to build up your current activity level, whatever it may be.

## BENEFITS OF EXERCISE

Being active has benefits for everyone. It improves sleep, concentration, energy and mood. Regular exercise can also help control blood pressure and cholesterol and may reduce your risk of many conditions, including heart disease, stroke, diabetes and depression. There are additional benefits for arthritis. Regular physical activity can help do all of the following:

***Relieve pain and stiffness and increase energy*** Regular exercise can triumph over two of the most common problems of arthritis — pain and lack of energy. Studies show that moderate-intensity aerobic and muscle-strengthening exercises can reduce pain and morning stiffness. Exercise improves your balance and boosts your endurance. It may also reduce inflammation.

***Protect bones and joints*** Within a relatively short period of time, regular exercise can strengthen the muscles surrounding your joints. This helps stabilize weakened joints and increases flexibility. Stronger muscles may even help compensate for cartilage loss and can improve your range of motion.

Over the long term, exercise can help slow bone loss that leads to osteoporosis — a condition that causes bones to become weak and brittle and susceptible to fractures. Physical activity helps you maintain bone density and offset bone loss that happens naturally as you age. Exercise also helps improve your posture and balance.

***Control your weight*** Combined with healthy food choices, regular exercise can help you lose weight or maintain a healthy weight. Keeping off extra weight has many health benefits, and it's important for your joints. Excess weight adds stress to your weight-bearing joints, which can aggravate pain, stiffness and inflammation.

***Reduce or delay disability*** Regular exercise helps you gain strength and agility that can improve your ability to do everyday activities, such as carrying grocery bags and climbing stairs. Keeping up better function helps you maintain your independence and quality of life.

Exercise may also improve some of the workplace limitations that go hand in hand with arthritis. In one study of people with arthritis in the workplace, participants in a six-week walking program saw significant improvements in many aspects of their jobs. They reported less trouble concentrating, crouching or bending, working in awkward positions, moving objects, and standing for long periods of time.

***Improve mood*** People with arthritis are at higher risk of anxiety and depression. Getting regular physical activity can help to reduce these mood disorders, relieve stress and improve your overall well-being.

You don't have to expend hours of hard work and sweat to get these health benefits. Any activity is better than no activity. And the more active you can be, the more it can help you.

## GETTING STARTED

If you haven't been active for a while, starting an exercise program may be a challenge. You may feel some pain and stiffness at the beginning. You may be worried about hurting yourself. Or you just may not have much confidence.

Luckily, you don't need a lot of equipment to be active and you don't have to log a lot of hours at the gym if that's not your thing. Your health care team can help design a simple program that caters to your needs, interests and capabilities.

Be patient with yourself. Your first few exercise outings may not be easy, but try to stick with it. For many people with arthritis, it takes six to eight weeks to establish a routine and to see the health benefits. With the following guidelines, you'll be on your way.

### Talk to your doctor

Before you begin or change an exercise routine, discuss your plans with your doctor. Your doctor can recommend specific exercises and precautions based on your abilities and symptoms. Your doctor may also suggest that you meet with a physical therapist or an occupational therapist. These professionals are trained to help people find ways to move effectively. A therapist who is experienced at working with people who have arthritis may be very helpful. He or she can show you how to modify exercises to make them work better for you.

## Gather your equipment

Choose activities that are fun for you, and select appropriate equipment. If you're planning to exercise on land (as opposed to in the pool), the most important piece of equipment is a comfortable, supportive pair of athletic shoes that are appropriate for the exercise you choose. Look for shoes with plenty of room in the toe box, especially if you have joint deformities such as bunions or hammertoes. Then check the sole. You want a thick, supportive sole for shock absorption. Some people with arthritis get a better fit with shoe inserts. Be sure to replace your shoes before they wear down and cause foot pain. This often occurs after walking or running approximately 500 miles.

Depending on what activities you enjoy, you may also benefit from specialized equipment, for example, a recumbent bike or special handles for golf clubs. You don't need to spend a lot of money on fancy equipment, though. Walking is free, and it's one of the best exercises for arthritis.

## Exercise at the best time of day

Generally speaking, exercise whenever it's best for you. Try to loosen up with gentle exercises first thing in the morning. It's usually best to avoid exercising right after you eat. Also, keep in mind that exercising at least five to six hours before bedtime may help you sleep better and feel less stiff in the morning.

## Start slow and focus on mechanics

Some people with arthritis are glad if they can take a step or two. Maybe you can easily walk several miles. Start wherever you are and build up gradually. Your goals will be different from those of someone else with arthritis.

If you haven't been physically active for a while, begin with five or 10 minutes of walking at a time. As you become more fit, increase the frequency, duration and intensity of your walks. Build slowly and gradually, allowing enough time for your body to adjust to each new level before adding more. Because of your arthritis, it may take you three or four weeks to adjust. Walking in a pool may help you build endurance, as the water relieves some of the pressure on your weight-bearing joints.

Keep your goals manageable. Perhaps you can walk only a minute each day at first. But if you add a minute each week, you'll be walking nearly an hour each day after a year. Meanwhile, doing several short sessions of activity throughout the day, such as three 10-minute walks, can have similar benefits to a longer exercise session.

Remember that body mechanics and positioning during exercise are very important. Poor positioning or body mechanics can make joints more painful or cause swelling. Some positions may be stressful to certain joints. Your doctor or physical therapist can show you how to adapt standard exercises so that they are comfortable for you.

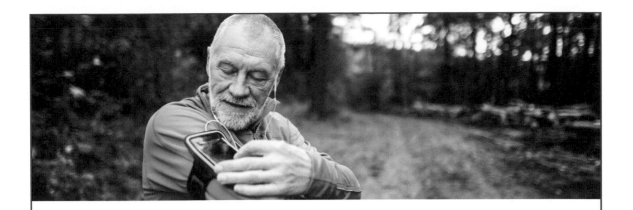

## INCREASING YOUR ACTIVITY LEVEL

Start with less intense activity and get accustomed to it before attempting more intense exercise. To build up, increase your exercise in this order.

*Frequency:* The number of days you exercise a week.

*Duration:* The length of each activity session.

*Intensity:* How hard you're working.

When you're ready, interval training is a good way to add intensity to your workout. This technique involves alternating short bursts of higher intensity activity with periods of lower intensity activity. For example, you might alternate walking at a leisurely pace for a few minutes with walking fast. If you're a swimmer, try alternating a couple of fast laps with a couple of slow laps. Start with just one or two higher intensity intervals a session, lasting only 30 seconds. Gradually build up to three to five higher intensity intervals a session on nonconsecutive days. You can also gradually increase the length of the higher intensity intervals to one to two minutes each.

Interval training is an especially effective way to build your cardiovascular fitness. And by adding bursts of higher intensity activity, you can reap the benefits of exercise in less time.

## Modify, modify, modify

Arthritis symptoms will tend to vary from day to day. On some days, you'll feel great — as if you could keep walking or swimming forever. On other days, you may feel like ditching your regular workout because you feel more pain and stiffness and have less energy due to fatigue.

On those tough days, try to modify your activity and stay as active as possible. It can be difficult to resume your routine after days of inactivity. So it's better to modify your plans than skip them entirely. For example:

- If you don't feel up to a 30-minute walk, try to accumulate 30 minutes of walking in shorter stints throughout the day.
- If it's painful to walk on a hard surface, try riding a bicycle or walking in a swimming pool.
- If you omit your walk, you can still do your flexibility exercises.
- Remember, any activity is better than no activity.

## Know when to slow down

It's important to listen to your body carefully when you have arthritis. You'll learn by trial and error how much exercise is too much. Pay attention to how you feel before and after each session. Do you feel the same or better? How about two hours — or two days — later?

It's normal to feel some new aches and pains in your joints and surrounding muscles

## WHEN TO CALL YOUR DOCTOR

Introduce new activities gradually, and pay attention to warning signs. Call your doctor if you experience:

- Pain that is sharp, stabbing or constant
- Pain that causes you to limp
- Pain that persists for a few days, despite rest, medication, or hot or cold packs
- Joints that are extremely swollen, red or "hot"

Seek emergency medical attention if you experience:

- Chest pain
- Severe shortness of breath
- Faintness or dizziness
- Nausea
- Discoloration in your arms or legs

during and after exercise, especially during the first four to six weeks of starting a new exercise program. However, if you have increased pain in the joints affected by arthritis or you experience new pain that lasts for two hours or more after you exercise, you may need to slow down a little and adjust your routine.

You can start by taking care of your acute symptoms. That may involve a little rest and taking an over-the-counter pain reliever as needed.

The next time you exercise, break the activity into smaller segments or reduce the intensity or number of repetitions. Also think about your mechanics. Are you performing an activity in a way that aggravates your condition?

To minimize pain, make sure you're using good equipment and good posture. Try changing your activity to lower the impact on your joints.

Be sure to do a proper warmup and cooldown every time you exercise. You can warm up your muscles with a warm shower or bath, heat packs, or massage to reduce stiffness before exercising. Just don't apply heat to an already inflamed joint.

At the end of each session, finish with slow, easy movements. After exercise, it may help to apply either heat or cold to affected joints for 10 to 15 minutes.

If you're not regularly taking an anti-inflammatory medication and heat and cold don't relieve your pain, you can try taking aspirin, ibuprofen (Advil, Motrin IB, others) or acetaminophen (Tylenol, others) one hour before exercise. These can help limit swelling and reduce pain. Just avoid mixing medications or overmedicating. You don't want to mask pain that warns you to stop.

If you're already treating arthritis pain with daily medications and you can't exercise without pain, you may need the help of a physical therapist. He or she can help develop an exercise plan that is best for you.

If exercise brings on a sharp cramp or muscle pain, gently rub and stretch the muscle until the pain subsides. Don't exercise joints that are tender, injured or severely inflamed.

Most people with arthritis can exercise safely. You don't have to give up on exercise at the first sign of discomfort. Adjust your routine and backtrack, as needed. But stay focused on your goal of regular activity.

## YOUR WEEKLY WORKOUT

To get relief from your symptoms and maintain strength and range of motion in your affected joints, you'll need to develop a well-rounded exercise program.

Your starting point may be nothing more than a walk around the block, but eventually, you should try to include the following components in your weekly routine:

***Aerobic exercise*** Work up to at least 30 minutes on most days (150 minutes of moderate-intensity aerobic exercise every week).

***Strength training and balance exercises*** Aim for at least three days a week, taking care not to work the same muscle group two days in a row.

***Flexibility exercises*** Stretch for 15 minutes every day.

Even if you can't always meet these activity goals, it's important to be as active as you can. And it's OK if you have to change your activity levels from week to week, depending on your arthritis symptoms.

## Aerobic exercise

When you're doing aerobic activity, you're repeatedly moving large muscles in your arms, legs and hips. You breathe faster and deeper, which maximizes the amount of oxygen in your blood. Your heart beats faster, which increases blood flow to your muscles.

For the greatest health benefits, the U.S. Department of Health and Human Services recommends that most adults get at least 150 minutes a week of moderate-intensity aerobic activity, or 75 minutes a week of vigorous activity. Aim for either goal — or an equivalent combination of moderate and vigorous activity — if your arthritis allows. If not, be as active as you can. Especially if you're older, it's important to know your limits for safe activity.

Regular aerobic activity provides both short-term and long-term benefits for arthritis. It can reduce pain and joint tenderness while improving aerobic capacity and mobility. Aerobic activity is also important for burning calories and controlling your weight.

Studies investigating the benefits of various types of aerobic activity, such as walking, running, cycling, aquatics and aerobic dance, have declared no clear winner for arthritis symptoms, so choose the activities that you like best.

Focus on joint-friendly activities that don't twist or pound your joints. Some people with arthritis are able to tolerate high-impact activities, such as running, basketball, tennis or aerobics class. But these activities may aggravate your symptoms. If you're just getting started, stick with activities that are easy on the joints, such as walking, bicycling, water exercise or dancing. Using elliptical machines and stationary bikes may also be good choices, if they're available.

Whatever activity you choose, always allow time to warm up with some gentle range-of-motion exercises. Begin with a slow, steady rhythm. Don't jerk or bounce. Maintain good posture while you exercise.

As comfortably as you can, work up to a pace that gets your heart pumping a little harder and makes your breathing a little faster — but still allows you to carry on a conversation. For the last five to 10 minutes, slow down and let your muscles and heart rate return to normal.

To meet the recommended aerobic activity goals, be creative about how and when to exercise. Walk on a treadmill or use an exercise bike while watching TV. Walk with a friend or your family after dinner. Schedule exercise into your day as you would an important appointment.

Although sustained, continuous exercise may provide the greatest benefit, you don't need to do all of your exercise at one time. Break activity into smaller sessions if you need to.

As mentioned earlier in this chapter, begin any aerobic exercise program gradually, slowly increasing the intensity and length of your workouts. Try to build up to at least 30 minutes of aerobic activity five or more days a week, adding a minute or two at a time.

If you're comfortable with your level of activity and want an additional challenge, gradually increase to 45 or 60 minutes five days a week. This level of activity provides additional health benefits.

It may help to use an exercise journal, a smartphone app or an activity tracker such as a watch to help you log your progress.

## Strength training and balance exercises

Another component of your program is to do muscle-strengthening and balance exercises two to three days a week. Always warm up first, with five to 10 minutes of stretching or gentle aerobic exercise. Be sure not to work the same group of muscles two days in a row so the muscles have time to recover.

Choose a mix of activities that build strength and balance. Some activities — such as yoga and squats — are good for both. Other activities are more targeted at one area of fitness than at another.

***Strength training exercises*** As muscles become stronger, they provide better joint support. Strong muscles can also take some of the pressure off painful joints and contribute to better overall joint function. People with arthritis who do regular strength training exercises report less pain and stiffness and a better quality of life.

Strength training is often done with free weights or weight machines. But strength training can also be done in your living room using inexpensive, lightweight resistance tubing, your body weight, or even canned goods from your pantry. Isometric exercises, which involve no movement, can be especially beneficial for people with arthritis. In the pool, the water can provide resistance for strength training. Talk to your health care team about the strength exercises that are best suited for your joints and symptoms.

***Balance exercises*** Tai chi, yoga, Pilates, backward walking, side stepping and standing on one foot are good examples of balance exercises, also called body awareness exercises. These activities can improve your posture, balance, sense of joint position, core strength and coordination. Some also provide stress relief and relaxation.

Balance exercises are particularly important if you are worried about falling or are at risk of falling because of your age, medical history or arthritis symptoms. If you have knee arthritis, the condition may cause muscle weakness that can increase your risk of falling.

Many group classes include some balance exercises. Or you can do balance exercises at home — even while brushing your teeth! For example, you can do the hip exercise on page 277 at your bathroom sink.

## Flexibility exercises

Flexibility exercises are at the core of a good exercise program for arthritis. These stretching and range-of-motion exercises counteract the stiffness that arthritis causes in your joints and spine.

Performing these exercises daily can help maintain or improve your flexibility in the affected joints and surrounding muscles. In turn, this helps reduce your risk of injuries and improve normal joint function, which makes daily activities and other forms of exercise easier.

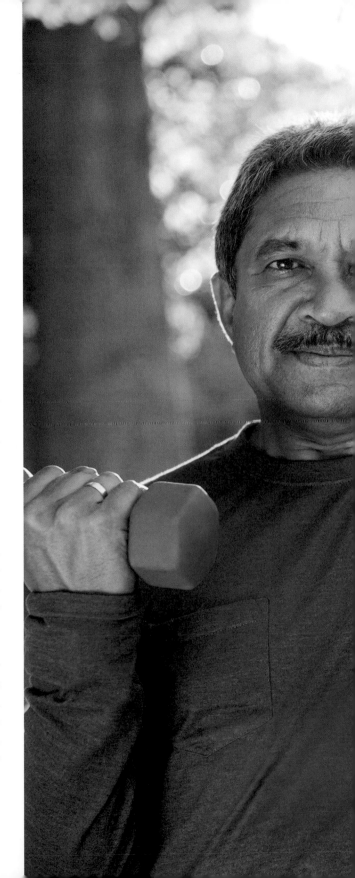

## MIX AND MATCH FOR BETTER HEALTH

Try to be active for at least 30 minutes on most days. Even three separate 10-minute bursts of activity can add up to a lot of calories burned. Bits of activity lasting less than 10 minutes can help improve your health, too — anything is better than nothing.

| Activity | Calories burned in 10 minutes of activity* |
|---|---|
| Ballroom dancing, slow | 37 |
| Basketball game | 97 |
| Bicycling (less than 10 mph, leisure) | 48 |
| Bowling | 37 |
| Elliptical trainer, moderate effort | 61 |
| Fishing | 43 |
| Gardening | 46 |
| Golfing (carrying clubs) | 52 |
| Jogging, 5 mph | 100 |
| Light housework, such as sweeping | 28 |
| Swimming laps, slow crawl | 71 |
| Swimming, treading water | 43 |
| Walking (2 mph, strolling) | 34 |
| Walking for exercise (3.5 mph, brisk pace) | 52 |
| Yoga (hatha) | 30 |

*Calories are based on a 160-pound person. If you weigh less than 160 pounds, you need to spend more time to burn the same number of calories. If you weigh more than 160 pounds, calories burned would be somewhat more.

Adapted from Ainsworth BE, et al. 2011 compendium of physical activities: A second update of codes and MET values. *Medicine & Science in Sports & Exercise.* 2011; doi:10.1249/MSS.0b013e31821ece12.

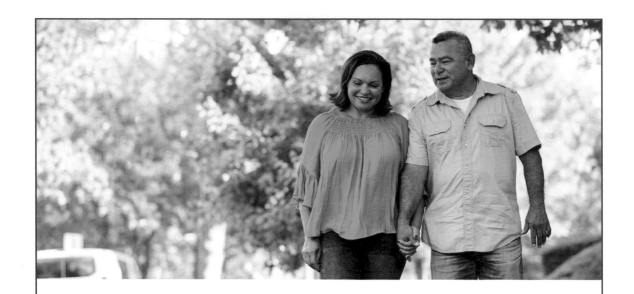

## EVERY MOVE COUNTS

Take advantage of opportunities to get up and move around throughout the day — normal daily activities add up. You get health benefits from carrying out the trash, cleaning, shopping, vacuuming, making the bed and mowing the lawn. But consider these activities a supplement to, not a substitute for, your regular exercises. And don't forget to balance these tasks with rest.

You can boost your exercise total by increasing physical activity in your routine daily tasks. Park your car farther away from your destination and walk a little farther. Or walk your dog farther than around the block.

Pick a regular time to do flexibility exercises at least once a day — for some people, doing them in the evening reduces morning stiffness the next day. You'll need five to 10 repetitions of each flexibility exercise once or twice a day to maintain your range of motion and flexibility.

If you're trying to increase range of motion and flexibility in a joint that has lost motion or is tight, you may need more repetitions or more daily sessions. Talk to your doctor or physical therapist if you need help.

# EXERCISE GUIDE

You may benefit from some of the exercises illustrated on the following pages. Your health care team can help identify the best set of exercises for your arthritis.

## Exercises for strength and balance

### Squats

Stand with a sturdy chair behind you. Hold on to a counter for support. Breathe out as you sit back and squat down as far as you can comfortably go. Keep your knees in line with your toes, making sure they don't fall forward. Hold the position for five seconds. Inhale as you return to standing. Relax and repeat. As you build strength, hold the squat for longer or squat down farther.

### Sit-to-stand

Sit in a sturdy chair that has arms. Keeping your spine straight, raise yourself up off the chair without using your arms or hands to assist you. Keep your knees over your toes during the motion. Relax and repeat. If your legs are weak, you may need to push your body up using your arms or hands to assist you. Skip this exercise if it causes pain to your hands, wrists or elbows.

*Toe lift*

Stand with your feet as wide as your hips. Hold onto a counter for support. Keeping your heels firmly planted, lift your toes as high as you can. Lower your toes and repeat.

*Heel lift*

Stand with your feet as wide as your hips. Hold onto a counter for support. Keeping your toes firmly planted, lift your heels as high as you can. Lower and repeat.

*Biceps strengthening*

Sit in a chair with a length of resistance tubing. Grasp one end of the tubing in each hand and place your hands on your knees, with palms up and arms straight. Pull upward with one arm. Slowly return to the starting position and repeat with the other arm.

*Triceps strengthening*

Grasp one end of the resistance tubing in each hand at shoulder height, with thumbs up and elbows bent. Straighten one arm toward your knee, keeping your elbow at your side. Slowly return to starting position and repeat with the other arm.

## Exercises for flexibility

### Neck stretch

Tilt your chin forward and down to your chest. Next, tilt your ear toward one shoulder and then the other, without raising your shoulders. Finally, keeping your neck, shoulders and spine straight, turn your face side to side.

### Overhead arm raise

Stand with your arms straight out at chest height. Gently raise your arms over your head. Lower them back to the starting position. Relax and repeat. For a variation, start with your arms out to the sides, palms facing forward.

### Behind-the-back stretch

Grasp one wrist behind your back. Gently pull your arm up until you feel a stretch in your shoulders. Relax and repeat. Switch arms.

### Shoulder blade squeeze

Place your hands on the back of your head. Pinch your shoulder blades together by moving your elbows back. Hold briefly. Relax and repeat.

## Cat stretch

Get on your hands and knees. Arch your back away from the floor and then let it sag toward the floor. Focus on your middle to lower back where the motion should be taking place. Don't arch your head backward too far. Relax and repeat. If you have hand or wrist arthritis, you may not be able to tolerate this position.

## Lumbar rotation

Lie on your back, with knees bent and feet on the floor. Place your hands behind your head. Gently roll your knees to the left, all the way to the floor if you can. Hold this position for a few deep breaths. Return to the starting position. Then roll to the right. Repeat.

## Lower back stretch

Lie on your back, with your knees bent and feet on the floor. Keeping your lower back on the floor, lift your right knee and hug it toward your chest, using your hands (left). Hold this position for a few deep breaths. Repeat with the left knee. Then hug both knees (right). If knee pain is aggravated by this exercise, place your hands behind the knee joints when pulling your knees toward your chest.

## Pelvic tilt

Lie on a firm, flat surface with your knees bent. Tighten your abdominal muscles to flatten the small of your back against the surface (lower left). Release tension in your abdominal muscles to arch the small of your back (lower right). Slowly return to the starting position.

### Knee bend

Stand with your feet as wide as your hips. You may want to hold on to a counter for support. Slowly bend one knee, bringing your heel up toward your buttocks, and hold for a few seconds. Return to the starting position and repeat with the other knee. To help improve balance, stand in place for progressively longer periods of time with your knee bent.

### Hip swing

Stand with your feet shoulder-width apart. You may hold on to a counter for support. Slowly swing one foot off the floor to the side, as far as you can, and hold. Keep your spine neutral and do not allow it to bend, twist or rotate during the hip-swing motion. Return to the starting position and repeat with the other foot. To work on balance, remove one hand from the counter.

*Standing march*

Stand between a counter and a sturdy chair. Hold on to the counter and chair for support, if needed. Keep your spine straight and slowly march in place, lifting your feet as high as you can.

*Ankle rotations*

Sit or lie down with your legs out in front of you and your heels on the floor. Bring the toes of one foot toward you, then push them away from you (top). Move your toes to one side and then to the other side (middle). Move your foot in a circle in one direction, then the other direction (bottom). Repeat with the other foot.

# Hand exercises

Arthritis is a cause of pain and deformity in the many small joints of your hands and fingers. Daily exercises can help maintain your strength, flexibility and range of motion in these joints.

### Thumb stretch

Hold your hand in a relaxed position with fingers straight. Bend your thumb across your palm, touching the tip to the base of your smallest finger. If you can't make your thumb touch, stretch it as far as you can. Return thumb to the starting position. Repeat and switch hands.

### Knuckle bend

Hold your hand straight with fingers close together. Bend the end and middle joints of your fingers. Keep your knuckles straight. Slowly return your hand to the starting position. Repeat multiple times, then switch hands.

### Fingertip touch

Hold your fingers straight and close together. Slowly form an O shape by touching your thumb to your index finger. Then follow with your middle, ring and smallest fingers. Repeat this exercise and switch hands.

### Thumb stabilization

Hold your hand straight with fingers close together. Gently curve your fingers into a C shape. Slowly return your hand to the starting position. Repeat and switch hands.

*Closed fist*

Hold your fingers straight and close together with the side of your wrist and hand resting on a tabletop. Close your fingers into a gentle fist, wrapping your thumb around the outside of your fingers. Don't squeeze. Slowly return your hand to the starting position. Repeat and switch hands.

*Forearm twist*

Hold your forearm out with your palm up. Slowly rotate your forearm, turning your thumb up and over. Rotate back to the starting position. Relax and repeat. Switch arms.

*Finger walk*

Rest your hand on a tabletop with your palm facing down. Move your thumb away from your fingers. Beginning with your index finger, move it toward your thumb. Follow with your middle, ring and smallest fingers one at a time. Repeat and switch hands.

*Wrist stretch*

Hold your wrist out away from your body with your thumb pointing toward the ceiling. Bend your wrist so that your palm is facing you. Hold briefly. Then bend your wrist so your palm is facing away from you. Hold briefly. Repeat and switch wrists.

## TAILORING YOUR PROGRAM

Your health care team can provide you with guidelines and recommendations for activity. These may be based on the type of arthritis you have, the severity of your symptoms and your health goals. Make sure you understand their recommendations and restrictions. (Ask questions until you do!) Then, choose workouts that you enjoy and that are convenient for you.

You'll be more likely to stay motivated if you figure out what it takes to get you moving. What interests you? What's fun? The following options are good choices for exercising with arthritis. Combine them to create a well-rounded exercise plan that meets all of your activity goals.

## Group exercise programs

Some people enjoy participating with others in exercise programs and classes designed for people with arthritis. Group programs may be a good fit for you if you're feeling hesitant to take charge of your own activity plan or would feel safer getting started under the guidance of a trained instructor. You'll also like these programs if you find support in working out with people who have similar symptoms and challenges to yours. Groups can be a great source of motivation and new friendships.

On the other hand, maybe you'd prefer to swim in solitude. Consider your personality and social comfort level before signing up for a group class.

## FINDING A GROUP PROGRAM

The Arthritis Foundation has developed several exercise programs for people with arthritis, including walking, tai chi and warm-water aquatic exercise. These programs are offered in communities across the country. Programs are led by Arthritis Foundation-certified instructors and can be modified to meet your needs. For more information or to find a program in your area, see *www.arthritis. org/living-with-arthritis/tools-resources/*.

Many kinds of exercise instruction are available online, through streaming services and on DVD. If there isn't an instructional class available in your community — or it doesn't work with your schedule — you can find videos you like and exercise from the comfort of your own living room.

Many communities offer a range of classes and activities tailored for people with arthritis, including special walking events, regular walking programs, tai chi, aquatic classes and more. Group exercise programs naturally vary — some meet once a week and others are more often. Some programs focus on aerobic exercise, while others combine a mix of activities.

Figure out how group exercise fits your weekly exercise goals, and plan other activities accordingly. Your doctor or physical therapist can provide information about options in your area.

## Walking

If you can walk comfortably, then a walking program is your best bet for a starter aerobic exercise. It's an excellent activity for overall conditioning. It improves cardiovascular health and bone density. Walking also helps to nourish your muscles and joints. And it leads to improved flexibility, strength and balance, which helps keep stumbles from becoming falls.

Walking is inexpensive and usually convenient — it can be done almost anywhere and anytime. At first, walk only as far or as fast as you feel comfortable.

Plan a route that's close by and accessible. Being able to step out the door to start your walk is both convenient and motivating. Use stores, downtown areas or public spaces as destinations. Or see if a local shopping mall caters to walkers. Many large malls allow walkers in the early morning hours before retail stores open their doors. This may be a good option when it's too hot, too cold, rainy or icy outside.

Choose a walking route that's varied. Make it interesting, but don't involve too many stops, turns and busy intersections. You'll benefit most from a sustained, steady stride. Note where there are uneven sidewalks, inclines, loose gravel or dirt paths to help you avoid falls.

Make personal safety a priority. Walk in the daytime or in well-lighted areas. Carry a cellphone or whistle with you.

## Tai chi

The ancient Chinese martial art of tai chi (TIE-CHEE) was developed more than 1,000 years ago. Today, people continue to use this exercise to relax and strengthen muscles and joints and reduce tension.

Tai chi combines slow, deliberate circular movements and postures with deep, regular breathing that can increase circulation, relax the mind and body, and ease chronic pain. Studies show that this practice may be particularly helpful for osteoarthritis of the knee.

When learned correctly and practiced regularly, tai chi is an excellent source of balance and flexibility exercises. But it will take a commitment of time and effort. You can use videos to learn tai chi or look for classes in your area. Local health clubs, recreational departments and martial arts centers may offer tai chi classes. Some are designed specifically for people with arthritis.

## Water exercise

If pain and stiffness make it difficult for you to exercise, a warm-water exercise program may do wonders for you. These programs typically take place in pools heated to between 83 and 88 F. The buoyancy of the water reduces the weight that your joints, bones and muscles have to bear. And the soothing warmth relaxes your muscles, which may decrease muscle spasms and tightness. Combined, these factors decrease joint pain while building strength, range of motion and aerobic fitness — all in one class.

Many health clinics, gyms and local swimming pools offer aquatic exercise classes. You don't have to be a good swimmer to participate. Once you're comfortable exercising in the water, you can ease your way into land-based activities.

## Sports and other activities

If you enjoy sports and are comfortable doing them, don't let arthritis slow you down. Discuss your interests with your health care team. You might enjoy swimming, biking, cross-country skiing, golfing or tennis. With good judgment and a little creativity, you can make many favorite activities work for you.

Just remember to modify the activities as needed. Ask your health care team for assistance. If you golf, you might try playing nine holes of golf instead of 18. Use a golf cart instead of walking. Play in a scramble tournament on a team so you're not hitting every ball yourself. If you have hand or finger arthritis, try using molded golf grips on your clubs. They provide cushion and surface tack for an easier grip and help absorb the impact of hitting a golf ball.

Mixing different athletic activities into your workout (cross-training) is a good way to keep exercise boredom at bay. Cross-training may also reduce your chances of injuring or overusing one specific muscle or joint.

## STAYING MOTIVATED

When you have arthritis, regular exercise isn't about having bigger biceps or enduring more miles. It's an essential therapy for minimizing stiffness and pain, maintaining or improving your range of motion, and building muscle strength around affected joints. These are important accomplishments!

The key to exercise motivation is that it has to be personal. The reasons that help you stay active day after day and week after week should be your reasons and not someone else's. How do you discover your inner motivation? Start by asking yourself a simple question: "What can exercise do for me?"

You may need exercise to help relieve your symptoms, such as pain and fatigue — that's the most common motivation. Perhaps there are specific tasks that you want to continue doing, for example, being able to raise your arms above your shoulders in order to brush your hair or grasp buttons when putting on a shirt. Maybe you're interested in maintaining a high quality of life for as long as you can, for example, to continue living independently at home.

Maybe the idea of living with a chronic disease has scared you a little bit. Use that emotion to your advantage — fear is a great motivator. The point is that there are no wrong reasons for going out to exercise, as long as they are your reasons. The best motivation comes from within you, and without that internal drive, any long-term goal will be difficult to achieve.

Be sure to note any changes that may occur in your symptoms or in your physical capabilities while you're active. And celebrate success when you reach your goals — even the minor ones.

Of course, there will be days when you feel frustrated, discouraged or unenthusiastic. Here are tips for sticking with your activity goals:

**Use realistic strategies** Set measurable activity goals at the beginning of each week, such as walking for 30 minutes on five days or attending your first water aerobics class.

Review your progress at the end of the week. Did you achieve your goals? If so, congratulate yourself and set new goals for the following week. If not, ask yourself if the goals you set were achievable. Then, set more realistic goals for the next week.

**Find an exercise buddy** Knowing that someone is expecting you to show up in the park or at the gym is a powerful incentive to get moving. Working out with a friend, co-worker or family member can bring a new level of motivation to your workouts.

**Enlist your family's support** You'll need your family's help to make time to exercise and to provide support on the days when you're feeling sluggish. Ideally, you'll be able to do things together, too. Plan family outings that include swimming or walking.

**Reward achievements** Reward yourself for small accomplishments. Treat yourself to a massage, an hour to yourself, a movie or a new book.

**Enjoy the outdoors** If you love fresh air and nature, go outside and be active. Check out different parks for walking or biking.

Finally, always have a Plan B to fall back on. The normal ebb and flow of arthritis symptoms can put a kink in your best-laid exercise plans. If you scheduled a tennis lesson for Wednesday morning or a bike ride for Friday afternoon, you may feel defeated if symptoms flare during these times and you can't stick with your commitments.

Flare-ups can also get in the way as you try to increase your level of physical activity. Every time you take two steps forward, it may seem that your symptoms push you two steps back.

This is an undeniable challenge that you'll likely face. It's how you respond to the challenge that makes all the difference. For long-term success, you may need several strategies at the ready to solve problems as they arise.

To do that, it helps to plan ahead. Try to identify the barriers that are most likely to stop you from exercise: Your work schedule is unpredictable, you struggle with motivation, you don't like to exercise alone or you worry about injury.

Once you've identified the most common barriers, try to come up with specific solutions that may remove or change them. Maybe you can carve out an extra period of time for exercise each week, in case your regular schedule suddenly fills up. Or maybe you can keep an easy exercise video to follow at home during times when you're not feeling well.

Come up with your own solutions to potential roadblocks. The benefits of physical activity are worth it.

# Eating a healthy diet

You might expect treatment for joint pain to involve your doctor's office, the pharmacy and perhaps physical therapy. But what about the grocery store? Or your daily lunch stop? The food choices you make can have a significant effect on your overall health and well-being, especially if you have arthritis.

To feel healthy, it's important to eat well. That doesn't mean you have to count calories or that you can never eat french fries or chocolate chip cookies. Rather, your focus is on choosing healthy foods most of the time.

Strive for a flavorful, balanced diet based on plant foods. It's your best bet for fighting inflammation, increasing your energy and controlling your weight — all of which can help to reduce your symptoms of arthritis.

## DIET AND ARTHRITIS

A healthy diet can increase your energy, brighten your mood, improve your job performance, and lower your risk of heart disease, high blood pressure and diabetes. It's also beneficial for arthritis. A healthy, plant-based diet, emphasizing fruits, vegetables, whole grains, low-fat dairy products and lean proteins, can help:

- *Minimize arthritis symptoms and medication side effects.* Fruits, vegetables and foods made from whole grains contain beneficial vitamins, minerals, fiber and compounds called phytochemicals. These healthy compounds are associated with reducing inflammation, which can be a primary cause of pain and discomfort. Fruits and vegetables are also naturally low in calories and sodium and high in potassium. That makes them a good choice if you're coping with side effects of arthritis medications, such as fluid retention and weight gain.

- **Support bone strength.** You're at increased risk of developing osteoporosis if you have a type of inflammatory arthritis or connective tissue disease, such as rheumatoid arthritis or lupus, or if you take corticosteroid medications. Getting enough calcium and vitamin D in your diet through low-fat dairy products may help slow bone loss and reduce your risk of fractures.

- **Promote a healthy weight.** Most plant foods are relatively low in calories, so a plant-based diet can help with weight control. Maintaining a healthy weight is good for your overall health, but it's especially important when you have arthritis. That's because excess weight adds stress to your weight-bearing joints, especially your knees, which can aggravate pain, stiffness and inflammation.

You'll learn more about these three benefits as you read this chapter. And you'll learn how to use the Mayo Clinic Healthy Weight Pyramid to help you make smart food choices to help control your arthritis. More-detailed information about the pyramid starts on page 292, but the basic idea is simple: Use the shape of the pyramid to help you select healthy foods. Eat most of your food from the food groups at the base of the pyramid and less from the groups at the top.

It's best to see your doctor before you begin any healthy-weight plan.

# REDUCING ARTHRITIS SYMPTOMS

For people with arthritis, the old saying "You are what you eat" tends to ring true. Many people with rheumatoid arthritis find that the food they eat plays a role in the severity of pain and other symptoms they experience.

Scientists and physicians have long suspected a connection between nutrition and arthritis, too. Early research dating back to the late 1920s looked for food allergies among people with arthritis. Today, research seems to indicate a direct link between diet and inflammation. Researchers have found different ways that some foods may offer protection against inflammation, while other foods may trigger or exacerbate the inflammation process.

A great deal of study is now focused on identifying particular foods that fall on either side of the inflammation equation. Researchers are still trying to understand exactly how foods may contribute to — or help — arthritis symptoms. Meanwhile, the following theories can help guide your eating choices.

## Protection against inflammation

Research shows that some fats and certain nutrients or compounds found in foods may reduce the pain, inflammation and joint tenderness caused by rheumatoid arthritis.

Foods considered to be the most beneficial are part of an overall healthy diet, so there's no reason to wait for conclusive studies before eating more of these foods. To help reduce inflammation and pain, eat foods that contain these substances:

**Omega-3 fats** Prepare more meals with cold-water fish, such as tuna, salmon, mackerel and herring, which are rich in omega-3 fatty acids. Walnuts, pecans, ground flaxseed and soy foods (tofu, edamame, and soy-based milk, yogurt or cheese) also are good sources of omega-3s. These inflammation-fighting unsaturated fats seem to modify the inflammatory process and may play a role in regulating pain. Although extra-virgin olive oil doesn't contain omega-3s, it's been shown to have anti-inflammatory properties, too. For information on omega-3s in fish oil supplements, see page 234.

**Antioxidants** Antioxidants are dietary substances that may help protect cells from damage. These substances appear to slow oxidation, a natural process associated with inflammatory arthritis that leads to cell and tissue damage. Common antioxidants include vitamins C and E, carotene, lycopene, and flavonoids.

In general, the most colorful vegetables and fruits have the highest levels of these substances. Think of spinach, kale, beets, blueberries and cherries. Studies have shown that blueberries, cherry juice and pomegranate juice — all rich in flavonoids — can improve knee arthritis pain and decrease inflammation. Other foods that are rich in antioxidants include beans, nuts, green tea, red wine, dark chocolate, cinnamon, ginger root and turmeric powder. However, supplements containing antioxidants don't seem to have a similar effect.

***Fiber*** Dietary fiber — found mainly in fruits, vegetables, whole grains and legumes — includes the parts of plant foods that your body can't digest or absorb. Fiber passes relatively intact through your digestive system, and it's probably best known for its ability to prevent or relieve constipation. But diets high in fiber can provide other health benefits as well, such as reduced inflammation. The fiber feeds bacteria in your digestive tract, improving the diversity and balance of gut bacteria. A healthier gut has been shown to help reduce inflammation in people with arthritis. In addition, eating high-fiber foods may help you reach or maintain a healthy weight and lower your risk of diabetes, heart disease and some types of cancer.

## Special diets

In addition to studying specific nutrients, scientists have been investigating whether certain diets can reduce the severity of rheumatoid arthritis.

## TESTING YOUR SYMPTOMS

Arthritis symptoms vary from day to day, so it can be difficult to determine if particular foods are affecting how you feel. In general, red meats, processed sugary foods and fried foods tend to be associated with inflammation. For a small number of people with arthritis, it's possible that sensitivities to certain foods — even foods considered healthy, such as dairy products or nightshade vegetables including potatoes and eggplant — may trigger or worsen symptoms.

If you believe that a particular food increases arthritis symptoms, you might try a test: Drop the item from your diet for a short time, and then resume using it again. Note whether the change affects your symptoms. However, don't omit whole food groups or a large number of foods without first consulting a registered dietitian or your doctor. Without proper guidance, you could become deficient in nutrients that are important to maintaining good health. This, in turn, could affect your arthritis symptoms. Be skeptical of any diet that eliminates an entire group of foods or stresses only a few foods while eliminating others.

Some research suggests that following a vegetarian or vegan diet may be beneficial. While research is ongoing, several studies have found that following a vegan diet for as little as three weeks is associated with lower levels of C-reactive protein, a marker of inflammation.

Researchers have also been exploring whether a gluten-free diet may help with arthritis. Some studies have found that after following a gluten-free vegan diet, people with rheumatoid arthritis had reduced symptoms or markers of inflammation. It's not clear if those effects are due to avoiding gluten, eating a vegan diet or other factors. Some people do notice improved joint symptoms after going gluten-free — including people with celiac disease. However, more study is still needed.

The Mediterranean diet is one of the most widely studied. Overall it's considered very healthy, and research has found many anti-inflammatory and disease-fighting benefits. This way of eating emphasizes vegetables, fruits, whole grains, nuts, fish, legumes and healthier types of oils such as olive oil. Meanwhile, it limits red meat and sugary or processed food. Studies suggest that the diet helps curb inflammation, which may relieve joint pain and stiffness. It has also been shown to protect against heart disease and other chronic diseases, including certain cancers, and it may even help you live longer.

Work with your doctor or a registered dietitian as you make the switch to a special diet or eliminate certain foods — to ensure that you're getting all of the nutrients you need.

## THE MAYO CLINIC HEALTHY WEIGHT PYRAMID

The Mayo Clinic Healthy Weight Pyramid is built on the underlying principle of energy density — the amount of energy (calories) in a given amount (volume) of food. Foods that form the base of the pyramid, such as fruits and vegetables, are low in energy density. Most of them have few calories in a relatively large amount of food. In contrast, foods at the top of the pyramid are high in energy density. They have a lot of calories in a relatively small amount.

The pyramid helps you focus on foods that provide a lot of volume and nutrients, without overloading on calories and unhealthy fats. As a result, you'll eat well and feel full while losing or maintaining weight. Plus you reap the benefits of the nutrient-rich foods that make up the bulk of the pyramid.

Here's a closer look at the six food groups that make up the pyramid.

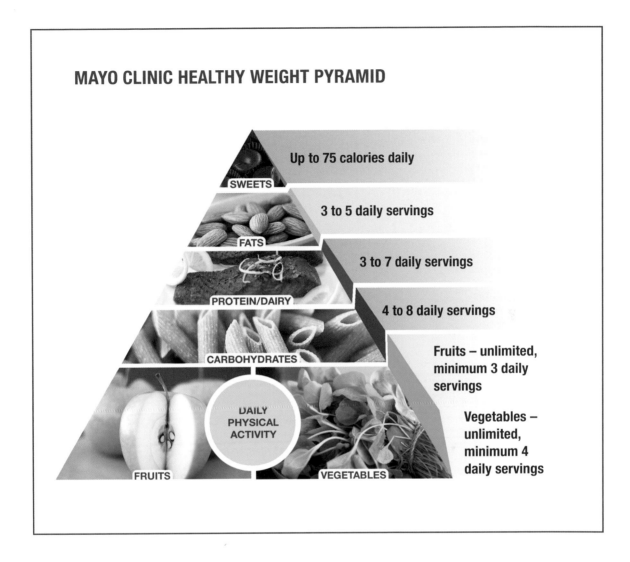

## MAYO CLINIC HEALTHY WEIGHT PYRAMID

SWEETS — Up to 75 calories daily

FATS — 3 to 5 daily servings

PROTEIN/DAIRY — 3 to 7 daily servings

CARBOHYDRATES — 4 to 8 daily servings

Fruits – unlimited, minimum 3 daily servings

Vegetables – unlimited, minimum 4 daily servings

DAILY PHYSICAL ACTIVITY

FRUITS

VEGETABLES

## Vegetables and fruits

Vegetables and fruits share many attributes. They offer a wide array of flavors, textures and colors, as well as many disease-fighting nutrients.

Most vegetables and fruits are also low in energy density. They are high in water and fiber, which provide no calories. You can improve your diet simply by eating more vegetables and fruits in place of other foods.

*Vegetables* Vegetables include a wide array of plant foods: roots and tubers, such as carrots and sweet potatoes; salad greens, such as lettuce and spinach; and broccoli, kale, cabbage and many more. Other plant foods, such as tomatoes, peppers and cucumbers, are included in this group, although they're

**Eating a healthy diet      293**

botanically considered fruits because they contain the seeds of the plant.

Vegetables contain no cholesterol, and they are naturally low in fat, high in dietary fiber and generally low in calories. In addition, they're low in sodium and high in essential minerals such as potassium and magnesium. This makes them a good choice to help offset fluid retention or weight gain that may be caused by arthritis medications.

Another benefit of vegetables is that many of them are great sources of inflammation-fighting antioxidants. In general, the more colorful the vegetable is, the higher its antioxidant levels. Good examples include red bell peppers, beets, tomatoes, carrots, and dark green vegetables, including kale, spinach, broccoli and Brussels sprouts.

Fresh, frozen, and canned vegetables are all good sources of nutrients. However, canned vegetables may be high in sodium because sodium is used as a preservative in the canning process. If you use canned vegetables, look for labels that indicate that no salt has been added, or rinse the vegetables before using them.

***Fruits*** Any food that contains seeds surrounded by an edible layer is generally considered a fruit. As with vegetables, you want to eat a variety of colorful ones. Strawberries, raspberries, blueberries, apples, oranges, peaches, plums, grapes, melons, mangos and papayas are all flavor-packed, nutritious powerhouses.

Like vegetables, fruits are great sources of fiber, vitamins, minerals and other phytochemicals. The most colorful fruits tend to have the most antioxidants. And since most fruits have a sweet or sweet-tart taste, they're good options as healthy snacks or dessert.

Fresh fruit is best, but frozen fruits with no added sugar and fruits canned in water or their own juices also are great choices. Because of processing, fruit juice and dried fruits, such as raisins or dehydrated bananas, can be a concentrated source of calories. They still provide some nutrients, but it's best to measure your portion.

## Carbohydrates

Carbohydrates are your body's main energy source, and they are found in a wide range of foods. Most carbohydrate foods are plant based. They include grain products, such as bread, cereals, rice and pasta. This food group also includes certain starchy vegetables, such as potatoes and corn.

Which kind of carbs should you eat? Think of all the carbohydrate-containing foods placed in a straight line. At one end are oats, brown rice and whole wheat flour. In the middle you'll find potatoes, white rice, white flour and pasta. And at the other end are highly processed products such as cookies, candies and soft drinks.

The foods in this lineup incorporate all three kinds of carbohydrates: fiber, starch and sugar. It's not hard to identify the healthiest and least healthy sections — less refined whole grains on one end, highly refined sugar on the other end.

The health benefits of many items in the middle aren't as clear. The nutrient value of foods such as rice, pasta, bread and potatoes vary and can shift depending on how they're processed and served.

Consider, for example, white and whole-grain breads. Both begin as nutrient-rich grains, typically wheat. With white bread, however, the grain's bran and germ are removed, taking away many natural vitamins and almost all of the fiber. That's why it's best to choose whole-grain breads, because most of the vitamins and fiber are retained. The same goes for whole-grain pastas and cereals as well as brown rice. Similarly, the edible skins often removed from potatoes and sweet potatoes are full of nutrients and fiber.

When choosing carbohydrates, the key term to look for on labels is whole. Generally, the less refined a carbohydrate food, the better it is for you. Whole grains are particularly important if you have diabetes or you take corticosteroid medications, because they can help slow down the rise in blood sugar as you digest them. Better control of your blood sugar may also help reduce inflammation, which can help improve arthritis symptoms.

## Protein and dairy

Protein is essential to human life. Your skin, bones, muscles and internal organs are made up of protein, and it's present in your blood, too. Protein is often associated with

## TIPS FOR USING THE PYRAMID

Although it may seem difficult at first to adapt to a new healthy-eating plan, it will become part of your routine with time and practice. Here are tips to make this new approach work for you:

- *Plan by the week.* You may find it more efficient and less stressful to plan menus for an entire week rather than figuring out what you're going to eat one day at a time — or at the very minute you step into the kitchen to start preparing a meal.
- *Focus on the produce.* If you're a meat-and-potatoes eater, the pyramid's focus on fruits and vegetables may be a challenge. Try filling the biggest part of your plate with vegetables at dinnertime while moving the meat to the side. Snack on vegetables and fruits that require little preparation, such as baby carrots, cherry tomatoes, bananas and grapes. Or try making your regular soups, pastas and casseroles with less meat or no meat. Try adding extra vegetables, beans or other legumes instead.
- *Make pleasure a priority.* You may have to cut back on some of your favorite foods to lose weight and curb inflammation. But you don't have to sacrifice your enjoyment of eating. Be sure to include the flavors, colors and textures you enjoy at every meal. If you have a sweet tooth, try satisfying it with naturally sweet fruit. If you're a chocolate lover, opt for small bits of dark chocolate, which has more antioxidants than milk chocolate does.

animal products, but it's also found in plants.

Choose proteins from animal products wisely. All meats, including chicken and fish, contain cholesterol. And many cuts of meat, as well as poultry products with the skin on, can be high in saturated fat, which can increase inflammation. Red meat has also been associated with inflammation. If you're used to eating a lot of red meat, try to eat it less frequently and only in small portions (about 3 ounces). Fill up on healthy foods such as vegetables, fruits and whole grains so that smaller portions of meat are enough.

You also get protein, as well as calcium, from dairy products. Low-fat dairy products have the same nutrients as whole-milk versions, but with less fat and fewer calories. Good

- *Adapt menus to the season.* Use the freshest foods available for your meals — asparagus, peas and cherries in the late spring, tomatoes, corn and peaches in the late summer. Recently harvested produce is often available at local farmers markets. And produce is generally cheapest when it's in season.

- *Look for shortcuts.* As you adapt to a new way of eating, make it as simple as possible. Try buying pre-cut vegetables and fruits, bagged salads, and precooked meats such as a rotisserie chicken or canned tuna. You can also try using shredded low-fat cheeses and frozen vegetables and fruits to save on prep time and see what works for you.

- *Don't forget convenience.* You don't have to cook every meal from scratch. Keep convenience foods, such as a favorite frozen entree or side dish, on hand for those days when there's little time to fix meals. Just be selective about what you choose. Read the nutrition labels carefully.

- *Be flexible.* Every food you eat doesn't have to be an excellent source of nutrition. It's OK to eat high-fat, high-calorie, inflammatory foods on occasion — sometimes it may be your only option. Your main goal is to choose foods that promote good health most of the time.

choices include vitamin D-fortified low-fat milk and yogurt. Vitamin D works with calcium to protect your bones, which is especially important when you have arthritis.

Of course, if you have a milk allergy or you're lactose intolerant, you'll want to get these nutrients from other sources, such as plant-based milks. Eating dairy increases inflammation in people with milk allergies.

Research has been somewhat mixed on how dairy foods affect arthritis in others. Saturated fat in cheese and high-fat dairy products is thought to increase inflammation. But in a recent large review, researchers found that eating dairy products actually had an anti-inflammatory impact overall.

Legumes, which include beans, peas and lentils, also are good sources of protein.

Legumes are typically low in fat, contain no cholesterol, and are high in protein, fiber, folate, potassium, iron and magnesium. They're a great substitute for meat in soups and stews. And they may help reduce inflammation.

Finally, fish and shellfish are good sources of protein, and some also contain omega-3 fatty acids. Omega-3s can help lower triglycerides — fat particles in blood that can raise your risk of heart disease. Omega-3s may also improve the function of your immune system, help regulate your blood pressure and reduce inflammation and arthritis pain. Research suggests that most people would benefit from eating at least two servings of fish a week.

## Fats

Fats are essential to the life and function of your body's cells. Along with providing reserves of stored energy, fats help maintain cell structure. They also play a role in immune system functioning and the regulation of many body processes, including some processes associated with inflammation. In short, you need some fat in your diet.

The key is that you want the right quantity and quality. The fat group near the top of the Mayo Clinic Healthy Weight Pyramid refers to fats that are typically added to foods during preparation, not the fat within foods in the other groups. These added fats include cooking oils, spreads and salad dressings. Some plant foods that are rich sources of fat also fit in this category, including avocados, olives, seeds and nuts.

There are several different kinds of fat in food. In terms of their healthfulness, not all fats are equal. Monounsaturated and polyunsaturated fats are the best choices. Look for products with little or no saturated fats, and avoid trans fats. Just remember that all fats are dense sources of energy — even the healthiest ones. So eat them in moderation.

**Monounsaturated fats** These fats are found in olive oil, flaxseed oil, peanut oil and canola oil, as well as most nuts and avocados. This type of fat helps reduce low-density lipoprotein (LDL) cholesterol and helps clear arteries by maintaining high-density lipoprotein (HDL) cholesterol. In addition, extra-virgin olive oil contains antioxidants, and canola and flaxseed oils and some nuts also contain omega-3 fatty acids — polyunsaturated fats that may help reduce inflammation.

**Polyunsaturated fats** These fats are found in plant-based oils such as safflower, corn, sunflower and soybean oils. Cold-water fish, such as salmon, provide omega-3s — a heart-healthy form of this fat.

**Saturated fats** Saturated fats are found in animal-based foods, such as meats, poultry, lard, egg yolks and whole-fat dairy foods.

## WHAT'S A SINGLE SERVING?

| Vegetables | Visual cue |
|---|---|
| 1 cup cut-up vegetables | 1 baseball |
| 2 cups raw, leafy greens | 2 baseballs |
| **Fruits** | |
| ¾ cup sliced fruit | 1 tennis ball |
| 1 small apple or medium orange | |
| **Carbohydrates** | |
| ½ cup whole-grain pasta or cereal | Hockey puck |
| ½ small whole-grain bagel | |
| 1 slice whole-grain bread | |
| **Protein and dairy** | |
| 2½ ounces chicken or 3 ounces fish | Deck of cards |
| 1½ ounces lean beef | ½ deck of cards |
| **Fats** | |
| 2 ounces low-fat hard cheese | 4 dice |
| 1½ teaspoons peanut butter | 2 dice |
| 1 teaspoon margarine or butter | 1 die |

## RECOMMENDED DAILY INTAKE OF CALCIUM AND VITAMIN D FOR MEN AND WOMEN

| Age (years) | Recommended calcium intake (mg/day) | Upper limit of calcium (mg/day) | Recommended vitamin D intake (IU/day) | Upper limit of vitamin D (IU/day) |
|---|---|---|---|---|
| 19 to 50 | 1,000 | 2,500 | 600 | 4,000 |
| 51 to 70 | 1,000 (men) 1,200 (women) | 2,000 | 600 | 4,000 |
| 71 and older | 1,200 | 2,000 | 800 | 4,000 |

Source: Institute of Medicine, 2010

Some postmenopausal women need a higher amount of calcium or vitamin D, depending on osteoporosis risk.

They're also in coconut oil, palm oil and other tropical oils, which are used in coffee creamers, snack crackers, commercial baked goods and other processed foods. Saturated fat is the main dietary culprit in raising blood cholesterol and narrowing the heart's coronary arteries. These types of fats are also associated with inflammation.

***Trans fats*** Small amounts of trans fats occur naturally in dairy and meat products. The main dietary sources of trans fat, though, are processed foods made with partially hydrogenated oil. This type of fat has been used in stick margarine and vegetable shortening and in foods made with them, including many cookies, crackers and cakes, as well as candies, snack foods and deep-fried foods. Trans fat raises "bad" (LDL) cholesterol levels and lowers "good" (HDL) cholesterol levels, along with other harmful effects. Like saturated fats, trans fats seem to be associated with increased inflammation.

In 2015 the Food and Drug Administration determined that partially hydrogenated oil is no longer generally recognized as safe, and it has been phased out of the production of foods. However, some foods that were manufactured before the ban took effect may still include trans fats.

## GOUT AND DIET

Gout is a complex form of arthritis characterized by sudden, severe attacks of pain, redness and tenderness in your joints. It occurs when there's too much uric acid in your blood, a condition called hyperuricemia. Your body produces uric acid when it breaks down purines. Purines are substances made naturally in your body. They're also found in certain foods, such as organ meats, anchovies, herring, asparagus and mushrooms.

Normally, uric acid dissolves in your blood and passes through your kidneys into your urine. But sometimes your body produces too much uric acid. In other cases, the kidneys don't get rid of enough uric acid.

To prevent gout attacks and to reduce the risk of other chronic conditions associated with gout, such as heart disease, try the following tips:

- *Limit red meats.* Red meats such as beef, pork and lamb can increase the level of uric acid in your blood. Organ meats (liver, brain and kidney) are particularly high in purines. Because all meat, including poultry, contains purines, limit meat to a few ounces daily. To get protein in your diet, eat low-fat dairy products, nuts, beans and peas.
- *Eat fish and seafood in moderation.* Although fish and seafood are heart healthy, both have been linked to higher uric acid levels and gout. Eating moderate (4-ounce) portions of fish and seafood twice weekly may have benefits overall. You can also get the benefits of omega-3 fatty acids found in fish from plant foods such as ground flaxseed, chia seeds, soy foods and walnuts.
- *Cut back on fat.* Saturated fat reduces the body's ability to eliminate uric acid. High-fat meals also contribute to obesity, which is linked to gout.
- *Reduce or avoid alcohol.* Alcohol interferes with the elimination of uric acid from your body. Beer and liquor have each been linked to an increased risk of gout attacks, even in moderate amounts. One recent study found that drinking wine also was associated with gout attacks, although previous research had not shown a link. To play it safe, limit or avoid all types of alcohol.

- *Drink plenty of fluids, particularly water.* Fluids help remove uric acid from your body. Aim for eight to 16 8-ounce glasses a day. There's also some evidence that drinking coffee in moderation is associated with decreased gout risk. But avoid sugary drinks high in calories.
- *Limit or avoid foods or beverages sweetened with high-fructose corn syrup.* Fructose, the type of sugar found in fruit and honey and used in high-fructose corn syrup, is known to increase uric acid. Avoid soft drinks and other beverages that include this common sweetener. It's smart to limit naturally sweet fruit juices, too.
- *Add cherries to the menu.* There is some evidence that eating cherries is associated with a reduced risk of gout attacks.
- *Get your vitamin C.* Vitamin C may help lower uric acid levels. Talk to your doctor about whether a 500-milligram vitamin C supplement fits into your diet and medication plan.
- *Lose weight if you're overweight.* Weight loss helps lessen the load on weight-bearing joints such as your knees and ankles, and it may also decrease uric acid levels. But avoid rapid-weight-loss diets, which could increase uric acid levels in your blood.

## Sweets

Foods in the sweets group include sugar-sweetened beverages, such as sodas, as well as candies, cakes, cookies, doughnuts and other desserts. And don't forget the table sugar you add to tea or coffee.

Sweets are typically a dense source of calories, mostly from sugar and fat. Yet they offer very little nutrition. In addition, sweets can cause spikes in blood sugar, which can lead to problems if you have diabetes or if you manage high blood sugar levels as a side effect of taking corticosteroid medications.

You don't have to avoid sweets entirely, but be smart about your selections and portion sizes. The pyramid recommends limiting sweets to 75 calories a day. When possible, select healthier desserts, such as a small amount of dark chocolate.

## FEED YOUR BONES

If your arthritis keeps you from getting regular exercise, you may be at an increased risk of osteoporosis — a condition that causes bones to become weak, brittle and susceptible to fractures. Weight-bearing exercise helps your body build and maintain bone. But if you aren't able to stay active, you may lose bone mass. Your risk of developing osteoporosis is also higher if you have a type of inflammatory arthritis or connective tissue disease such as rheumatoid arthritis or lupus, or if you take corticosteroid medications.

## A RISK OF BEING UNDERWEIGHT

Being overweight can worsen the symptoms of arthritis, but for people with rheumatoid arthritis there's also a risk in being too thin. In a study conducted at Mayo Clinic, researchers found that people with rheumatoid arthritis who had a low body mass index (BMI) were three times more likely to die of cardiovascular disease than were individuals without rheumatoid arthritis who had a normal weight. It's likely that people with the most severe forms of rheumatoid arthritis have an active and extensive inflammatory response, which can be associated with weight loss. For these individuals, the best course of action may be finding a doctor who will pay close attention to cardiovascular disease prevention and care.

If your BMI is normal or low, it's also important to be careful as you make healthy changes to your diet or eliminate foods that seem to trigger your symptoms. Sometimes, these changes can result in unexpected weight loss. Talk to your doctor or dietitian if you lose weight without trying.

To reduce your risk, it's important to get enough calcium in your diet. This mineral is one of the building blocks of bone, and it may help slow bone loss. You also need adequate vitamin D to help keep your bones strong. You get some vitamin D from food. You also get this vitamin from sunlight — your body makes vitamin D when your skin is exposed to the sun's rays. Still, you may need a vitamin D supplement if you don't get enough calcium and vitamin D in food or you don't get much direct sunlight outdoors.

How much calcium and vitamin D you need depends on your age and sex. (See the chart on page 301.) The best way to get these nutrients is with a balanced diet. You probably know that dairy products are rich in calcium. You can also get a healthy dose of calcium from tofu, salmon, fortified cereal and dark leafy greens such as kale. What about vitamin D? Milk and yogurt are often fortified with it, to help with calcium absorption. Other good sources include fish such as sockeye salmon and canned tuna, fortified orange juice, and eggs.

If you think your diet frequently misses the mark, check with your doctor or registered dietitian to see if you should take a calcium or vitamin D supplement. In some instances your doctor may also recommend medications to prevent osteoporosis, especially if you're taking steroid medications long-term to treat your arthritis.

For most people, the best way to keep your bones strong — along with getting those essential nutrients — is through regular weight-bearing exercise and strength (resistance) training. Even going for a walk can help. The greater the demands you place on your bones, the stronger and denser they become.

## BENEFITS OF A HEALTHY WEIGHT

Research has shown that being overweight or obese increases your risk of osteoarthritis of the knee. Being overweight or obese also tends to worsen the signs and symptoms of arthritis. Excess weight adds stress to your weight-bearing joints, especially your knees, aggravating pain, stiffness and inflammation. Being obese can even cause pain in the neck and hands.

As a result, it's important to lose weight if you're overweight. And if you're at a healthy weight, it's critical to avoid weight gain.

Weight loss is especially important if you and your doctor are considering joint surgery as a treatment option for arthritis, because excess weight can make surgery more difficult and risky. In fact, some surgeons insist that their patients who are overweight lose weight before they undergo elective operations.

The good news is that if you have osteoarthritis or rheumatoid arthritis and you're carrying extra weight, shedding some of those excess pounds can reduce the stress on your back, hips, knees and feet — all places where you may develop arthritis pain. In fact, weight loss has been shown to improve symptoms and reduce the need for knee surgery no matter how much structural damage has occurred in the knee. A loss of 5% to 10% of your total body weight may:

- Decrease pain
- Provide a sense of control
- Increase mobility
- Increase ability to exercise
- Increase energy level
- Improve balance

All of these benefits, in turn, help decrease fatigue, prevent falls and improve your self-image.

And if you have pounds to lose, greater results may reap bigger rewards. A recent study found that people who lost 20% of their total body weight helped reduce pain and improve walking function significantly more than those who lost 5% to 10% of their body weight.

### Weight-control basics

At first glance, the basic formula for weight control seems simple. If you burn more calories than you consume from food, you'll lose weight. If you take in more calories than you spend (through daily activity, exercise and basic body functions), you'll gain weight, which can worsen arthritis pain. However, it can be challenging to implement a practical, effective and sustainable weight-loss plan.

You may need to make changes to what you eat in order to control your weight, but it shouldn't be at the cost of good health, taste and practicality. The diet you choose should be simple, inexpensive, enjoyable and satisfying so you'll stick with it. Adding regular moderate physical activity also is important.

Even with arthritis, you have many physical activities to choose from that can help burn calories and increase muscle mass. You don't have to lift heavy weights to counteract muscle loss as you age. You can exercise your muscles with resistance bands or by using the weight of your own body, as in pushups, lunges and standing squats. Normal daily activities such as cleaning, shopping and doing laundry help you burn calories, too.

The more active you are, the easier it is to maintain and even increase your muscle mass and maintain a healthy weight. (See Chapter 15 for more guidance on exercise.) On days when you're not feeling well, try to stay active with lower intensity activities.

## Guide for weight loss

Before starting a weight-loss plan, it's important to work with your doctor. However, you can use the Healthy Weight Pyramid as your guide to making smart eating choices. The pyramid ensures that you're getting a balanced diet — including foods that may help reduce inflammation but won't overload you with calories and unhealthy fat. It's a great plan for lifelong healthy eating.

## WHAT'S YOUR BMI?

Body mass index (BMI) is a tool for indicating your weight status. For most people, BMI is a reasonably accurate measure of body composition and indicator of whether they're at a healthy or an unhealthy weight. To determine your BMI, find your height in the left column. Follow that row across to the weight nearest yours. Look at the top of that column for your approximate BMI.

Whatever your BMI, you will benefit from a discussion about your weight and overall fitness with your doctor.

| BMI | Normal | | Overweight* | | | | | Obese | | | | |
|---|---|---|---|---|---|---|---|---|---|---|---|---|
| | 19 | 24 | 25 | 26 | 27 | 28 | 29 | 30 | 35 | 40 | 45 | 50 |
| Height | Weight in pounds | | | | | | | | | | | |
| 4'10" | 91 | 115 | 119 | 124 | 129 | 134 | 138 | 143 | 167 | 191 | 215 | 239 |
| 4'11" | 94 | 119 | 124 | 128 | 133 | 138 | 143 | 148 | 173 | 198 | 222 | 247 |
| 5'0" | 97 | 123 | 128 | 133 | 138 | 143 | 148 | 153 | 179 | 204 | 230 | 255 |
| 5'1" | 100 | 127 | 132 | 137 | 143 | 148 | 153 | 158 | 185 | 211 | 238 | 264 |
| 5'2" | 104 | 131 | 136 | 142 | 147 | 153 | 158 | 164 | 191 | 218 | 246 | 273 |
| 5'3" | 107 | 135 | 141 | 146 | 152 | 158 | 163 | 169 | 197 | 225 | 254 | 282 |
| 5'4" | 110 | 140 | 145 | 151 | 157 | 163 | 169 | 174 | 204 | 232 | 262 | 291 |
| 5'5" | 114 | 144 | 150 | 156 | 162 | 168 | 174 | 180 | 210 | 240 | 270 | 300 |
| 5'6" | 118 | 148 | 155 | 161 | 167 | 173 | 179 | 186 | 216 | 247 | 278 | 309 |
| 5'7" | 121 | 153 | 159 | 166 | 172 | 178 | 185 | 191 | 223 | 255 | 287 | 319 |
| 5'8" | 125 | 158 | 164 | 171 | 177 | 184 | 190 | 197 | 230 | 262 | 295 | 328 |
| 5'9" | 128 | 162 | 169 | 176 | 182 | 189 | 196 | 203 | 236 | 270 | 304 | 338 |
| 5'10" | 132 | 167 | 174 | 181 | 188 | 195 | 202 | 209 | 243 | 278 | 313 | 348 |
| 5'11" | 136 | 172 | 179 | 186 | 193 | 200 | 208 | 215 | 250 | 286 | 322 | 358 |
| 6'0" | 140 | 177 | 184 | 191 | 199 | 206 | 213 | 221 | 258 | 294 | 331 | 368 |
| 6'1" | 144 | 182 | 189 | 197 | 204 | 212 | 219 | 227 | 265 | 302 | 340 | 378 |
| 6'2" | 148 | 186 | 194 | 202 | 210 | 218 | 225 | 233 | 272 | 311 | 350 | 389 |
| 6'3" | 152 | 192 | 200 | 208 | 216 | 224 | 232 | 240 | 279 | 319 | 359 | 399 |
| 6'4" | 156 | 197 | 205 | 213 | 221 | 230 | 238 | 246 | 287 | 328 | 369 | 410 |

Source: National Institutes of Health, 1998

*Asians with a BMI of 23 or higher may have an increased risk of health problems.

Each food group in the pyramid comes with a recommended range of servings. How many servings you should eat depends on a variety of factors, including your weight, activity level and sex. If you're trying to lose weight, you'll want to aim for servings in the lower range for each food group rather than in the higher range. It's important, however, that you eat at least the minimum daily servings for each food group to maintain good health. Your doctor or dietitian can also help you find the right number of servings.

It's also important to remember that a serving is not the same thing as a portion. A serving is an exact amount of food defined by common measurements, such as cups, ounces and tablespoons. A portion is the amount of food put on your plate. And if you're used to restaurant-sized portions, one meal often contains several servings of each food.

You can use common visual cues to estimate servings. Check out the table on page 300 for helpful examples.

## Appetite control

Long-term use of some arthritis drugs may increase your appetite, making it more difficult to keep your weight under control. Eat slowly and stretch mealtimes to a minimum of 20 to 30 minutes to allow your natural appetite-control mechanism to work.

Increasing the amount of high-fiber foods in your diet can help you feel full more quickly. To get more fiber, try whole-grain breads instead of white bread, fresh fruit instead of juice, and raw vegetables and fruits in place of salty snacks. These tips also may help you curb an overactive appetite:

- *Eat a healthy breakfast.* Make breakfast a high-fiber cereal, whole-grain bread and fresh fruit so you're less tempted to eat unhealthy snacks throughout the morning. Starting the day with a good breakfast can also set you up for eating a more-balanced lunch.

- *Be sure you're hungry.* Are you eating because you're stressed or bored? On those occasions, try reading, being active or calling a friend in place of eating.

- *Eat slowly.* Savor the flavor and texture of individual foods to boost your satisfaction. Remember, it takes about 20 minutes for your brain to receive a signal that you're full. Make sure your meals last at least this long.

- *Ride out the urge.* Cravings generally pass within minutes, maybe even seconds. If you're not actually hungry, busy yourself with an activity unrelated to food until the desire to eat passes.

- *Start small.* If you feel you always need to finish what's in front of you, start with half the amount of food on your plate that you normally eat. You may find that a smaller amount is still enough. To make less food seem like more, serve your main course on a salad or dessert plate.

- *Enjoy a treat now and then.* Keep tempting treats out of the house so you don't overindulge. But allow for an occasional ice cream cone or small piece of apple pie when you're out.

## STRATEGIES FOR SUCCESS

Whether you're trying to lose weight or eat more healthfully to improve arthritic symptoms, the following strategies may help. Healthy eating isn't just about adding up calories and eating servings of salmon and kale. It's about organization, planning and practicality — at restaurants, in the grocery store and in your own kitchen.

### Make a menu

You'll be more likely to stick with a healthy diet if you have a plan. With the right ingredients on hand, healthy meals come together from scratch almost as fast as they do with processed convenience foods.

Try planning your meals one week at a time. Consider your calendar as you plan. If you're invited to a friend's house for dinner on Saturday, cross that meal off your list. If you're volunteering on Wednesday evening and that will delay dinner, pencil in leftovers or an extra-quick meal that won't take much time and energy to prepare. Make sure your plan includes healthy options for breakfast, lunch and snacks, too. And don't forget to take it with you to the store.

Menu planning may take a little getting used to. But it's one of your best defenses against unplanned, unhealthy eating — such as grabbing chips or cookies when you need a break at work or arrive home hungry. Planning also helps you get a healthy meal on the table when your energy is low or you're in pain.

***Plan for leftovers*** Make a double batch of chili so it stretches over two dinners instead of one. Prepare two lasagnas and freeze one for later. Or roast a chicken and turn the leftover meat into a stir-fry later in the week. No matter how you do it, preparing for two meals at once is always a timesaver.

***Cook ahead*** Make Tuesday night's stew during a free Sunday afternoon. Prep your vegetables in the morning so they're ready to use at dinnertime. Prepare a simple balsamic vinaigrette while you're talking on the phone. You may find many occasions when you can do small tasks in advance, making cooking less daunting later on.

*Look for shortcuts* When you go to the grocery store, feel free to purchase pre-cut fruits and vegetables, meats cut for stir-fries, and other items that save you time in the kitchen. They may cost a little more but can be worth it when you're not feeling well. Even prepared foods from the grocery store are generally less expensive than take-out or restaurant foods of similar nutritional value.

*Keep a list of menu ideas* Make a file of recipes that include few ingredients and take 20 minutes or less to make. Refer to the list as you plan weekly menus, or pull it out when an unexpected event disrupts your day and you can't stick to your original meal plan.

*Include family members* Ask family members what they'd like to eat that's different and healthy. They may be more willing to assist and experiment along with you.

## ADDING NUTRITION TO CONVENIENCE FOODS

It's OK to eat convenience foods, such as frozen entrees or side dishes, on busy days. Just be selective about what you choose. Look for items that are relatively low in fat, calories and sodium. Then, give them a nutritional boost:

Add spinach, fresh peppers, grated carrots, mushrooms and onions to prepared spaghetti sauce to increase fiber, nutrients and flavor.

Top frozen pizza with fresh tomatoes or thinly sliced peppers before heating. Or add a handful of arugula and a drizzle of olive oil or lemon juice after heating.

When preparing packaged whole-grain (brown) rice, toss in vegetables (peas, broccoli, corn) or fruit (raisins, apple, apricots).

Serve fruits and vegetables as side dishes when eating convenience foods, such as frozen microwave dinners.

## Create a kitchen that really cooks

When you have arthritis, the time you have for meal preparation and the amount of effort you're able to manage can be major factors in deciding what foods you serve. Help yourself by making your kitchen efficient and easy to use.

***Tools for organization*** Arrange your kitchen so the most common or important things that you use are within easy reach. Make use of energy-saving storage devices such as Lazy Susans. You may also want to buy easy-to-open containers to keep food and equipment handy.

If you have the space, it may help to have a small, wheeled cart for tasks that involve moving supplies from one place to another, to minimize the loads you have to carry. For example, use the cart to gather ingredients from the refrigerator and pantry or while setting the table. Arrange one complete place setting at a time and work your way around the table. You can also use the cart to clear the table and carry items to the sink for cleanup.

***Lightening your workload*** Keep utensils nearby as you cook, to save steps and motions. Use a small electric food processor to chop and dice foods and grate cheese. Rinse dirty cooking utensils and equipment immediately so that cleanup will be easier later on.

Here are a few other tips for cooking with ease:
- Use utensils with fat handles that are easy to grip.
- Keep your knives sharpened for easy cutting.
- Slide heavy objects along the counter rather than lifting them.
- Serve hot items from the stove directly on the plates rather than lifting heavy pots and pans to serve in large serving dishes.
- Cook and serve in the same dish whenever possible.
- Use a slotted spoon to remove vegetables from water instead of lifting the kettle and pouring the contents into a colander.
- Place a nonslip pad or wet cloth under a mixing bowl to help hold it stationary without gripping.

## Tips for eating out

You can dine out and still stay true to your dietary goals. The following tips can help you stay on track when you're eating away from home:

***Choose restaurants carefully*** Look for places that offer lots of variety, where you can find a healthy meal that's appealing. Restaurants that prepare the food you order from start to finish are more likely to accommodate special requests. Many restaurants post menus and nutritional information on their websites, so you can look for healthy options and decide what to order beforehand.

***Keep hunger under control*** Don't skip meals on days you're eating out. If you're ravenous when you go into a restaurant, you're more prone to order too much food.

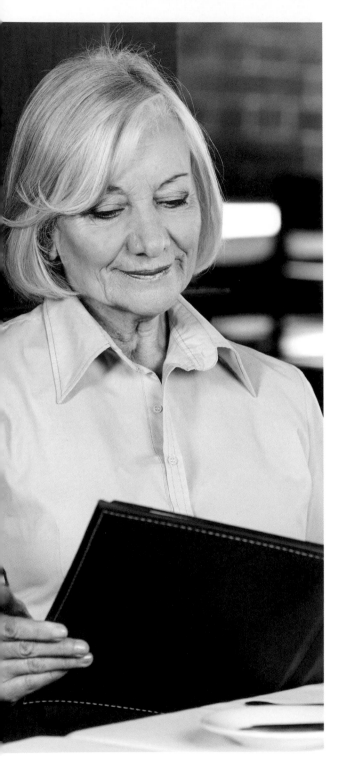

In fact, you may want to have a light snack of vegetables or fruit an hour or so before the meal to avoid overeating.

**Look for plant-based options** Many restaurants have special listings for healthy eating. However, foods in the diet or light section may still be a heftier meal than you think. Look for items that contain small amounts of meat, poultry or fish, and lots of vegetables and low-fat carbohydrates — for example, a baked potato, brown rice or a slice of whole-grain bread.

**Order wisely** If you can't find a healthy dinner item, order a la carte. Make a meal out of a broth-based (not creamy) soup or a salad and one appetizer. Choose something that's broiled, baked or steamed, not fried. Also consider sharing the meal with a companion or asking for a take-home box to come with your food so you can immediately save half to take home for another time.

**Speak up** Ask your server to clarify any unfamiliar terms or explain how a dish is prepared. Request smaller portions and substitutions, such as fresh fruit for french fries. Ask whether items can be broiled instead of fried.

**Cut out the condiments** Taste your food before instinctively adding salt, butter, sauces and dressing. Well-prepared food often needs only minimal enhancement. Ask for sauces or dressing on the side. Dab your fork in the sauce before using it to pick up your food. This allows you to enjoy the sauce but limits the amount.

## FOOD AND DRUG INTERACTIONS

You may have heard that certain foods you eat can alter the effectiveness of some medications. On the flip side, some arthritis medications can interfere with how well your body uses certain nutrients. So you may need higher amounts of some vitamins or minerals to help make up for their reduced effectiveness.

Make sure you understand how your medication should be taken. Some of the drugs used to treat arthritis are most effective if you take them on an empty stomach. Others should be taken with food to prevent stomach irritation. Carefully follow the instructions from your health care team.

Two of the most common side effects of arthritis medications are heartburn and stomach upset, often described as a gnawing pain or empty feeling in the stomach. These symptoms might be caused by the food or the medication or a combination of both.

To help prevent the symptoms, sit upright for at least 15 to 30 minutes after eating meals or taking medications. Try to avoid eating for at least one hour before bedtime. Limit foods that tend to trigger reactions, such as alcohol, caffeine, cola, spicy foods, fried foods and black pepper.

Be sure to discuss your medications with your doctor. Learn whether you need to avoid any foods because of medications, if you have any need to take supplements, and what is the most effective way to take the medication. In the end, it's important that your medications and your healthy-eating plan are working together. Both play important roles in helping you live well with arthritis.

# Your mind and your health

Your mind is a collection of thoughts, feelings, beliefs and emotions — the infrastructure that processes and supports the continuous flow of information through your brain. It's a subtle yet powerful tool guiding your conduct in daily life. The health and vitality of your mind is extraordinarily important to maintaining your physical health and allowing you to live a balanced, satisfying life.

Thoughts and feelings you have about yourself and your place in life can powerfully influence your perception of and ability to cope with a condition like arthritis. How well you're able to manage your joint pain may be based on whether you're an optimist or pessimist, whether you feel confident or insecure about yourself, and whether or not you feel in control of your own life.

Put simply, positive or optimistic thoughts can have health-enhancing benefits. Negative or pessimistic thoughts can intensify stress and pain. In general, optimists are convinced they can change and make things work out. They tend to react to adversity by taking action. Having a positive attitude may provide a buffer from stress, and you face life's difficulties with a greater sense of hope.

The mind-body connection works in various ways. For example, if you believe your life is under control, you tend to take better care of yourself — such as eating right, exercising and getting enough rest — than if you think nothing you do matters. Feelings of helplessness, meanwhile, may weaken your immune system by inhibiting the response of certain cells to invading bacteria, viruses and tumor cells. People with a pessimistic outlook also may isolate themselves from the proven, health-enhancing benefits of companionship, love and support from family and friends.

With arthritis, how well you manage the condition depends at least as much on your own actions as on the skill of your health care team. If you believe you can manage arthritis — if you believe that you can handle pain and fatigue — you're more likely to use medical resources more effectively than people with less faith in their coping skills. Between two people with the same level of physical impairment, the one with better coping skills is likely to experience less pain and have less difficulty functioning.

Research has proven certain ways the powerful link between mind and body can affect your health. If you're convinced that you're doomed to live in pain with arthritis, you may be subjecting your body to extra stress and feelings of helplessness, making day-to-day activities more of a struggle.

But if you believe in yourself and your abilities, you're already giving yourself a boost that will help you learn how to manage arthritis while living a full and satisfying life.

## YOUR BODY AND STRESS

For years, scientists have closely studied the complex interactions involving emotions, stress and disease, and the body's immune system and nervous system. It's the job of your immune system to maintain your health and facilitate healing by warding off invaders, such as bacteria and viruses, and abnormal cells.

Your nervous system provides communication links between organs that are part of your immune system, such as the spleen, lymph nodes and thymus. The nervous system also regulates hormones — body chemicals that control the immune response.

Stress can have a powerful impact on these functions. When you're under stress, your brain triggers the release of hormones as your body gears up to face the challenge. It's what you feel when you're scared or excited. Your heart beats faster, your breathing speeds up and your muscles tense.

These physiological reactions can be a positive thing, giving you an energy boost that's necessary to pass a test, give a speech or perform onstage. They can also "rev up" your immune system, preparing your body to heal injury or fight infection.

There's a downside to this process. Research shows that when stress is ongoing, or chronic, the continuous release of hormones begins to suppress your immune system, making you more susceptible to illness. If you're older or already have an illness, you become more prone to stress-related changes.

With a chronic condition such as arthritis, stress makes it harder to manage your symptoms. One of the most negative effects of stress is increased pain resulting from muscle tension and fatigue. The pain, in turn, reduces your stamina, causes feelings of helplessness, and intensifies anger, anxiety and frustration. As a result, you may become depressed and feel more and more helpless.

Stress is a part of life that can't be avoided. While you can control many stressful occurrences, you can't control all of them. Accidents or illness occur. Even positive events in your life, such as a job promotion or wedding, may cause you stress.

For most of us, minor stressors are more common than major ones. Research indicates that these minor events can have a significant impact on how you feel day to day. Stress can also be generated from within — your reaction to an event is often what determines the amount of stress you experience. This reinforces the stress cycle of pain, reduced coping abilities and depression.

## Heed the warning signs

The first step in breaking the stress cycle is learning to recognize when you're under stress. People experience stress differently in varying combinations of physical symptoms, emotional changes and behavioral changes.

Physical effects of stress may include:
- Headaches
- Chest pain
- Heart pounding
- High blood pressure
- Shortness of breath
- Muscle aches or pain
- Clenched jaws
- Teeth grinding
- Tight, dry throat
- Indigestion
- Constipation or diarrhea

- Stomach cramping or bloating
- Increased perspiration, often causing cold, sweaty hands
- Fatigue
- Insomnia
- Weight gain or loss
- Diminished sex drive
- Skin problems, such as hives

Emotional effects of stress may include:
- Anxiety
- Restlessness
- Worrying
- Irritability
- Depression
- Sadness
- Anger
- Mood swings
- Feelings of insecurity
- Lack of concentration
- Confusion
- Forgetfulness
- Resentment
- Assigning blame to others
- Guilt
- Pessimism

Behavioral effects of stress may include:
- Overeating
- Loss of appetite
- Poor anger management
- Increased use of alcohol and drugs
- Increased smoking
- Withdrawal or isolation
- Crying spells
- Changes in close relationships
- Job dissatisfaction
- Decreased productivity
- Burnout

If you experience any of these changes, try to determine if they may be caused by something other than stress, possibly with the help of your doctor or psychologist. If your symptoms appear to be stress related, try to figure out what's triggering them. Obviously, situations such as divorce or a death in the family are major stressors. But what about the day-to-day occurrences that rev up your stress reactors?

Take note of the things that make your heart beat faster and neck muscles tighter. Is it arguing with a co-worker, sitting in rush-hour traffic, juggling too many commitments or maybe all of these? Keeping a written log for a few weeks can give you a better handle on what sets your nerves on edge.

If you can identify your symptoms and what triggers them, you may be able to better control stress, by avoiding the triggers, changing the circumstances, if possible, or altering your reaction to the events.

## FOCUS ON THE POSITIVE

OK, so you have arthritis. That's no reason to think of yourself as hopeless, alone or unhealthy.

Remember, you have choices. Taking care of yourself by eating well, exercising and getting enough rest can go a long way toward making you feel better and staying active. But what if you believe you're not in control of your situation? Chances are your thoughts are working against you.

## DEPRESSION AND ARTHRITIS

Depression is more than just feeling down or blue. It's a biochemical imbalance of the brain, causing certain symptoms that, if extreme, can be life-threatening. When you have arthritis, it's not unusual for you to become depressed.

Depression can lead to many emotional and physical problems. Symptoms may include persistent sadness, irritability, anxiety, loss of interest or pleasure in life, neglect of personal care, changes in eating or sleeping habits, persistent fatigue, loss of energy, and feelings of worthlessness or guilt. Symptoms of depression tend to magnify the pain and discomfort of arthritis.

Please see a medical professional if you think you may be depressed. The condition usually requires long-term treatment involving medication and psychological counseling.

If you're reluctant to seek treatment for depression, consider this: It may actually help reduce pain. Research has found that for older adults with both arthritis and depression, taking antidepressant medications or attending therapy sessions reduced the symptoms of both conditions. The individuals also reported better joint function and overall health.

Self-talk is rapid-fire or automatic thoughts that pass through your brain constantly, although you may not be aware of it. If you pause for a moment and listen to what's going through your mind, you might be surprised by how negative your self-talk can be.

For example, you start a walking program and instead of focusing on the benefits the activity brings, you chide yourself for being out of shape. Or before you give a presenta-tion, you tell yourself, "I'm lousy at speaking under pressure."

Negative self-talk may underlie some (or most) of the stress you're feeling. Cognitive behavioral therapy, a common type of talk therapy, may help you transform that self-talk from negative to positive. It can be an effective tool for anyone wishing to learn how to better manage stressful life situations such as arthritis.

To use cognitive behavioral therapy, you'll work with a counselor (psychotherapist), who will help you become more aware of your inaccurate or negative way of thinking. Therapy allows you to view challenging situations clearly and respond to them in a more effective manner.

Therapy is generally focused on specific problems — for example, the struggles you may be having with mobility or your worry about the appearance of a deformed finger joint — using a goal-oriented approach. Sessions help you to:

- Identify the difficult situations
- Become aware of your thoughts, emotions and beliefs about these situations
- Identify the negative or inaccurate thoughts you have
- Challenge your negative or inaccurate thinking

Your therapist will encourage you to consider whether your view of a situation is based on actual fact or based on your inaccurate perception of what's going on. This can be difficult if you have long-standing ways of thinking about your life and yourself. With practice, your ability to develop positive thinking and behavior will become a habit and won't take as much effort.

Instead of thinking, "I'll never be able to do anything I enjoy," you can tell yourself, "I'll take good care of myself so I can still do many things" or "I may have to slow down, but I don't have to give up." By changing your outlook, you'll find more constructive ways to cope with arthritis.

## REDUCE STRESS

In addition to redirecting negative thoughts, there are other strategies for managing stress. You may talk about your problems with others, listen to soothing music or take a short evening walk. Even if you usually do pretty well in getting through life's crises as they arise, at times you may need a little extra help.

The following tips may help you better manage stress:

- ***Try to be more tolerant.*** Learn to be more accepting of yourself and of situations over which you have no control. A starting point is the recognition that you'll always experience a certain amount of stress — and that is normal.
- ***Plan your day.*** Having a plan may help you feel more in control of your life. Keep a schedule of daily activities and appointments so that you're not faced with conflicts or last-minute dashes to get somewhere on time.
- ***Get organized.*** De-clutter living and work spaces so that you don't have to spend time and energy searching for misplaced items.
- ***Manage your time.*** Often, stress is a result of too much to do and too little time. Setting priorities and practicing simple time management skills may go a long way toward depressurizing your day.
- ***Take occasional breaks.*** Periodically during the day, take time to relax, stretch or walk.
- ***Get adequate sleep, stay physically active and eat well.*** A healthy body

promotes good mental health. Sleep reinvigorates you. Physical activity burns off stress-related tension. And a balanced diet provides energy to handle daily stress.

- **Discuss your concerns.** Talking with a family member or friend may help to relieve stress and cast events in a different light.
- **Get away.** Take a break from your normal routine. You might benefit from a change of scenery or a different pace of life.
- **Enjoy a good laugh.** It's healthy to spend time with people who have a positive outlook, don't take themselves too seriously or have a sense of humor. Laughter helps reduce or relieve tension.

If self-help measures don't reduce stress, help from a counselor, psychiatrist, psychologist or clergyperson may be what you need. Many people mistakenly believe that seeking outside help is a sign of weakness. But it takes strength and self-awareness to realize that you need help — and good judgment to seek it.

## LEARN TO RELAX

Relaxation helps reduce the muscle tension that can increase pain. If you need help relaxing, there are a number of relaxation techniques you might try. Finding one that works for you helps decrease pain and increase your comfort level.

Relaxation techniques typically need to be learned, which means initially following some direction and then practicing them regularly. Yoga, tai chi and other techniques that involve defined postures and repetitive movements can help you relax. Prayer and meditation, especially when kept simple, familiar and repetitive, also may help.

These quiet, reflective exercises can help you reverse the mental arousal from stress. Regular practice of relaxation techniques may also reduce stress by changing your thought patterns. It can be another powerful means of shifting thoughts from negative to positive.

Following are several relaxation techniques, although these are by no means all of them. If you wish to try one, there are many instructional products on the market, streaming videos or classes that may help you. Pick a quiet time and place where you won't be disturbed. Practice regularly, preferably daily, for a minimum of 15 to 20 minutes. And try to be patient — it may take several weeks to get the hang of it and start to see some benefit.

## Meditation

This ancient practice has been called an altered state of consciousness and a unique state of relaxation. There are almost as many ways to meditate as there are people who meditate.

The basic premise of meditation is to sit quietly and focus on the rhythm of your breathing or on a simple word or phrase repeated over and over. When distracting thoughts arise — and they will — you simply notice them and let them go, always returning to your focus. With meditation, you enter a deeply restful state that reduces your body's stress response.

There are different types of meditation, including mindful meditation, relaxation response and transcendental meditation. All forms work similarly. By meditating often, you can learn to relax your breathing, slow brain waves, and decrease muscle tension and your heart rate. Like other relaxation techniques, meditation can help lessen your response to the chemicals that your body produces when you're stressed, such as adrenaline. Too much adrenaline on a regular basis can be harmful.

## Guided imagery

With this practice, also known as visualization, you enter a relaxed state brought on by meditation or self-hypnosis. In this state, you employ all your senses to imagine a setting that helps alleviate the physical symptoms of stress.

Studies of guided imagery suggest that when you imagine something, the same parts of your brain are stimulated as when you actually experience it. When you visualize a calming environment, your brain receives messages of relaxation that are passed on to your autonomic nervous and endocrine systems, which regulate key functions such as heart rate and blood pressure.

## Progressive muscle relaxation

This relaxation technique works on the theory that to learn how to relax your muscles, you must first know how they feel when they're tensed. Therefore, progressive relaxation is a series of exercises that takes you through each of the major muscle groups from head to toe — tensing and releasing tension as you go. Along the way, you focus on how the relaxed muscles feel compared with the tense muscles.

A similar technique to progressive muscle relaxation is called body scanning. You systematically focus on each muscle group, noting any tension and then letting it go without tensing the muscles. Instead of physically tensing and relaxing muscles, you focus on the sensations in each part of your body.

## Self-hypnosis

Self-hypnosis is an induced state of relaxation that enhances your focus and helps make you more open to act on suggestions given to you — or that you give to yourself — in a hypnotic state. Self-hypnosis alters brain wave patterns in much the same way as other relaxation techniques. This stress-relieving result may be why it works to ease pain and stress and alter behavior.

## Massage therapy

Massage therapy involves the manipulation of soft tissues of your body. There are several forms of massage, including the traditional kneading and rubbing of Swedish massage and the application of pressure at specific points of the body, which characterizes acupressure (shiatsu) massage.

Massage can reduce your heart rate, increase blood circulation, relax muscles, improve range of motion and increase endorphins, which can help relieve pain. Massage can also be effective at relieving stress, depression and anxiety. It can decrease the perception of pain and has been shown to reduce arthritis pain.

The environment in which you receive massage is important. A warm, quiet area, free from distracting noise or interruption, can help relieve muscle tension. Low-volume sound or music also relaxes muscles. Your massage therapist may use a mineral oil to reduce friction, contributing to smooth, effective massage strokes.

## Keep a journal

Writing down your thoughts and feelings can help you blow off steam, increase self-awareness, solve problems and put things in perspective. By writing regularly, you can also create a record of your symptoms, see patterns in their occurrence, gain a better understanding of your disease and find wording to better communicate about your condition. You may also be able to determine whether medications are affecting your mood or whether your arthritis flares when you're under stress.

Some research has even suggested that for people with chronic illnesses such as rheumatoid arthritis, writing about their stressful experiences may be linked to improved symptoms. One theory is that the emotional processing involved in the act of writing can help to reduce stress.

## SEEK SUPPORT

Having friends and loved ones to talk to can help you feel less alone and overwhelmed, and more able to cope. This may be especially true when you're dealing with the pain and fatigue of arthritis. Having people who care about you also makes you more likely to take better care of yourself.

In addition, having support may help to improve your physical functioning. Receiving daily doses of friendliness and understanding from others may improve your psychological well-being. And having social companionship — being asked to join in — appears to be beneficial both physically and psychologically. In short, staying connected and maintaining close relationships is good for your health.

Support groups may offer benefits similar to individual support. In fact, in a group of relative strangers, you might actually feel more comfortable expressing your deepest fears and daily concerns without worry of scaring or burdening your loved ones. Depending on the nature of the group, you can deal with difficult problems, share experiences, learn how others cope with the same challenges and change your perspective.

You may get the most benefit from a support group if you're interested in learning about the experiences of others and if you're willing to share your thoughts and feelings. To find a group, talk to your doctor, your local Arthritis Foundation chapter or others you know who have arthritis.

If you're not comfortable in a group setting but feel a need to express and process your feelings about arthritis, you might consider individual counseling. A therapist can also help you learn meditation or self-hypnosis to practice on your own. Talk to your doctor for a recommendation.

## INTIMACY

Sexuality is a natural, healthy part of living, and part of your identity. When the chronic pain of arthritis invades your life, the pleasures of sexuality often disappear. You may be concerned that sexual intercourse will cause physical pain, especially if you have arthritis in your back or hip. You may be worried that your partner finds you less attractive because of pain or swollen joints. Or you may have simply lost interest in sex as a result of the symptoms.

It doesn't have to be this way. You can have a healthy and satisfying sexual relationship while managing arthritis. The key is honest communication. It also helps to be creative and willing to change.

No matter what your health condition is, it's important not to lose sight of your sexuality.

Here are strategies for enhancing your sex life and achieving greater satisfaction:

- **Communicate openly.** Talk with your partner about how you feel, what you want or need from the relationship, and how to be intimate in a way that's enjoyable for both of you. If you have unspoken fears regarding sexual contact, tell your partner about them. Talking openly together can ease your concerns and open the door for creative problem solving.

- **Rekindle your romance.** Go on a date, plan a picnic, send flowers or just spend extra time together. Set the stage for sexual intimacy with dinner by candlelight or holding hands during an evening stroll.

- **Prepare your body.** Do gentle range-of-motion exercises for a few minutes before having sex. This may help prevent pain and stiffness. A warm bath or shower with your partner also may help relax your muscles and prepare you for intimacy. Taking a pain medication or muscle relaxant before sex might be another option — but first, talk with your doctor about which type of drug and what dose is right for you.

- **Expand your definition of intimacy.** For many people with arthritis, it's the act of intercourse that causes the most problems. Consider alternatives that might be more comfortable and fulfilling, including cuddling, fondling, sensual massage, masturbation, oral sex or use of a vibrator.

- **Experiment to make intercourse more comfortable.** Instead of a conventional posture that may be painful, try a different position, for example, lying side by side, kneeling or sitting. Many good books are available that describe different ways to have intercourse.

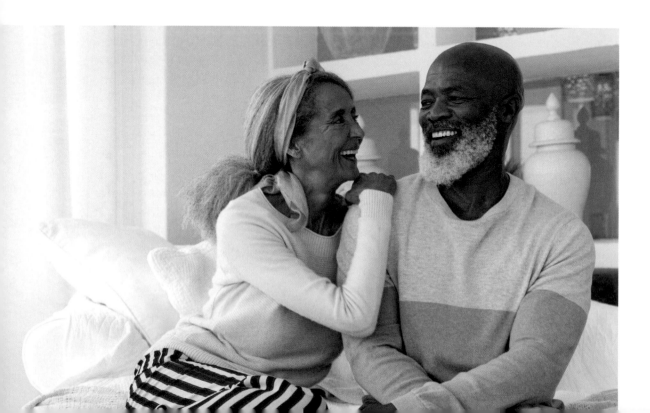

- *Change your routine.* Many people have higher pain levels in the evening. If this is true for you, try being intimate in the morning — when you're refreshed from a good night's sleep and may have the most energy.

If you continue to have sexual problems, talk with your doctor. Describe when and how your sexual desire or performance has been affected by arthritis. Pain and fatigue can reduce your libido, but many medications, including glucocorticoids and antidepressants, also can reduce your sex drive. Your doctor may be able to change your medication, change the dosage or recommend other strategies to enhance your sex life.

However, even if you suspect a medication may be affecting sexual performance, it's important that you don't stop taking it without first consulting your doctor.

In all partnerships, it takes effort to maintain what is good and to correct what isn't. Be willing to make that effort. A healthy sexual relationship can positively affect all aspects of your life, including your physical health, self-esteem and productivity.

Remind yourself that problems can also be opportunities. In your efforts to become more intimate again, you may discover something about your partner that you otherwise might have missed. The relationship you recover may be even better than the one you had before you developed arthritis.

## SIMPLIFY YOUR LIFE

We live in an era of multitasking — doing (or trying to do) several things at once. Yet many people seem to long for a simpler, slower paced, more meaningful life. Arthritis may force you to slow down and focus on single tasks. That may not mean quitting your job or hobbies, but you may need to allow more time for rest and self-care. As a result, you might pay more attention to the things in your life that give you satisfaction and pleasure.

The following suggestions can help simplify your life.

*Reassess success* Living a fast-paced, competitive lifestyle is exciting at times, but it may not always be the right choice for you. You may make more money and have a better golf score or higher profile in your community than you'd have with a less demanding job or lifestyle. But consider whether it's worth the added stress. Maybe it is — or maybe you'd gladly trade having more money or prestige for having more free time.

*Accept things you can't change* Maybe you can't do all of the things you did before you had arthritis. If you have rheumatoid arthritis, the wax-and-wane nature of your disease might make it difficult to plan ahead, and you may be too tired to pursue every interest. Don't fight it. Decide what's important. Give top priority to those things you must do and you want to do. For the rest, delegate them, drop them or ask for help.

**Take a breath** When you're stressed, your breathing is rapid and shallow. Relaxed breathing is slow and deep. By slowing your breathing, you can decrease the stress response and force your body into a relaxed state. Practicing relaxed breathing for at least 15 minutes a day may even help you control conditions such as high blood pressure.

Here's one way to practice deep breathing: Inhale slowly to a count of four, then exhale slowly to a count of four. Do this whenever you're under pressure — when you're waiting in line or working on a deadline.

**Learn to say no** You can't do everything, especially when you have arthritis. The next time someone asks for help, think twice before you say yes. Do you have the time? Are you already overcommitted? Is this a project you really want to work on? Are you feeling overwhelmed or worn out?

For some people, saying no may make them feel like failures for not living up to their

---

## LEARNING TO HELP YOURSELF

The Chronic Disease Self-Management Program teaches people with different chronic conditions, such as heart disease, lung disease and arthritis, how to take better care of themselves, tackle problems such as pain and fatigue, and use medications wisely. Two trained leaders facilitate the small-group workshops, which typically meet once a week for 2½ hours over a six-week period. Often, one or both leaders are non-health-care professionals and have some form of chronic disease.

These self-management workshops take place in communities across the nation. You can locate the nearest workshop by visiting the National Council on Aging (NCOA) website at *www.ncoa.org/ncoa-map*.

The Arthritis Foundation sponsors fitness programs designed to help you reduce pain and increase strength and flexibility. Certified instructors lead separate group classes for walking, tai chi, aquatics and low-impact exercise. You can locate a program by visiting the Arthritis Foundation website at this address: *www.arthritis.org/living-with-arthritis/tools-resources*.

own high standards. They try to do things as they would have before having arthritis, which leads to fatigue.

There's no need to feel guilty — it's OK to say no. Cognitive behavioral therapy is an excellent way to learn how to accept your condition without feeling like you've somehow failed. Besides, you won't be very helpful to anyone if you're tired and running on empty.

**Own less, clean less** Unless it's edible, just about everything you bring into your house requires time and energy-consuming maintenance. Perhaps you once enjoyed souvenirs or trinkets that now just serve as dust collectors.

Apply the "pleasure principle" to your possessions. Do they really make you happy? Consider getting rid of anything that doesn't significantly add to your life. If you haven't used it in a year, maybe you should put it in storage or give it away. And avoid buying things you don't need.

## GET YOUR REST

Throughout this chapter, you've read about simple steps you can take to reduce stress and gain control over arthritis. Certainly another key step is getting adequate rest. Modern society tends to push a busy lifestyle at the expense of rest. Achievement is often valued over health and quality of life. For some, it's a source of pride not to get much sleep or need much sleep.

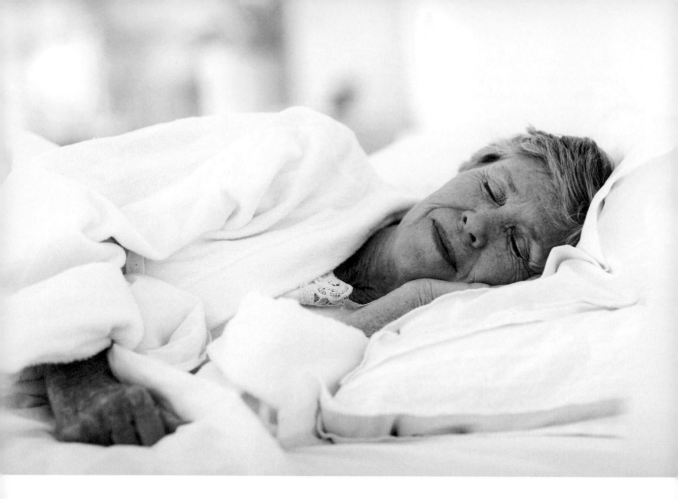

When should you get rest? Whenever you're tired. Arthritis, particularly rheumatoid arthritis, makes you more prone to fatigue. This condition makes it imperative that you listen to your body and give it what it needs, especially when it comes to rest.

Know your limits. Your energy is a limited resource to be budgeted. Let's say you have $10 to spend each day, and you can choose how you want to spend it — but you may not use tomorrow's money today, or tomorrow will be a very bad day. Learning to budget your resources is an important part of having a chronic disease. If you need to rest in a comfortable chair or nap during the day to reserve your energy, allow yourself to do it.

Be sure to get a good night's sleep. According to the Centers for Disease Control and Prevention, around one-third of U.S. adults usually don't get the recommended amount of sleep. Chronic sleep deprivation impairs your attentiveness, coordination and reaction time. It also increases your risks of obesity, high blood pressure, heart attacks, diabetes and depression.

Sleep as many hours as you need, not as many as you think you can survive on. There are no prizes awarded for getting by on only four hours a night, and you could aggravate your arthritis by not sleeping enough.

Most adults need between seven and nine hours of sleep each night. You can tell if you're getting quality sleep if you can awaken in the morning without an alarm clock and feel refreshed, alert, and able to carry out daily activities without being tired or dozing off. One caveat: It's possible to sleep too much. If you're depressed, you might seek refuge in sleep.

Midday naps are fine as long as they don't affect your sleep at night. Try to avoid napping after 3 p.m. And keep naps relatively short — generally about 10 to 30 minutes. It may be that all you need to do is sit down and take a break from activity. Find a comfortable chair and rest without falling asleep. It's OK to be a little tired. And be sure to intersperse rest periods with periods of exercise and other activity.

## STAY IN CONTROL

*Self-efficacy* is a term that describes your ability to take action and achieve goals. It's based on believing that you can have control over things that affect your life and that you have confidence to succeed in particular situations.

Research shows that self-efficacy is the best predictor of success in health outcomes, in-

cluding how well you cope with arthritis. A strong sense of self-efficacy means that you can look at the challenges of living with arthritis as tasks you take control of. It means that you remain committed to achieving these goals and have the ability to bounce back from setbacks.

At this moment, you may be feeling overwhelmed by your symptoms or just don't have confidence that you can change things for the better. You can increase your self-efficacy in small steps. Developing a more positive outlook, learning a relaxation technique or including short rest breaks during periods of activity to prevent fatigue — these are all steps that can increase your self-efficacy.

Use the power of your thoughts, feelings, and beliefs about your illness and your life to help manage arthritis.

# Protecting your joints

You wouldn't intentionally overload one of your joints — particularly if you have arthritis. The joint may already be stiff and painful, and injury would limit it even more. But it's easy to overload or injure your joints through daily movements. The good news is that you can learn ways to protect your joints throughout your day.

The goal of this chapter is to help you preserve your joints and protect them from harm. Much of permanent joint damage is due to chronic inflammation, which you can take steps to reduce. Medications are an important part of this but are not your only tool.

Joint protection starts with your posture — the positions that you hold your body in when you're standing, sitting or lying down. Good posture means that whether you're stationary or in motion, you're putting the least amount of strain on your bones and supporting muscles, tendons and ligaments. It means there's less wear on your joint surfaces.

If you have poor posture, that means your joints are not ideally aligned. For example, when you sit with your shoulders rolled into a slouch, your head, neck and back may be curved forward. The supporting muscles and ligaments need to work harder at keeping you upright and balanced. This effort causes extra wear on your joints, which may lead to arthritis and associated symptoms such as fatigue.

Good posture evenly distributes the weight of your body and maintains the natural curvature of your spine. Staying in one position for a while should feel almost effortless. See the illustrations on page 348 for good stand-ing and sitting posture.

If you're trying to improve your posture, it may feel a little stiff at the beginning. Don't worry! Keep practicing good posture, and it will soon start feeling natural.

## BASICS OF JOINT PROTECTION

The following principles can help preserve your joints and protect them from damage.

### Use proper body mechanics

Body mechanics are the actions you take in order to function in daily life. These move-ments include lifting, carrying, pushing, pulling, and getting out of a chair or bed, as well as using tools for jobs such as vacuum-ing, shoveling, raking, and writing with a pen. The mechanics for some of these ac-tions are illustrated on pages 349–353.

Using good body mechanics follows the principles for good posture. Better move-

### TRIM EXTRA POUNDS

If you weigh more than what is a healthy weight for you, you have plenty of com-pany. Most adults in the United States fall into this category. Being seriously overweight has significant implications for your health and for your joints.

If you're overweight, you're more likely to develop osteoarthritis of the knee or hand. Extra pounds can speed the breakdown of cartilage in the joint. Other joints, including the back, hips, ankles and big toes, also can be damaged by extra weight. Being overweight increases the risk of developing rheumatoid arthritis, too.

Of course, many factors may contribute to the development of arthritis. One is heredity — the genes you inherit from your parents. A previous joint injury can make arthritis more likely, as well. There's also the wear and tear on a joint over time. Being overweight can accelerate the process.

Losing even a few pounds can reduce your chances for knee pain and disability. Good nutrition and proper exercise are keys to weight control. For more details on exercise and nutrition, see Chapters 15 and 16.

ments allow you to work efficiently, conserve energy, maintain balance and reduce stress on your joints. Stressful body mechanics may cause muscle strain, which can lead to pain and increase the wear on your joints.

Whatever the task, use the largest joint possible to accomplish it. That means if you can use your elbows rather than fingers and wrists to power or perform a job, do so — or, if it turns out that you can use your shoulders rather than elbows, adjust your mechanics accordingly.

The better way to lift and carry something cradled in your arms is by allowing your hips and knees to do most of the work, with the object tucked close to your body.

Avoid placing constant or excessive pressure on your joints. For example, break the habit of resting your chin on the knuckles of your hand. Use a briefcase with a shoulder strap or wheels to avoid carrying heavy objects with your hands.

Avoid remaining in the same position for long periods of time. For example, if you're driving a car or seated at a desk, take frequent breaks to move around and flex your joints.

To preserve the joints in your fingers and hands, avoid tasks that require tight grasping, pinching or gripping. Assistive devices can help you do these tasks with less strain on the joints. These devices are described later in the chapter.

## Get active

Reducing arthritis pain doesn't mean avoiding activity. In fact, regular exercise is one of the most effective ways to protect your joints, extending their life and usefulness.

Exercise can strengthen the muscles surrounding your arthritic joints, providing much-needed support. It increases joint flexibility and range of motion. And it reduces fatigue, boosts energy levels and helps you lose weight, thereby reducing the load on your joints.

The following tips can help you get more active. If you're not accustomed to physical activity, check with your doctor first. He or she can advise you on the best way to get started.

You may also be referred to an occupational therapist or physical therapist for guidance. They can help you learn the best ways to exercise with your particular joint pain.

***Warm up and cool down*** Before any exercise, warm up joints and muscles with a heating pad or hot pack, with massage, or by gently walking in place for a few minutes. A warm bath or shower also may help.

Hot packs, applied for 20 minutes, should feel warm and soothing but not uncomfortably hot to the touch. Because heat may increase swelling and pain, don't apply it to an already warm, swollen joint. After exercise, it may help to apply cold to the arthritic joints for 10 to 15 minutes.

**Start slowly** To maintain mobility without damaging your joints, it's important to move each joint through its full pain-free range of motion — all the directions it can comfortably move in. Your pain-free range may vary from day to day or throughout the day.

Gently stretch the muscles around affected joints at least once a day, perhaps in the morning when you get up. You may also want to stretch before you exercise and at the end of your exercise routine. If you have time and energy for only limited stretching, save it for after activity.

Always warm up for a few minutes before stretching, and take care not to overdo it, especially if you have rheumatoid arthritis. Gentle stretching loosens your muscles and increases a stiff joint's range of motion. Sudden jerking or bouncing may be harmful to your joints, so aim for slow, fluid motions.

**Step it up gradually** Start exercising at a comfortable level. That might be no more than a walk to the end of your driveway and back. If that's all you can do at the moment, start with that. Once you're reasonably comfortable, increase the distance that you walk a little at a time.

Try exercising at different times of the day. Find a time when you feel the least amount of pain and stiffness.

**Know your limits** The kind of exercise you do and how hard you do it will depend on what type of arthritis you have, and how strong your symptoms are from day to day.

If you have rheumatoid arthritis, consider the amount of wear and tear the activity may have on affected joints. Non-weight-bearing activities, such as swimming or riding a stationary bike, are probably best. A low-impact activity such as walking also may be a good option. If the affected joint is not painful and a particular activity is not causing pain during or after the exercise, it's probably OK to proceed. If the activity causes pain, stop and consider an alternative exercise. For example, if riding an upright stationary bike seems to aggravate hip pain, try using a recumbent stationary bike.

If you have osteoarthritis of the hip or knee and the bones and cartilage of the affected joint aren't too worn down, then a low-impact activity such as walking might be what you need. However, if the bones and cartilage of the joint are significantly worn down, walking may cause even more damage. Nonweight-bearing activity may be a better choice.

Setting up a personal exercise program to suit your needs is discussed in more detail in Chapter 15.

## Organize and prioritize

Planning your daily schedule is a good way to reduce strain on your joints. Start by prioritizing tasks. Get the important jobs done before you get tired or overwork yourself. Recognize which tasks require the most effort. You may need assistance for those.

You can also tailor your workspace to your needs. Adjust the height of a desk and chair to levels where you can sit comfortably and aren't required to stretch or strain. Keep frequently used tools and supplies within arm's length to minimize straining to reach them.

If you're on your feet a lot, make sure you're wearing shoes that fit well and provide firm support. Use long-handled versions of tools, such as a dustpan or garden trowel, for tasks that would usually involve bending and stooping. Move bags, boxes and equipment on wheeled carts or baskets whenever possible.

## Respect pain

Learn to tell the difference between the general discomfort you feel from arthritis and the pain that comes from overusing a joint, such as from exercising too much or too hard.

Adjust your level of activity or work method to avoid excessive pain. You're more likely to damage a joint when it's painful and swollen. Don't overwork tender, injured or badly inflamed joints. Pain is considered excessive if it alters your breathing pattern — you find that you're holding your breath or breathing more rapidly than normal. Excessive pain also doesn't subside when you stop an activity.

If pain increases, lasts more than an hour or two after the activity, or comes on more quickly day after day, chances are you're doing too much activity or moving in a way you shouldn't be.

## BE KIND TO YOUR JOINTS

An important rule of joint protection is simply avoiding situations that aggravate your condition — increasing inflammation and wear on your joints. But how do you put that advice into practice? Try these tips:

- When writing, use good posture and lighting. Relax your hand often and stretch your neck often. Use a pen with a wider barrel or special grip. Nylon-tip or rolling-ball pens require less pressure than pencils and ballpoint pens.
- Install lever-type handles instead of knobs on the doors in your home.
- When you're moving lawn supplies or groceries and doing other household tasks, use a utility cart to transport heavy items and to avoid extra trips.
- When traveling, use luggage with built-in wheels.
- During an activity, sit (with good posture) instead of standing when possible.

## Get your rest

This concept may seem confusing: On one hand, you're told to be active. On the other hand, you're supposed to take frequent rest breaks.

In fact, it's a delicate balance to keep. At times, you'll need rest to restore your energy. At other times, you'll need exercise to maintain strength and stay reasonably flexible.

There are two forms of rest: joint rest and whole-body rest. It's important for you to give your body both.

***Joint rest*** Using a joint affected by arthritis helps keep it strong and flexible. Even so,

the joint can easily become fatigued, swollen or painful after heavy exertion. When the muscles around a joint feel tired, that's usually a signal to sit down and rest.

If a joint is injured or badly inflamed, it will need recovery time. For example, you may need to wear a splint to keep the joint stationary. As the inflammation dies down, the splint can be removed and you can gradually start moving the joint.

***Whole-body rest*** If you have arthritis, especially rheumatoid arthritis, a well-rested body is an important goal to reach every day. Rheumatoid arthritis makes you especially vulnerable to fatigue. Joint pain can cause you to lose sleep or prevent you from sleeping well. The pain may cause you to change positions frequently to take weight off the affected joints.

Fatigue associated with arthritis is a deep-down exhaustion. It can make virtually everything you do seem like too great an effort, leaving you feeling almost helpless. When you're exhausted, you may not feel like doing much. But if you don't engage in enough physical activity, your muscles only get weaker, and you'll find it even more difficult to get started with physical activity.

Alternatively, you may tend to keep going until a job is done, regardless of discomfort — whether walking to the corner or finishing the laundry. That strategy may not be the best either. When you exercise too strenuously without breaks, you can strain muscles and joints and risk injury.

The key is to get rest before you become too tired. Pace yourself. Don't try to push through periods of feeling extra tired. If you experience a surge of joint inflammation (flare), you'll need to schedule more time to rest your joints.

Try dividing any exercise or work activity into short segments with frequent breaks. Plan 10 minutes of rest for every hour during periods of physical exertion. On the surface, that approach may sound disruptive, but it can help you get more done without pushing your joints to their limit.

**Protecting your joints    341**

From time to time during each day, find a comfortable position and relax for a while. An easy chair, couch, bed or reclined seat in your parked car are all potential options. You don't need to sleep, but you do need to give your body a break.

When it's bedtime, go to bed. Avoid the temptations of watching TV or reading. A good night's sleep gives your joints the rest they need. It can also help restore your energy and enable you to deal more effectively with pain.

If you have rheumatoid arthritis, set a goal of eight or nine hours of sleep each night. If you have trouble sleeping, talk to your doctor about it promptly. When sleep disturbances are treated, fatigue usually improves.

## ASSISTIVE DEVICES FOR DAILY TASKS

Putting the basic principles of joint protection into practice can help you extend the life of your joints. But even if you're doing your best to reduce wear and tear, proper activity, body mechanics and rest may not be enough. That's when you may look for help from assistive devices — tools and technology that have been adapted to help you perform daily tasks.

For example, your painful knee may need a brace to support it — that's a form of assistive device. Or you may opt for using a cane to help you walk. If your hands are affected by arthritis, special grips may be added to a toothbrush handle or pen that allow you to hold them securely.

How do you know what kind of assistive device to look for or how to use it? That's typically the result of an in-depth evaluation by your team of care providers, which may include your doctor, physical therapist, occupational therapist and other specialists. They will evaluate your condition in relation to how well you're able to function in daily life and match a specific device to your needs. You may want to keep a list of activities that are difficult, to discuss with your providers.

The team also provides specialized training in the care and use of a device. And they provide follow-up, evaluating how successfully the device helps you and making adjustments as your condition changes.

People sometimes avoid assistive devices, refusing to believe they need any help, or they think the use of special tools is a form of weakness. Some people worry that using an assistive device such as a cane will make them look old or lead to a loss of function.

In reality, assistive devices allow you to be more independent. In that way, they play an important role in helping you manage your arthritis. Think about it like this: Few people think twice about getting into a car to drive across town. But the car is an assistive device. It makes it easier for you to get from one place to another quickly and comfortably.

Assistive devices are simply a means to an end. They make it easier and safer for you to perform many everyday activities, such as opening a stubborn jar or taking a shower, without making your condition worse.

Medical supply houses and catalogs and many pharmacies offer a wide variety of assistive devices that are practical and affordable. Sometimes, a little creativity is all you need. For example, you can use plastic foam tubing — the kind used to insulate plumbing — to make sleeves that fit on all kinds of handheld tools and utensils, making them easier to grasp. The foam insulation also reduces vibration.

Here are tips for selecting and using some of the many assistive devices available.

## Hand-held aids

If you have arthritis in your hands, avoid making a tight fist or tightly pinching an object. Most pencils and pens, for example, have thin handles that force you to grasp them tightly. This position puts painful stress on the joints of your fingers, thumb and wrist. Keeping your fingers and thumb unclenched is less physically stressful. So, look for grips or clips you can use with writing utensils to give them a wider grip.

## Grooming and personal hygiene

If you have limited range of motion, you may opt for long-handled brushes and combs. Bathing aids such as long-handled sponges and brushes can help you reach all parts of your body with less effort and pain. Use an electric toothbrush or one with a specially designed handle. Try mirrors with foam rubber handles for an easier grasp. Bath benches, grab bars and toilet seat risers provide greater ease, safety and independence with personal hygiene.

## Getting dressed

If you have trouble reaching to your feet, look for a shoehorn with an extension handle or a stocking aid that allows you to pull on hosiery without bending forward.

Use special tools that help you grip buttons and zippers securely. Attach elasticized fabric fasteners in place of buttons on cuffs, or sew the buttons with elasticized thread that stretches as you slip your hand through the sleeve.

Select pants or skirts with a stretch waist if a limited range of motion makes dressing a

A buttonhook can help you grasp and fasten buttons on your clothes if pinching buttons is difficult for your fingers.

challenge. You might use clip-on neckties for convenience, or with a regular necktie, leave the knot tied and slip the tie over your head.

## In the kitchen

Organize your work area. Make sure the items you use often are within easy reach. Store frequently used cookware and utensils in cabinets at hip-to-shoulder height. Seldom-used items may be stored in less convenient spots.

A single-lever sink faucet can make the numerous tasks you perform at the sink less taxing on your finger joints. Operating an electric can opener puts less stress on your joints than a manual opener. In addition, use

An L-shaped knife allows your hand and wrist to stay in a more neutral position, avoiding the pinch grip that you have to use with traditional knives.

an electric jar opener or an opener that can be mounted under a cabinet or countertop.

If you have a hard time opening a refrigerator door with your hand, try looping a strap through the door handle. Pass your arm through the strap to pull the door open.

An electric knife can ease routine slicing and trimming tasks. You may also work on a cutting board with tiny raised spikes that hold food firmly in place as you cut it. If you use a nonelectric knife, buy one that's L shaped with a wide-diameter vertical handle. Grasp the handle like a dagger and cut with a sawing motion without applying much pressure.

In the grocery store, it may help to select foods that don't require slicing and dicing. For example, cut-up fruit and vegetables in the produce section may cost more but save you time and effort.

## Doing housework

For cleaning, use a long-handled mop, dustpan and broom. Work with long, smooth strokes. Use a rocking motion while working with long-handled tools. Shift body weight onto the front foot when making a forward stroke. Then shift weight to the rear foot when making a backward stroke.

Fill a bucket only half-full to help avoid heavy lifting. Wash windows with a firm sponge that allows you to hold it with an open hand. Kneel close to the side of the bathtub, maintaining a balanced posture, and use a long-handled brush to scrub the other side. Store cleaning supplies on each floor and within easy reach so that you don't need to transport them everywhere.

Do laundry on a regular basis to avoid having heavy loads accumulate. Place a table that's a comfortable height near the washer for sorting and folding clothes. If you have a front-loading washer or dryer, place it on blocks for easier access. Protect your back by avoiding unnecessary bending or stooping whenever you can.

### In the shop

For some tasks, there's no alternative to using a manual tool, which may require gripping, pushing or lifting. But often, there's a power alternative that puts less stress on your joints than a manual tool does. For example, a power nail driver or screwdriver may be easier on your joints. Where appropriate, look for lighter weight versions of tools or handle extensions that can improve the leverage for turning a tool.

## ASSISTIVE DEVICES FOR MOBILITY

Devices such as braces, canes and walkers help you move about safely and maintain your balance, both inside and outside. They can offer you a more independent lifestyle and allow you to accomplish many tasks that you might otherwise require assistance

with. At the same time, these devices provide extra support, stability and protection for painful joints.

### Using a brace

If you have osteoarthritis in a knee, wearing a brace can provide pain relief. It may also help correct a slight misalignment of the joint that could be contributing to your condition. Pain symptoms often improve in many cases of mild to moderate osteoarthritis.

The brace wraps around the joint, helping to relieve pressure on the affected parts and reduce pain and swelling. Any brace, especially a knee brace, should fit properly. It's important to work with your team of care providers to get a good fit. Depending on the type of brace, it may offer a long-term solution to the problem of pain.

### Using a cane

When properly adjusted to your height and grip, a cane greatly improves your balance and mobility. A poorly fitted cane, by contrast, throws you off balance, makes you less stable on your feet and increases your arthritis symptoms.

It's a common mistake to choose a cane that's too long. This pushes one side of your body up, putting extra strain on your shoulders and arm muscles. On the other hand, a cane that's too short causes you to lean forward, putting extra pressure on your wrist.

**Select the right style**  When buying a cane, don't base your decision on looks alone. A distinctive cane may add fashionable flair, but there are more important factors to consider. For example, a lightweight cane is easier to lift than a heavy one. A physical therapist can recommend a cane to best meet your needs and can teach you to walk with it so it feels natural.

## Fitting a cane

Elbow bent about 20 to 30 degrees

Cane lines up with wrist crease when arm is straight down

It's important that a cane fits properly. With the cane in your hand, the bend in your elbow should be about a 20- to 30-degree angle.

**Consider length**  To determine the proper length of a cane, stand up straight with your shoes on. Hold your arms at your sides. The length should equal the distance from the crease in your wrist to the floor. When you hold your cane while standing, your elbow should bend at a comfortable angle, about 20 to 30 degrees.

If you walk in different shoes that have heels of varying heights, make sure you have an adjustable cane. Nonadjustable canes can only be cut one time to fit.

**Get a good grip**  Choosing a grip is generally a matter of personal preference. A good grip relieves unnecessary stress on your joints, while numbness or pain in your hand or fingers may signal a poor fit.

A handle with a large diameter is generally easier to hold for extended periods. Make sure your fingers and thumb don't overlap when you grip the handle. If you have trouble grasping with your fingers, ask your doctor or physical therapist for advice.

The traditional candy-cane-style grip may not be the best choice because it doesn't center your weight over the staff. Instead, consider one with a swan-neck grip or with a grip that straddles the pole part of the cane.

**Check the tip**  The end of your cane should have a supple rubber tip that grips the floor. The tip provides traction and safety while you use the cane. Check the tip regularly — maybe about once a month. Replace the tip before it wears down and becomes smooth.

**_Learn proper technique_** Hold your cane with the hand opposite your weaker leg. Stand tall and look ahead, not down at the floor. Pick up and move your cane in unison with the weaker leg. Keep the cane in place as you move the stronger leg forward.

Put as much weight on your cane as necessary to make walking comfortable, stable and smooth. Don't place the cane too far

**Walking with a cane**

If you use a cane to assist one of your legs, grip the cane in the hand opposite the affected leg. Move the cane in unison with your affected leg.

ahead of you. Be careful when walking on uneven ground or on ice or other wet, slippery surfaces.

When going up stairs, remember "up with the strong" and lead with your stronger leg. Then pick up and move the cane at the same time you move your weaker leg up to the step.

When going down stairs, it's "down with the weak." Pick up and move the cane at the same time you move your weaker leg down the step. Then bring your stronger leg down to the step. When using stairs in either direction, use your free hand to hold the handrail if there is one.

If you're receiving Medicare, the program will share the cost of a cane. But your doctor has to write a prescription for the cane, indicating that it is "needed for walking." Most other health insurance plans also provide coverage if a cane is prescribed.

Once you've found a cane that fits and you've used it for a while, decide if the assistive device is a help or hindrance. If you've fully recovered from joint replacement surgery, you can retire your cane — and relearn to walk without it.

## MOVING IN THE RIGHT WAYS

The following pages demonstrate how to tailor your everyday movements to protect your joints. Follow these tips to ease arthritis pain and avoid further joint damage.

# GUIDE TO JOINT-FRIENDLY POSTURE AND MOVEMENT

*For good standing posture:*

- Hold your chest high, keeping your shoulders back and relaxed.
- Gently pull your bellybutton toward your spine. Hold the position while breathing normally and looking straight ahead.
- Keep your feet parallel, with your weight evenly balanced on both feet.
- Keep your knees straight — not bent or in a locked position.

*For good sitting posture:*

- Rest both feet flat on the floor, keeping your knees level with your hips.
- Sit with your back pressed firmly against the chair. If necessary, support your lower back with a small cushion or rolled towel.
- Keep your upper back and neck comfortably straight, tucking your chin in slightly.
- Keep your shoulders relaxed — not elevated, rounded or pulled backward.

*To properly lie down in bed:*

- Start by sitting on the bed so that your head will hit the pillow when you lie down.
- Using your arms for support, slowly lower yourself onto the bed while bringing your legs up to a side-lying position.
- When sitting up from lying down, first bend your knees and then roll to your side. Slide your feet over the edge of the bed as you use your arms to push your body up to a sitting position.

*To properly lift objects:*

- Keep your back straight and your feet apart, as in the standing position.
- Lower your body to get close to the object. Bend from your hips and knees. Do not bend at the waist.
- Hold the object by putting your hands around it, keeping it close to your body.
- Keeping your knees bent and your back straight, lift the object using your arm and leg muscles. Do not use your back muscles.
- If the object is too heavy, ask for help.

**Protecting your joints    349**

*To properly push and pull objects:*

- Keep your feet apart, as in the standing position.
- Keep your back straight.
- Lower your body to get close to the object. Bend from your hips and knees. Do not bend at the waist.
- Use the weight of your body to help move the object.
- If the object you're moving is too heavy, ask for help.

*To properly use long-handled tools:*

- Maintain a balanced posture with your back straight.
- Use a rocking motion, shifting your body weight from your front foot to your rear foot.
- Move your arms and legs rather than your back.
- Use long smooth strokes rather than short, choppy motions.

*Holding a book*

There are better and worse ways to hold a book, when considering your joints. A pinching grip (left) can strain your finger joints and cause pain. Instead, rest the book comfortably on your palms to ease pain (right).

*Getting up from a chair*

When rising from a seated to a standing position, slide forward in the chair, but don't move your feet forward. Keeping your feet slightly apart, use your legs to stand up. If possible, push up on the arms of the chair with your palms as you rise.

**Protecting your joints      351**

*Devices that support and protect your joints*

Hand-held devices can help you perform many simple tasks. Large-barrel implements such as pens (upper left), toothbrushes (upper right) and eating utensils can reduce the stress on your finger and thumb joints. Squeezing a doorknob can be hard on finger joints. A lever attachment (lower left) makes it easier to open the door. A special turning tool (lower right) features a collection of collapsible metal pins that mold around objects such as oven knobs and keys.

**352    Chapter 18**

*Helpful kitchen tools*

Kitchen tools, such as vegetable peelers, can be purchased with wider handles (upper left). A cutting board equipped with nail pegs and a raised ledge (upper right) helps secure food during meal preparation, reducing the amount of force you need to hold food while chopping. When faced with a stubborn jar lid or bottle cap, different types of opening devices can reduce the amount of stress placed on your hand joints (lower left). Spring-loaded scissors (lower right) open automatically, reducing joint strain in your fingers and thumb.

# Traveling with arthritis

Travel can be stressful even when you're healthy. But if you have arthritis, the thought of carrying luggage, changing planes or walking long distances can be enough to give you second thoughts about taking a trip.

However, having arthritis doesn't mean that you're stuck in one place. In fact, today it's easier to travel with a disability than ever before. Thanks to laws such as the Americans with Disabilities Act and the Air Carrier Access Act, the travel industry, including airlines, hotels and cruise ships, has made travel more accommodating for people with special needs.

In addition, both new and established companies have recognized the growing market for travel clients with mildly to severely limited abilities. Special tours, vacation packages and activities are available for people with arthritis.

## PLANNING A TRIP

Where in the world do you want to go? Maybe you dream of visiting the Louvre Museum, in Paris, or hiking part of the Appalachian Trail. Or maybe your employer just needs you to solve a problem in Cleveland. The key to any successful trip starts with planning. With the right preparations, the world is yours to explore.

Naturally, you must be honest about your capabilities. Rock climbing might not be the best choice for you, but a mountaintop helicopter excursion might be an alternative. White-water rafting could be extremely painful with a neck condition, but a week in a riverside cabin might let you appreciate the water without discomfort.

Choose a vacation that has flexibility. Consider how you'll spend the day if your companions take on more-strenuous activities or extensive sightseeing. Remember, frequent rest periods may be the most important ingredient of a satisfying trip.

Doing research before your trip is important. Read travel guides and websites, including those geared toward people with disabilities. Librarians at your public library may be able to point you toward helpful information. Search for tour companies that offer vacations that appeal to you. You might even request information directly from locations you want to visit.

In addition, talking with people who've taken similar trips helps you know what you can expect when you arrive. And make sure to get your doctor's advice when planning a trip. He or she may have good insight into how much you can handle and how you accomplish your travel goals.

### Calling in the pros

Many people rely on travel agents and tour operators. Agents are professionals who can save you time and money, and they often don't charge for their services. Instead, they may receive commissions from the airlines and hotels they book with. Tour operators generally combine several travel compo-

nents, such as airline tickets, hotels and ground transportation, into one package that's usually less expensive than what you would pay if you put them together yourself. The fees of tour operators are usually included in these expenses.

To select a travel agent, start by asking friends and relatives for referrals. You can also call agencies and ask about their experience in arranging trips for travelers with physical limitations.

Choose an agent with whom you're comfortable discussing your needs, and make sure he or she is willing to spend the time required to arrange for those needs. Treat your agent as a travel partner who wants to continue working with you after the basic decisions have been made about your destination.

## CHOOSING WHERE TO STAY

Where you sleep at night can make or break your trip, so keep your physical needs in mind when choosing lodging. You may be able to book an "accessible" room on a hotel's website, but it's best to communicate directly with the hotel to make sure it will suit your needs. Be sure to specify what you'll require well in advance of your travel date. Always get written confirmation of any guaranteed arrangements.

There are many questions you might ask about your lodging. For example, find out how close you'll be to other destinations,

## SHOULD YOU BUY TRAVEL INSURANCE?

Without some form of travel insurance, hotels and airlines may refund your money if you become ill and can't make the trip or have to go home early. But it's probably best to purchase trip cancellation insurance if you think there's a chance you'll be unable to travel. Such policies are generally available from your travel agent, tour operator, booking website or AAA club. You may also want to search an independent website that lets you compare travel insurance options before buying. And your credit card may already provide some insurance for trips you've booked with it.

If you need to make a refund request, be sure to send a doctor's statement with the request. Be aware that trip cancellation insurance may not pay if you cancel because of a preexisting condition, so check on the coverage before buying.

Review your medical insurance coverage before you travel. Policies sometimes include costs of a medical illness while you're away from home, including travel back home if you become seriously ill, but many plans don't include this coverage. Again, some policies exclude preexisting conditions, so be certain to read the fine print.

such as the convention center, restaurant or beach. Ask what floor you'll be on, where the elevators are located in relation to your room, whether the bathrooms have handrails, whether the doors and faucets have levers instead of hard-to-grasp knobs, and whether the hotel has a shuttle that can be used by someone with physical limitations.

You might also ask if the hotel has porters to help carry your luggage and how you can arrange taxicab service if you're going to need it. You may want to inquire about handicapped parking, fire exits and access ramps. If you'll be there awhile, you may want to check on the availability of laundry and other services at the hotel.

In many cases, hotels are equipped to offer a range of special amenities and services, such as tours in accessible vans, heating pads for those unexpected flare-ups or in-house spas with whirlpools. It pays to ask as many questions as possible before you book.

You're not limited to the major hotel chains either. An increasing number of bed-and-breakfasts, inns and privately owned vacation rentals can host guests with disabilities. Travel guidebooks and websites may include designations to indicate accessible rooms. And on some vacation rental websites, you can even filter your search results for lodging with accessible features. That way, you'll only see options that work for you. To be safe, you may still want to contact the company or host to ask specific questions.

## PACKING YOUR BAGS

- Pack as few items as possible. Lay out the essentials in front of you. Choose articles of clothing that are easy to layer or combine with other items. Remove any duplicates or extras unless absolutely required.
- Travel with lightweight luggage that has sturdy wheels, telescoping handles and cross-body straps. Attach identification tags to all luggage.
- Airlines often allow one carry-on bag and one personal item, such as a purse, small backpack, personal computer or briefcase, onboard with you. Size matters — the smaller your baggage, the easier it will be to hoist into an overhead bin and the less likely it is to be checked at the gate. Also, make sure you're familiar with the baggage policies of the airline you're flying. Many charge fees for carry-on bags as well as checked luggage.
- In carry-on luggage, liquids, gels and aerosols are permitted in 3-ounce containers, placed in a quart-size, clear plastic, zip-close bag. One bag is allowed per traveler.
- Prescription medications and medical supplies will not count against your carry-on allowance, but if they exceed 3 ounces or cannot fit into a zip-close bag, you'll need to declare them to a security officer.
- Check with your airline or travel agent regarding the checked baggage policy, including the number of pieces you may bring and size and weight limitations.

## WHAT TO TAKE

Packing light is good advice for all travelers, but especially for people with arthritis. Try to plan carefully so that you'll have enough clothing, plus the important items that make your arthritis more manageable, without packing extra things you won't need.

Don't forget to bring any aids you use daily, such as a raised toilet seat, long-handled reacher, special pillow or heating pad. If you have electrical appliances and are traveling to a foreign country, you may need to pack a plug or voltage adapter.

To minimize strain on your joints, use lightweight luggage that's easy to transport. Check to see if porters and taxicabs will be available at your destinations, and ask the porters and drivers to carry your luggage whenever possible. At the airport, check your bags at the curb. Be sure to carry small bills for tipping the people who assist you.

Check weather forecasts for your destination to decide what type of clothing is most appropriate. Dressing in layers allows you to adapt easily to weather changes. You may be most comfortable wearing loose or stretchy clothing so that you can move around easily, whether traveling or enjoying your destination. Sunscreen, sunglasses, a hat (either for sun protection or warmth) and comfortable shoes also are essential.

When packing medications, you may not be able to "pack light." It's smart to take a supply that's more than enough for your trip, and carry medications in original containers. Keep them in your carry-on luggage, in case you're separated from the bags you've checked — although some travelers pack a duplicate supply in their luggage. If you need medications to be kept cool, most attendants will gladly store them in a refrigerator for you, although you may prefer carrying them separately in a vacuum flask or insulated container.

Along with your medications, bring copies of your prescriptions, contact information for your doctor, a summary of your medical history and a complete list of all the drugs you're currently taking. It's a good idea to leave copies of this information at home with a friend or relative, too, in case your doctor is unavailable. If you have other medical problems in addition to arthritis, you might consider wearing a medical alert bracelet or necklace.

## TRANSPORTATION

You'll want to take certain steps to ensure an enjoyable trip, depending on the form of transportation you use. The good news is that over the years travel companies have become more accommodating to people with disabilities, including arthritis.

### Traveling by air

Thanks to a U.S. law called the Air Carrier Access Act, regulations make it illegal to discriminate against disabled air travelers. These regulations clearly state the responsibilities of travelers, carriers, airport operators and contractors. For people with arthritis, the rules mean more time for boarding, accessible terminal parking and accessible restrooms, among other things.

Still, you must do your part. When you make airline reservations, state your special needs, such as seating or storage capacity for oversized arthritis aids. Allow extra time to get through the airport, request an airport wheelchair or other terminal transport if you need it, and check your luggage through to your final destination.

At all airports in the United States with scheduled airline service, passengers must go through a pre-boarding screening process for security. The Transportation Security Administration (TSA) has suggestions for people with disabilities and medical conditions to help make the screening process go smoothly. Those suggestions include:

- If you need assistance moving through the airport, contact your airline. The airline can provide someone to assist you through the terminal and screening line.
- If you require a companion or assistant to accompany you through the security checkpoint and to the boarding gate, request a gate pass for your companion from the airline. Do this before reaching the security checkpoint.
- The limit of one carry-on and one personal item doesn't apply to the medical supplies, equipment, mobility aids or assistive devices that you may require.
- Pack your medications and medical documentation in a separate bag to help speed the inspection process. Make sure the medication container isn't too densely filled and that it's clearly labeled.
- You may present any medical documentation about your condition to the screener. But such material isn't required, and having it won't exempt you from the screening process.
- Tell the screener about any special equipment or devices that you're using or about any devices located in or on your body.
- Make sure that all your carry-on items, equipment, mobility aids and assistive devices have identification tags attached.
- Items such as wheelchairs, scooters, crutches, canes, walkers, prosthetic devices, braces and orthopedic shoes are permitted through the security checkpoint.
- If your prosthetic device requires tools for removal, the TSA recommends bringing them along in case you need to remove the prosthesis for any reason.

- If you have a medical device either inside or outside your body, check with your doctor to learn if it's safe to pass through a metal detector or to be hand wanded. If your doctor says it's unsafe, request a pat-down inspection from the screener.
- If a personal search is required, you may request a private area for screening. You may request a private area at any time during the screening process.
- Ask the screener for assistance if you need help as you proceed through the screening, including walking through the metal detector.
- Certain times of the day are less congested at airports, making the process easier to negotiate. A travel agent or airline representative may be able to suggest less crowded flights.
- If you'll need to change planes, find out whether you'll have to change terminals and whether a shuttle between terminals is accessible to you. If not, ask for suggestions on how to reach your destination.

## Traveling by train

Trains generally provide a good transportation option for people with disabilities. Throughout Europe, rail travel is relatively easy and accessible, with many trains accommodating disabled travelers on international routes. In the United States, Amtrak offers special assistance for disabled passengers and their travel companions.

When making Amtrak reservations online or on the phone, you can request an accessible seat or room and space to store a mobility device. Have written documentation of your disability ready at the ticket counter and when boarding the train. This may include a letter from your doctor or membership card from a disability organization.

Most train stations have personnel to provide baggage assistance and to help get passengers from the station entrance onto the train. Amtrak suggests that you make any requests for assistance when you make your reservations.

Amtrak can supply you with a wheelchair. If you have your own wheelchair, it must not exceed 30 inches wide and 48 inches long and should have a minimum ground clearance of 2 inches. It must weigh no more than 600 pounds occupied.

## Traveling by bus

Many bus lines can provide assistance with boarding and getting off vehicles. The driver may also be able to help with stowing and retrieving your luggage and mobility devices. Most coach bus aisles aren't wide enough for wheelchairs. If you use a wheelchair or have trouble using stairs, make the arrangements for assistance with customer service. Try to make your request at least 48 hours before your departure.

Bus travel is often slower, so you may want to schedule trips for the middle of the week, when fewer people travel. Keep medications and bottled water with you. If you'll have a long ride, take a pillow and snacks, too.

## Traveling by car

When you travel by car, you'll enjoy more freedom than with other forms of transportation. You can stop whenever you want, you'll have more room to stretch out, and you can take along anything that fits in your vehicle.

There are ways to make the trip even more enjoyable. Be sure to stop frequently, getting out to stretch and move around. Keep medications, snacks, maps, an emergency kit and first-aid supplies in the car.

For safety, make sure your cellphone is charged before starting out, or carry a charger that can plug into the car. Make hotel reservations in advance, or stop early enough to find a place to stay. Don't let yourself get tired before finding lodging for the night.

If you're renting a car, ask for amenities that will make driving more comfortable, such as hand controls, a transfer board if you use a wheelchair, swivel seats, a padded or built-up steering wheel, or a spinner knob on the steering wheel that allows easier turning. To get a car with special features, you may need to reserve your vehicle two to three business days in advance.

## Traveling by ship

You may find travel onboard a cruise ship particularly relaxing. A number of design changes have been made to U.S. ships in recent years, such as the widening of passageways, doorways and elevators, and the addition of accessible staterooms for wheelchair travelers. Special meals and exercise plans may be available, too.

Keep in mind that while the ADA requirements generally apply to all ships operating in U.S. waters, cruise lines operating in other countries may not have the same accessibility requirements. So before booking, make sure you check to see that the cruise will have the accommodations you need.

Before booking a particular cruise, ask your travel agent or a cruise line representative about the ship's design and accessibility. You may want to consider which onboard amenities you'll use most — such as restaurants, meeting rooms, pools or sun decks — and try to book a room nearby. It's difficult to arrange having all of them close by.

When choosing a cruise, also consider where it stops. Cobblestone streets or ancient stone stairways may make it difficult to enjoy a destination if you have arthritis. Find out how passengers embark and disembark at each destination, too. At some ports of call, a ship may anchor at sea and shuttle passengers to shore on smaller boats. If you anticipate difficulty with embarking or disembarking the ship, you may want to choose a cruise that has fewer stops, or plan to stay onboard soaking up the ship's ambience while your companions go ashore.

Choices abound these days in cruises geared for the leisurely traveler, and many shore excursions now accommodate those with an unhurried pace. Most ships employ doctors, but their pharmacies are usually limited. You'll want to take along more than enough medication to get you through the trip.

## TRAVELING ABROAD

Whether you're touring Australia or Italy, Venezuela or Singapore, arthritis should not prevent you from having an enjoyable, stimulating adventure.

You may need to see a doctor before travel, depending on your general health and on your destination. If you're visiting a developing country, you should plan to consult your doctor or a travel medicine clinic. This consultation should take place at least four to eight weeks before the journey to ensure that any necessary medications can be prescribed and that vaccinations have time to take effect.

Services at travel medicine clinics vary widely. Some offer vaccinations and general information. Others offer comprehensive overviews of the health hazards along your itinerary, with detailed advice on how to stay well. The clinics are typically affiliated with medical centers or universities. Check the directory at the International Society of Travel Medicine website: *www.istm.org*.

In addition, the International Association for Medical Assistance to Travellers offers a free information packet detailing its services. These include free climate and sanitation information and advice on international disease and immunization requirements. You can learn more about this organization at *www.iamat.org*.

Although health care has improved in many world destinations, be sure you're carrying ample medications on overseas trips, and pace yourself so that you won't need a doctor to attend to a routine flare-up.

No matter where you're headed, take all reasonable precautions to keep yourself safe and healthy. Then relax and have fun. You can travel — and travel well — with arthritis.

# On the job

Having arthritis is no reason to put a career on hold or start planning early retirement. Focusing on what you can do instead of what you can't do may help you discover an inner strength you never thought you had and come up with creative solutions to the demands you face at work.

Your success in the workplace depends greatly on having a positive attitude, the confidence to work toward your goals, and the will to get on with life and not dwell on every obstacle that appears in your path.

One of the initial challenges you may face on the job will be deciding whether or not to inform your boss and co-workers about having arthritis. Many people are reluctant to share this — and there may be good reason. In some cases, this knowledge may raise questions in your employer's mind about whether you're physically able to do the job.

Some supervisors consider arthritis to be just aches and pains, and they may wonder whether you're using the disease as an excuse for special treatment. And in some situations, unspoken discrimination shows up as denied opportunities, such as promotions you deserve but don't get.

For reasons such as these, many experts recommend that you say nothing about the disease if you can answer no to both of the following questions:
- Is your arthritis obvious?
- Do you need special accommodations or resources to do your job?

If you answer yes to either question, it's usually best to inform your employer and co-workers that you have arthritis. Otherwise, they may come to believe that you're not doing your share of the work — and may resent you for it.

Choosing not to disclose your arthritis may also have consequences for you. If you decide to say nothing, you'll also probably ignore your body's warning signs and push yourself beyond your limits to maintain the secrecy. This will only make matters worse by increasing the pain and fatigue so common to arthritis.

If you decide that you need to tell your boss about your condition, schedule a meeting with care. Pick a time when distractions and job pressures for both of you are lower than usual. Be prepared to give a short course on the disease. If you have rheumatoid arthritis, you might explain that when pain flares up or fatigue sets in, these are signs that your affected joints need rest and repair.

At this meeting, have suggestions prepared for changes that will help you do your job better. If you need more rest breaks while at work, for example, you could note how that will help your productivity the rest of the time. Discuss work responsibilities with your doctor or occupational therapist, too. They may have ideas to help you perform certain tasks more easily, perhaps with the aid of assistive devices — even some as simple as putting armrests on your chair. They can also recommend exercises to increase your dexterity and range of motion for repeated movements you'll do during the workday.

## KNOW YOUR RIGHTS

The Americans with Disabilities Act was passed by Congress in 1990. It's the most extensive bill of rights for people with disabilities that has ever been signed into law.

This law bans discrimination against people with disabilities and requires companies of 15 or more employees to make reasonable changes to help individuals do their jobs. In fact, a wise employer who values your experience will be willing to provide the tools necessary for you to do your job well.

Reasonable accommodations might include the following:

- Providing or modifying equipment to help you do certain tasks, such as a wheeled cart to carry supplies, a headset instead of a hand-held phone or a chair with good back support. The cost of some assistive devices may qualify your employer for tax benefits.
- Installing a ramp if you have difficulty with stairs. Note that the employer can't make you pay for special equipment or accommodations like this. An exception would be if the changes place undue hardship on the employer, in which case you may be asked to share some of the cost. But what constitutes undue hardship is judged on a case-by-case basis.
- Adapting workplace furniture to suit your needs — for example, adjusting the height of your desk, allowing a stool for long periods of standing or providing a chair that ensures proper positioning.
- Allowing break periods for rest.

- Changing work responsibilities, eliminating tasks you have difficulty performing that aren't essential to your job.

If you believe that your employer treats you unfairly and is unwilling to make reasonable changes to help you do your job, you can file a formal complaint with the Equal Employment Opportunity Commission (EEOC).

You can order free publications about the Americans with Disabilities Act and anti-discrimination legislation at the EEOC website: *www.eeoc.gov*. The state where you live (or work) also may have laws protecting you from discrimination. If you have questions about your legal rights, talk with a lawyer who specializes in employment law.

## PROTECT YOUR JOINTS

Finding ways to reduce activities that irritate, inflame or damage your joints can help keep you off disability and in the workforce. Here are some ideas:

- Arrange your work area to reduce the need for lifting, walking or other movements that may be painful.
- Find the most comfortable positions, sitting or standing, for doing work. See tips for working at a computer on page 373.
- If you perform repetitive motions, such as typing or assembly work, rest the affected joints every 20 to 30 minutes by stopping the activity and stretching your muscles. In fact, even if you don't perform repetitive motions, try to take a

short break every half-hour or hour to change positions, stretch and relax.

- If a task is always painful, search for other ways to do it. Occupational therapists specialize in solving such problems. Or ask a co-worker for help in exchange for your assistance with something else.
- Use special tools or assistive devices that reduce the strain on your joints: electric staplers, dictation services, chair leg extensions (to make it easier to get up), and enlarged grips for pencils and pens.
- Don't be afraid to ask for help if you need it.

## Exercise

Maintaining muscle strength around your joints helps keep the joints stable and functional. Your doctor and physical therapist can design an exercise program that allows you to strengthen the joints that you use most often in your job. Some of the exercises can be simple and inconspicuous enough that you can do them during your lunch break or in momentary rest breaks. For example, if you work a lot with your hands, take a few seconds to bend your fingers, wrists and elbows as far as you can, then stretch them back out.

## Relax

Job stress can aggravate arthritis pain, which, in turn, intensifies job stress. You can break the cycle by learning relaxation techniques.

The following are a few ideas:

- Let your mind wander to recall a happy memory.
- Look out a window and enjoy the scene.
- Listen to a recording of relaxing sounds, such as gentle rain.
- Take a short walk or sit outside.
- Lie down or sit quietly for a few minutes.

## Conserve energy

You can help avoid the fatigue caused by arthritis by pacing yourself. Do the most important projects of the day during your time of peak energy. For example, if you know that you're a morning person, spend the morning doing the work that requires the most energy. Vary your schedule by alternating more difficult tasks with easier ones. If possible, take a rest break of about 10 minutes every few hours.

## COMMUTE WISELY

For some people with arthritis, the trip to work can be a painful, exhausting gantlet of obstacles: driving in heavy traffic, riding in a vehicle that isn't equipped for people with restricted movement, walking from a distant parking lot, and then going up a flight of stairs to an office or workstation. Each of these factors can cause arthritic pain to flare up and sap your energy before the workday even begins. These ideas may help make getting to work easier:

- Share rides with a co-worker. Pay for the service, or take turns driving.

- Use public transportation. It's usually slower but less exhausting than driving in bumper-to-bumper traffic. The Americans with Disabilities Act requires that accessible public transit vehicles be available to individuals with disabilities.
- If you need to drive, install equipment that minimizes the discomfort: a backrest, special mirrors, steering wheel modifications. Some automakers give you rebates if you install this equipment in new cars. They may also provide a list of local companies that do the installation.
- If you have trouble walking, talk to your employer about possibilities for parking near the building entrance.
- You may be able to get a disabled parking permit from your state transportation department. You'll need to present a letter from your doctor to get it. The permit allows you to use parking spaces reserved for people with disabilities.
- If you have difficulty with stairs, you may ask for a ramp leading into the building. You may also request a work space closer to the entrance.
- If you can manage stairs with handrails, make sure rails are installed on the stairs close to your work area. If not, request them. The addition can be beneficial to the general public and enhance public safety.

## GET COMFORTABLE WITH YOUR COMPUTER

Working at a keyboard for many hours can worsen the pain and fatigue of arthritis. If you work for most of the day at a computer, consider these tips for having better posture and position:

- As you sit in your chair, lean back slightly so that your lower back is firmly supported by the backrest. Keep your feet flat on the floor, with your knees bent at about 90 degrees. If you don't have firm back support, request a chair that allows you to adjust the backrest to different heights and angles.
- Move close to the keyboard so you aren't reaching for it. The keyboard should be about 3 to 6 inches from your lap. Both keyboard and monitor should be directly in front of you. The top of the screen should be at eye level.
- A padded bar between the keyboard and your lap can provide wrist support. While you're typing, your wrists should be straight, with your forearms parallel to the floor. Chairs with armrests offer support for the forearms, and wrist braces can help keep your wrists comfortably aligned. If your wrists are unsupported and usually bent as you type, you can develop carpal tunnel syndrome, which produces pain or numbness in your hands.
- Learning the proper technique for typing may be much easier on the joints than the hunt-and-peck method, which tends to put more pressure on individual joints.
- If typing is too difficult, use a mouse as much as possible. Voice-activated software is another option now available on many computers and smart devices.
- Take short breaks from the computer to stretch your legs, arms and fingers. Don't forget to give your eyes a break by focusing on an object at a distance.

## KEEP AN OPEN MIND

Despite all that you and your employer do to accommodate for your arthritis, the nature of your job or progression of your condition may require you to cut back on the number of hours you work or to find another line of work.

If your job requires heavy physical labor, such as construction, your doctor may refer you to an occupational therapist or to a vocational rehabilitation agency. These specialists can help you build strength and determine how much weight you can safely lift.

If physical restrictions are such that there's no work you can satisfactorily do at your company, a vocational rehabilitation agency can help you find other employment. Sometimes, employees in these circumstances transition to a related profession or industry. A former construction worker, for example, may join a company that sells equipment to the construction industry.

## JOB INTERVIEW TIPS

Although employers aren't allowed to ask if you have a disability, they may ask if you're able to perform specific job functions. A sample interview question might be: "Do you have any physical limitations that would hinder your performance of the job you're applying for?" Such questions can put you in an awkward situation if you think you'll actually need some kind of assistance in doing the work.

Some career counselors advise that you shouldn't disclose that you have arthritis. They suggest that doing so could eliminate you as a candidate with no chance to discuss the matter. In this line of reasoning, you should respond to the question with a no, under the presumption that the employer will provide the legally required reasonable accommodations if that becomes necessary. Another possible response, if you're not sure how arthritis will affect your job performance, is to answer *will discuss* on an application.

If your arthritis will be obvious at the interview, consider hinting about it during the interview setup (most likely in a phone conversation). But do so only after you make the interview appointment, and only if the person you're talking to is the one who will be interviewing you. Possible hint: "I sometimes have trouble with stairs. Do you have an elevator?" Hints like this may help reduce surprise, making it easier for the interviewer to concentrate on your needs.

Perhaps the most popular interview question is, "Tell me about yourself." As friendly as it may seem, this open-ended question is more than a pleasant icebreaker to conversation. It has the potential to be the most dangerous question of the day for you — or the most beneficial.

Law prohibits employers from basing their hiring decisions on age, sex, race, religion, health or nonfelony arrests. They aren't supposed to ask, "How's your health?" But by describing yourself in response to their open question, you may reveal more than you intend. If you're prepared ahead of time, you can answer the question honestly and, at the same time, avoid revealing your condition — unless you want to do so.

During the interview, summarize the assets you would bring to the job, such as your education, certification or previous employment experience. Relate your personal strengths to the kinds of tasks you may be required to do. For example, highlight the fact that you're organized and thorough, or good under pressure, or an excellent team player. You could add that your experience, desire to excel and eagerness to accept new challenges has led you to apply for the job.

If your condition will be obvious at the interview, you may want to refer to it briefly. But don't shift the focus to your limitations. Remain focused on your strengths.

Talk about the adjustments you've made that allow you to stay productive at work. For example, you can say something like this: "I understand that you're legally prohibited from asking about my arthritis, except for questions about how I would perform specific tasks required for the job. I'd be happy to answer any questions because I'm certain I can do the work."

If your arthritis isn't obvious at the interview but will require job accommodations, you face a tough dilemma that has no easy solution. Should you say nothing until you receive a job offer? If so, you can be certain that you won't be ruled out of employment

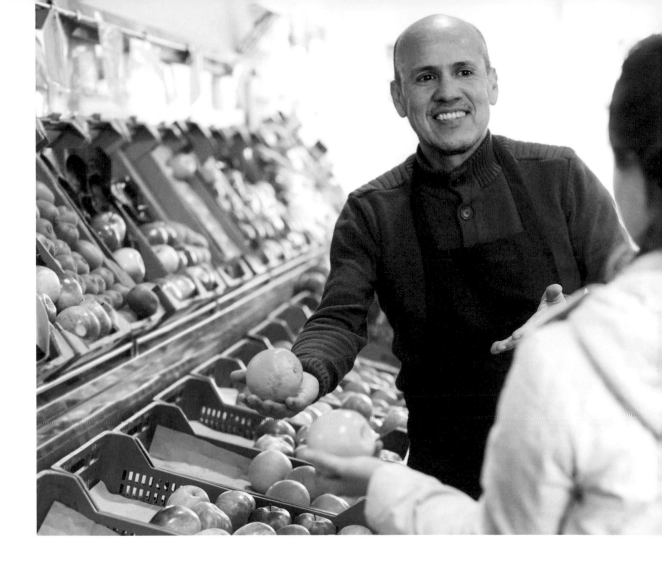

because of a disability. At the same time, the employer might feel misled. And this could generate hard feelings and a shaky start to your new job.

An alternate approach would be to tell the employer about your arthritis, especially if you're aware of aspects of the job in which you'll need some accommodation soon. If you decide this is the best solution for you, mention that the accommodations are usu-ally inexpensive. You can also include a re-minder of your qualities and experience that make you particularly strong candidate for that role.

When you have a positive outlook and make thoughtful preparations, you have ev-ery right to be hopeful about your future in the workplace.

# Your immune system and arthritis

Living with arthritis comes with challenges. As you've seen in previous chapters, there are many ways to overcome these challenges and make life easier. Finding a health care team you trust is key. This team — including your primary doctor or care provider, a rheumatologist, and other specialists — can guide you through treatments. They can also suggest exercises and lifestyle changes to help relieve arthritis pain and get back to your normal activities.

Along with relieving joint pain, the main goal of your health care team is keeping you healthy overall. For example, they'll work with you to keep your bones strong to prevent osteoporosis and lower your risk of fractures. Exercise, diet, and calcium and vitamin D supplements can all improve bone strength. Medications may help too.

Another important way your health care team can help you stay healthy is by working with you to prevent infections. Arthritis — as well as medications used to treat it — can weaken your immune system. That leaves your body at increased risk for an invading illness. And if your body can't fight back normally, a disease that typically isn't serious can take a larger toll on your health. It becomes especially important to prevent the spread of germs. In certain cases, your doctor may prescribe an antibiotic to lower your risk for some infections.

The following sections discuss ways to boost your immune system while you're living with arthritis. By taking preventive measures such as these, you can give yourself the best chance of staying healthy and strong so you can live a fulfilling, productive and enjoyable life.

## GET VACCINATED

For people of any age, the most effective way to prevent infectious diseases is to stay up to date on vaccinations. This is especially important for people with arthritis who are on medications that suppress, or weaken, the immune system. If you are taking biologics, kinase inhibitors or daily prednisone, you may be considered immunosuppressed.

The Centers for Disease Control and Prevention recommends certain schedules of vaccinations for children as well as adults. You can find these schedules and more information at *www.cdc.gov/vaccines*.

It's important to talk with your doctor about your vaccination history and how arthritis affects your risk of disease. You may need to consult a specialist if a vaccine is in question.

## Types of vaccines

For people who are immunosuppressed, vaccines are typically safe unless they contain live vaccine material. Live-attenuated vaccines use a weakened (attenuated) form of a live virus. In healthy people, this prompts the immune system to develop antibodies against that virus, but it doesn't typically make them sick. However, if your immune system isn't healthy to begin with, it may not be able to fight off even the weakened virus from a live vaccine. You should avoid being around others for at least a week if they have received a live vaccine.

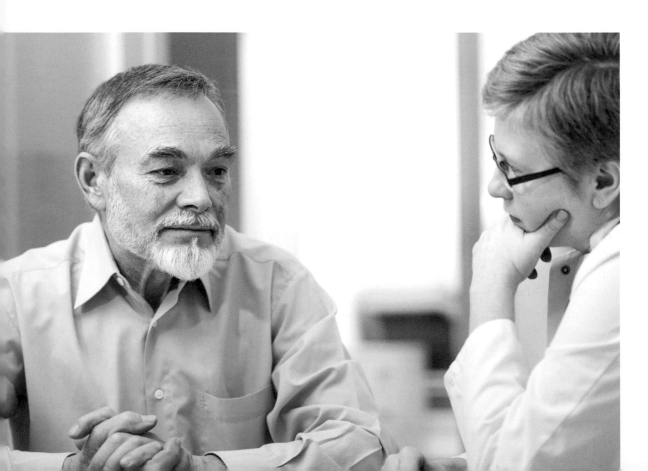

## LIVE VACCINES

Live-attenuated vaccines include a weakened version of a live germ. If you have a weakened immune system because of arthritis medications or other health conditions, you'll likely need to avoid these vaccinations. Because of the risk of infection, anyone who lives with an immunocompromised person should also avoid these vaccinations.

Live vaccines include:
- Chickenpox (varicella)
- Nasal spray flu vaccine (not the flu shot)
- Measles, mumps and rubella (MMR)
- Oral polio (not the polio shot), not used in the United States
- Oral typhoid (not the typhoid shot)
- Yellow fever
- Zostavax for shingles (not Shingrix, a newer shingles vaccine)

The rotavirus vaccine can be administered to infants ages 2 to 7 months who live with someone who is immunocompromised. However, for at least four weeks after an infant receives the rotavirus vaccine, an immunocompromised person should not handle the infant's diapers.

If you have any questions about vaccinations or exposure to certain diseases, talk with your doctor.

Common live vaccines include those for measles, mumps and rubella (MMR), chickenpox (varicella), and the nasally inhaled flu vaccine. Other live vaccines are given in special circumstances, usually for travel. See the sidebar above for more-detailed information about live vaccines and other common examples.

Many vaccines are inactivated, meaning they use a dead version of the disease-causing germ. Others use just a part of the germ or a product of it. There's no risk of transmitting the disease with these types of vaccines. But they can still train your immune system to recognize certain invaders and quickly build up antibodies to defend against them. Vaccines that are generally safe for most people, including those with weakened immune systems, include the following:

- Diphtheria
- Flu (shot only)
- Hepatitis A
- Hepatitis B
- Human papillomavirus (HPV)
- Meningococcal disease
- Pneumococcal disease
- Polio
- Rabies
- Shingles (Shingrix, not Zostavax)
- Tetanus
- Whooping cough (pertussis)

Ideally, vaccinations should be given before immune-suppressing medications are prescribed. If possible, they should be given two to three weeks before starting medications that weaken the immune system, so they have time to become fully effective. Alternatively, they may be given three months after immunosuppressing drugs are stopped. If you're breast-feeding, you can still receive vaccinations.

## KEEP YOUR IMMUNE SYSTEM HEALTHY

Another key to staying healthy is caring for your immune system itself. As you age, your immune system ages, too. Your body's capacity to respond to infections slowly weakens over time. That leaves older adults more susceptible to inflammation, potentially increasing the risk for autoimmune dis-

eases and other illnesses. Thus, improving and maintaining the health of your immune system is one of the most important steps you can take to live a long, healthy life.

Healthy living and behavioral choices are the cornerstones of immune health. To create the strongest foundation for your body's defense system, optimize your diet, exercise, sleep, and mental and spiritual health.

Just as making healthy choices in these areas can bolster your immune system, less healthy lifestyle factors can stress your body and hinder its ability to fight off attacks. Previous chapters have discussed many of these factors in more detail. To keep your defense system strong, make any of the following lifestyle changes that aren't already part of your routine.

***Stop smoking*** If you smoke, quitting now is one of the most powerful ways you can help your body fight illness. Smoking is the single greatest negative influence on immune health.

**Limit alcohol consumption** While some alcohol such as red wine is thought to be beneficial in moderation, avoid excess alcohol and all illicit or recreational drugs. These can compromise your health in general.

**Manage your weight** If you're carrying extra pounds, like many adults, losing some weight can improve your health in a number of ways. There is abundant data to suggest that being significantly overweight contributes to increased inflammation and a compromised immune system. Keep an eye on your weight as you get older, too. The body's natural metabolism tends to slow down with age, making it easier to gain weight.

**Watch what you eat** Foods that have anti-inflammatory effects, such as in the Mediterranean diet, may help maintain your immune system. On the other hand, processed foods and diets high in sugar, alcohol and red meat have all been shown to negatively affect immune cells and processes. So eating for immunity may be as simple as a healthy, plant-based diet. Eat more fruits and vegetables, nourishing fats such as mono-unsaturated fats, a variety of whole grains, and lean protein. In addition, staying well hydrated can help your body flush out toxins, curbing inflammation.

**Exercise** You already know that being active is important for your health. Exercise is one of the best medicines for life, and it's perhaps even more vital for people with arthritis. In fact, research shows that exercise benefits the immune system, boosting its function to fight disease. Frequent activity may even change how the immune system ages. Find a fun way to incorporate exercise into your daily routine. If you've avoided exercise because high-impact activity hurts your joints, try Tai Chi, dancing, yoga, gardening or walking.

***Get better sleep*** Missing out on sleep can make you more likely to get sick after being exposed to a virus. During sleep, your immune system releases cytokines, which help the body fight infection or inflammation. Sleep deprivation may decrease production of cytokines. In addition, infection-fighting antibodies and cells are reduced during periods when you don't get enough sleep. To stay healthy, make sleep a strict part of your to-do list. Schedule a "pre-sleep buffer" before bed to prepare for a good night's sleep — cut out nighttime caffeine, put down your phone, turn off the TV or computer, and create a dreamy sleep environment.

***Manage stress*** Daily life is often stressful and busy. But it pays to manage your stress effectively, as studies show that stress contributes to health decline. You can take steps to lessen the toll stress takes on your body by trying mind-body interventions such as listening to music, spending time on your hobbies, meditating, doing yoga and getting out in nature. You might also benefit from counseling, focusing on time management and exercise. See Chapter 17 for more information on stress relief.

***Avoid harmful environmental exposures*** What are your environmental risks? To keep your immune system healthy, avoid carcinogens — substances that cause cancer. This includes avoiding excessive sun exposure, limiting your exposure to smoke, staying safe from harmful chemicals that may be around your work or home, and other environmental factors that can be avoided.

## STAY UP AND RUNNING

Maintaining a healthy immune system is important for everyone. But especially for people with arthritis and on medications that suppress the immune system, helping this complex system stay strong and functional is key. Avoiding sickness helps you feel well enough to engage with family and friends, thrive at work, and keep up the activities you enjoy.

Researchers are continually making discoveries that give a deeper understanding of how immune cells and processes work. But there's no question that the steps in this chapter can help boost your immunity. As you take steps to gain control of your joint pain, keeping your whole body healthy overall is vital to your progress.

# Additional resources

## WHERE TO GET MORE HELP

You can find a lot of health information on the internet and social media. Some of it is very good advice, but some of it is downright bad. Don't believe everything that you find. The online environment has a way of making all health information appear of equal quality. The key is making sure to get information from trusted sources.

Carefully read reports and check if the information comes from respected publications, organizations or medical professionals. If something you find seems questionable or conflicts with conventional wisdom, you have the right to be skeptical.

Also beware of fraudulent medical products or information promising an arthritis cure. At worst, the products may actually be dangerous. Even vitamins can be harmful if they're taken in large doses. Watch out for glowing testimonials or medical treatments described as *secret, miracle, foreign, breakthrough* and *overnight*.

Listed here are resources and organizations that you can depend on for quality information on arthritis and guidance on living an active life with joint pain. Your medical care team may be able to point you to others.

### *American College of Rheumatology*
*www.rheumatology.org*
The website of this organization for health care professionals in rheumatology contains information on causes, symptoms and treatments for many forms of arthritis.

### *Americans with Disabilities Act (ADA)*
800-514-0301 (toll-free)
*www.ada.gov*
This website and toll-free number can help you find official information on the ADA, receive technical assistance or file a complaint.

### *Arthritis Foundation*
*www.arthritis.org*
The Arthritis Foundation is an excellent resource for knowledge and support. This national organization provides self-help materials and can lead you to local support groups, classes and medical care providers who are experienced in working with people who have arthritis. The Arthritis Foundation's magazine, *Arthritis Today,* features current news and advice for easing symptoms.

### *Choose PT*
*www.choosept.com*
This website from the American Physical Therapy Association offers information on how physical therapy may help you recover from many conditions, including arthritis.

### Equal Employment Opportunity Commission (EEOC)

*www1.eeoc.gov/eeoc/publications/index.cfm*
Find fact sheets about discrimination, information on your legal rights in the workplace, guidance on the ADA for employers and more on the EEOC's website.

### Job Accommodation Network

800-526-7234 (toll-free)
*https://askjan.org*
Provided by the Office of Disability Employment Policy, this resource offers free guidance on workplace accommodations and disability employment issues.

### Mayo Clinic

*www.MayoClinic.org*
Visit Mayo Clinic's website for additional information on many health conditions, medications and other treatments.

### National Institute of Arthritis and Musculoskeletal and Skin Diseases

*www.niams.nih.gov*
This organization, also known as NIAMS, is part of the National Institutes of Health. Its website offers more information on many forms of arthritis and related conditions, including who's at risk, what a diagnosis may involve and types of treatment.

### Go4Life

*go4life.nia.nih.gov*
Go4Life, from the National Institute on Aging, provides information and resources to help people age 50 and older incorporate exercise and physical activity into their daily lives.

### National Rehabilitation Information Center (NARIC)

*https://naric.com*
This database is the library of the National Institute on Disability, Independent Living, and Rehabilitation Research (NIDILRR). Visit the website to search for articles and guides on independent living, technology and more from research projects funded by NIDILRR.

### Office of Disability Employment Policy (ODEP)

*www.dol.gov/odep*
This federal agency of the Department of Labor works to improve employment opportunities for people with disabilities. Its website provides information on relevant laws and many other resources.

### Your local library

Your public library may offer helpful books related to arthritis, as well as online access to information from around the world. Ask a librarian about the best way to search for the information you need — for example, the latest update on clinical trials or product reviews before you purchase equipment.

# Index

synovial, 12
types of, 181
**journal, keeping,** 326–327
**juvenile dermatomyositis,** 108

# K

**Kawasaki disease,** 110–111
**kinase inhibitors,** 143, 171–172
**kitchen assistive devices,** 344, 353
**knee braces,** 215
**knee osteoarthritis,** 24
**knee replacement**
 first weeks after, 195–196
 illustrated, 195
 partial, 196–197
 procedures, 194
**knee surgery**
 debridement, 193–194
 joint fusion, 194
 joint replacement, 194–196
 minimally invasive, 196–197
 osteotomy, 194
 partial replacement, 196
 synovectomy, 194
 *See also* surgery

# L

**laboratory tests**
 anti-cyclic-citrullinated peptide (anti-
  CCP) antibody, 126–127
 antinuclear antibody (ANA), 126
 C-reactive protein (CRP), 126
 creatinine test, 126
 erythrocyte sedimentation rate (ESR),
  127
 hematocrit (HCT) and hemoglobin
  (Hgb), 127

HLA tissue typing, 127–128
liver enzyme tests, 128
Lyme serology, 128
muscle enzyme tests, 128
platelet count, 128
rheumatoid factor (RF), 128
uric acid, 128–129
white blood cell count, 129
*See also* evaluations
**leflunomide,** 160–161
**Legg-Calvé-Perthes disease,** 111–112
**legumes,** 297–298
**ligaments,** 12
**live vaccines,** 379
**liver, rheumatoid arthritis and,** 55
**liver enzyme tests,** 128
**localized osteoarthritis,** 23
**low back pain, mechanical,** 93–95
**lungs, rheumatoid arthritis and,** 54–55
**lupus.** *See* systemic lupus erythematosus
**Lyme disease,** 83–84
**Lyme serology,** 128

# M

**magnetic therapy,** 241
**marijuana,** 237–238
**massage,** 216, 241–242, 325–326
**Mayo Clinic Healthy Weight Pyramid**
 carbohydrates, 295
 fats, 298–301
 fruits, 294–295
 illustrated, 293
 produce focus, 296
 protein and dairy, 295–298
 servings, 300, 310
 sweets, 304
 tips for using, 296–297
 vegetables, 293–294

planning, 355–356
to the workplace, 371–372
**travel agents,** 356
**travel insurance,** 357
**treatments.** *See specific forms of arthritis;*
medications; surgery
**trigger finger,** 45
**trochanteric bursitis,** 35
**turmeric,** 236–237

## U

**ultrasonography,** 133–134
**underweight,** 305
**uric acid,** 128–129
**uveitis,** 65, 103, 104

## V

**vaccines,** 378–380
**vasculitis**
defined, 75, 109
giant cell arteritis (GCA), 75–77
Henoch-Schönlein purpura (HSP),
109–110
Kawasaki disease (KD), 110–111
**vegetables,** 293–294
**vegetarian/vegan diet,** 291
**viral infections,** 83
**vitamin D,** 305
**vitamins,** 235–236

## W

**walking,** 282
**water exercise,** 283
**weight, arthritis risk and,** 12, 22
**weight loss**
appetite control and, 310

guide to, 307–310
importance of, 306
in joint protection, 336
**weight management**
basics, 306–307
diet and, 288
exercise and, 260
immune system and, 381
**whiplash injury,** 93
**white blood cell count,** 129
**willow bark,** 239
**workplace**
arthritis disclosure and, 367–368
commuting to, 371–372
computer and, 372–373
job interview tips, 373–375
joint protection and, 370
reasonable accommodations, 369–370
rights, 369–370
success and, 366
**wrist surgery,** 182–184

## X

**X-rays,** 133

## Y

**yoga,** 230–231

# IMAGE CREDITS

The individuals pictured are models, and the photos are used for illustrative purposes only. There is no correlation between the individuals portrayed and the subjects being discussed.

All photographs and illustrations are copyright of MFMER, except for the following: